# Maternal-Newborn Nursing

## Reviews & Rationales

**Mary Ann Hogan, RN, CS, MSN**

Clinical Assistant Professor
University of Massachusetts, Amherst

**Rita S. Glazebrook, RN, CNP, PhD, MS, BSN**

Director, Minnesota Intercollegiate Nursing Consortium
Department Chair, St. Olaf College
Northfield, Minnesota

Prentice Hall

Upper Saddle River, New Jersey 07458

**Publisher:** Julie Levin Alexander
**Executive Editor:** Maura Connor
**Managing Development Editor:** Marilyn Meserve
**Development Editor:** Jeanne Allison
**Director of Production and Manufacturing:** Bruce Johnson
**Managing Production Editor:** Patrick Walsh
**Production Liaison:** Danielle Newhouse
**Production Editor:** Jessica Balch, Pine Tree Composition
**Manufacturing Buyer:** Pat Brown
**Design Director:** Cheryl Asherman
**Design Coordinator:** Maria Guglielmo
**Interior Designer:** Jill Little
**Cover Designer:** Joseph DePinho
**Electronic Art Creation:** Precision Graphics
**Marketing Manager:** Nicole Benson
**Production Information Manager:** Rachele Triano
**Media Editor:** Sarah Hayday
**New Media Production Manager:** Amy Peltier
**New Media Project Manager:** Stephen Hartner
**Composition:** Pine Tree Composition, Inc.
**Printer/Binder:** Courier/Westford

Pearson Education Ltd., *London*
Pearson Education Australia Pty. Limited, *Sydney*
Pearson Education Singapore, Pte. Ltd.
Pearson Education North Asia Ltd., *Hong Kong*
Pearson Education Canada, Ltd., *Toronto*
Pearson Educaión de Mexico, S.A. de C.V.
Pearson Education—Japan, *Tokyo*
Pearson Education Malaysia, Pte. Ltd.
Pearson Education, Upper Saddle River, New Jersey

Prentice Hall

10 9 8 7 6 5 4 3 2 1
ISBN 0-13-030456-5

# Contents

# Preface

## INTRODUCTION

Welcome to the new Prentice Hall Reviews and Rationales Series! This 9-book series has been specifically designed to provide a clear and concentrated review of important nursing knowledge in the following content areas:

- Child Health Nursing
- Maternal-Newborn Nursing
- Mental Health Nursing
- Medical-Surgical Nursing
- Pathophysiology
- Pharmacology
- Fundamentals and Skills
- Nutrition and Diet Therapy
- Fluid, Electrolyte, & Acid-Base Balance

The books in this series have been designed for use either by current nursing students as a study aid for nursing course work or NCLEX-RN licensing exam preparation, or by practicing nurses seeking a comprehensive yet concise review of a nursing specialty or subject area.

This series is truly unique. One of its most special features is that it has been authored by a large team of nurse educators from across the United States and Canada to ensure that each chapter is written by a nurse expert in the content area under study. Prentice Hall Health representatives from across North America submitted names of nurse educators and/or clinicians who excel in their respective fields, and these authors were then invited to write a chapter in one or more books. The consulting editor for each book, who is also an expert in that specialty area, then reviewed all chapters submitted for comprehensiveness and accuracy. The series editor designed the overall series in collaboration with a core Prentice Hall team to take full advantage of Prentice Hall's cutting edge technology, and also reviewed the chapters in each book.

All books in the series are identical in their overall design for your convenience (further details follow at the end of this section). As an added value, each book comes with a comprehensive support package, including free CD-ROM, free companion website access, and a Nursing Notes card for quick clinical reference.

## STUDY TIPS

Use of this review book should help simplify your study. To make the most of your valuable study time, also follow these simple but important suggestions:

- Use a weekly calendar to schedule study sessions.
  - Outline the timeframes for all of your activities (home, school, appointments, etc.) on a weekly calendar.
  - Find the "holes" in your calendar—the times in which you can plan to study. Add study sessions to the calendar at times when you can expect to be mentally alert and follow it!
- Create the optimal study environment.
  - Eliminate external sources of distraction, such as television, telephone, etc.
  - Eliminate internal sources of distraction, such as hunger, thirst, or dwelling on items or problems that cannot be worked on at the moment.
  - Take a break for 10 minutes or so after each hour of concentrated study both as a reward and an incentive to keep studying.
- Use pre-reading strategies to increase comprehension of chapter material.
  - Skim the headings in the chapter (because they identify chapter content).
  - Read the definitions of key terms, which will help you learn new words to comprehend chapter information.
  - Review all graphic aids (figures, tables, boxes) because they are often used to explain important points in the chapter.
- Read the chapter thoroughly but at a reasonable speed.
  - Comprehension and retention are actually enhanced by not reading too slowly.
  - Do take the time to reread any section that is unclear to you.
- Summarize what you have learned.
  - Use questions supplied with this book, CD-ROM, and companion website to test your recall of chapter content.
  - Review again any sections that correspond to questions you answered incorrectly or incompletely.

## TEST TAKING STRATEGIES

Use the following strategies to increase your success on multiple-choice nursing tests or examinations:

- Get sufficient sleep and have something to eat before taking a test. Take deep breaths during the test as needed. Remember, the brain requires oxygen and glucose as fuel. Avoid concentrated sweets before a test, however, to avoid rapid upward and then downward surges in blood glucose levels.
- Read each question carefully, identifying the stem, the four options, and any key words or phrases in either the stem or options.
  - Key words in the stem such as "most important" indicate the need to set priorities, since more than one option is likely to contain a statement that is technically correct.
  - Remember that the presence of absolute words such as "never" or "only" in an option is more likely to make that option incorrect.

- Determine who is the client in the question; often this is the person with the health problem, but it may also be a significant other, relative, friend, or another nurse.
- Decide whether the stem is a true response stem or a false response stem. With a true response stem, the correct answer will be a true statement, and vice-versa.
- Determine what the question is really asking, sometimes referred to as the issue of the question. Evaluate all answer options in relation to this issue, and not strictly to the "correctness" of the statement in each individual option.
- Eliminate options that are obviously incorrect, then go back and reread the stem. Evaluate the remaining options against the stem once more.
- If two answers seem similar and correct, try to decide whether one of them is more global or comprehensive. If the global option includes the alternative option within it, it is likely that the more global response is the correct answer.

## THE NCLEX-RN LICENSING EXAMINATION

The NCLEX-RN licensing examination is a Computer Adaptive Test (CAT) that ranges in length from 75 to 265 individual (stand-alone) test items, depending on individual performance during the examination. Upon graduation from a nursing program, successful completion of this exam is the gateway to your professional nursing practice. The blueprint for the exam is reviewed and revised every three years by the National Council of State Boards of Nursing according to the results of a job analysis study of new graduate nurses (practicing within the first six months after graduation). Each question on the exam is coded to one *Client Need Category* and one or more *Integrated Concepts and Processes*.

### Client Need Categories

There are 4 categories of client needs, and each exam will contain a minimum and maximum percent of questions from each category. Each major category has subcategories within it. The *Client Need* categories according to the NCLEX-RN Test Plan effective April 2001 are as follows:

- Safe, Effective Care Environment
  - Management of Care (7–13%)
  - Safety and Infection Control (5–11%)
- Health Promotion and Maintenance
  - Growth and Development Throughout the Lifespan (7–13%)
  - Prevention and Early Detection of Disease (5–11%)
- Psychosocial Integrity
  - Coping and Adaptation (5–11%)
  - Psychosocial Adaptation (5–11%)
- Physiological Integrity
  - Basic Care and Comfort (7–13%)
  - Pharmacological and Parenteral Therapies (5–11%)
  - Reduction of Risk Potential (12–18%)
  - Physiological Adaptation (12–18%)

### Integrated Concepts and Processes

The integrated concepts and processes identified on the NCLEX-RN Test Plan effective April 2001, with condensed definitions, are as follows:

- Nursing Process: a scientific problem-solving approach used in nursing practice; consisting of assessment, analysis, planning, implementation, and evaluation.

- Caring: client-nurse interaction(s) characterized by mutual respect and trust and directed toward achieving desired client outcomes.
- Communication and Documentation: verbal and/or nonverbal interactions between nurse and others (client, family, health care team); a written or electronic recording of activities or events that occur during client care.
- Cultural Awareness: knowledge and sensitivity to the client's beliefs/values and how these might impact on the client's healthcare experience.
- Self-Care: assisting clients to meet their health care needs, which may include maintaining health or restoring function.
- Teaching/Learning: facilitating client's acquisition of knowledge, skills, and attitudes that lead to behavior change.

More detailed information about this examination may be obtained by visiting the National Council of State Boards of Nursing website at http://www.ncsbn.org and viewing the *NCLEX-RN Examination Test Plan for the National Council Licensure Examination for Registered Nurses.* \*

## HOW TO GET THE MOST OUT OF THIS BOOK

### Chapter Organization

Each chapter has the following elements to guide you during review and study:

- Chapter Objectives: describe what you will be able to know or do after learning the material covered in the chapter.

### OBJECTIVES

▌ Review basic principles of growth and development.

▌ Describe major physical expectations for each developmental age group.

▌ Identify developmental milestones for various age groups.

▌ Discuss the reactions to illness and hospitalization for children at various stages of development.

- Review at a Glance: contains a glossary of key terms used in the chapter, with definitions provided up-front and available at your fingertips, to help you stay focused and make the best use of your study time.

## REVIEW AT A GLANCE

**anticipatory guidance**  *the process of understanding upcoming developmental needs and then teaching caregivers to meet those needs*

**cephalocaudal development**  *the process by which development proceeds from the head downward through the body and towards the feet*

**chronological age**  *age in years*

**critical periods**  *times when an individual is especially responsive to certain environmental effects, sometimes called sensitive periods*

**development**  *an increase in capability or function; a more complex concept that*

*is a continuous, orderly series of conditions that lead to activities, new motives for activities; and eventual patterns of behavior*

**developmental age**  *age based on functional behavior and ability to adapt to the environment; does not necessarily correspond to chronological age*

- Pretest: this 10-question multiple choice test provides a sample overview of content covered in the chapter and helps you decide what areas need the most—or the least— review.

## Pretest

**1** The nurse discusses dental care with the parents of a 3-year-old. The nurse explains that by the age of 3, their child should have:

(1) 5 "temporary" teeth.
(2) 10 "temporary" teeth.
(3) 15 "temporary" teeth.
(4) 20 "temporary" teeth.

**2** The mother of a 6-month-old infant is concerned that the infant's anterior fontanel is still open. The nurse would inform the mother that further evaluation is needed if the anterior fontanel is open after:

(1) 6 months.
(2) 10 months.
(3) 18 months.
(4) 24 months.

- Practice to Pass questions: these are open-ended questions that stimulate critical thinking and reinforce mastery of the chapter content.

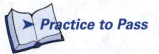

**Practice to Pass**

What would you explain as normal motor development for a 10-month old infant?

- NCLEX Alerts: the NCLEX icon identifies information or concepts that are likely to be tested on the NCLEX licensing examination. Be sure to learn the information flagged by this type of icon.

**NCLEX!**

- Case Study: found at the end of the chapter, it provides an opportunity for you to use your critical thinking and clinical reasoning skills to "put it all together;" it describes a true-to-life client case situation and asks you open-ended questions about how you would provide care for that client and/or family.

**Case Study**

A 6-month-old female infant is brought into the pediatric clinic for a well-baby visit. You as the pediatric nurse will be assigned to care for this family.

❶ Identify the primary growth and development expectations for a 6-month-old.

❷ What type common behavior is expected of this 6-month-old towards the nurse?

❸ What immunization(s) are recommended at this age to maintain health and wellness?

*For suggested responses, see page 406.*

- Posttest: a 10-question multiple-choice test at the end of the chapter provides new questions that are representative of chapter content, and provide you with feedback about mastery of that content following review and study. All pretest and posttest questions contain rationales for the correct answer, and are coded according to the phase of the nursing process used and the NCLEX category of client need (called the Test Plan). The Test plan codes are PHYS (Physiological Integrity), PSYC (Psychosocial Integrity), SECE (Safe Effective Care Environment), and HPM (Health Promotion and Maintenance).

## Posttest

**1** When using the otoscope to examine the ears of a 2-year-old child, the nurse should:

(1) Pull the pinna up and back.
(2) Pull the pinna down and back.
(3) Hold the pinna gently but firmly in its normal position.
(4) Hold the pinna against the skull.

**2** To assess the height of an 18-month-old child who is brought to the clinic for routine examination, the nurse should:

(1) Measure arm span to estimate adult height.
(2) Use a tape measure.
(3) Use a horizontal measuring board.
(4) Have the child stand on an upright scale and use the measuring arm.

### CD-ROM

For those who want to practice taking tests on a computer, the CD-ROM that accompanies the book contains the pretest and posttest questions found in all chapters of the book. In addition, it contains 10 NEW questions for each chapter to help you further evaluate your knowledge base and hone your test-taking skills. In several chapters, one of the questions will have embedded art to use in answering the question. Some of the newly developed NCLEX test items are also designed in this way, so these items will give you valuable practice with this type of question.

### Companion Website (CW)

The companion website is a "virtual" reference for virtually all your needs! The CW contains the following:

- 50 NCLEX-style questions: 10 pretest, 10 posttest, 10 CD-ROM, and 20 additional new questions
- Definitions of key terms: the glossary is also stored on the companion website for ease of reference
- In Depth With NCLEX: features drawings or photos that are each accompanied by a one- to two-paragraph explanation. These are especially useful when describing something that is complex, technical (such as equipment), or difficult to mentally visualize.
- Suggested Answers to Practice to Pass and Case Study Questions: easily located on the website, these allow for timely feedback for those who answer chapter questions on the web.

### Nursing Notes Clinical Reference Card

This laminated card provides a reference for frequently used facts and information related to the subject matter of the book. These are designed to be useful in the clinical setting, when quick and easy access to information is so important!

# ABOUT THE MATERNAL NEWBORN NURSING BOOK

Chapters in this book cover "need-to-know" information about maternal newborn nursing, including family-centered care during normal and complicated experiences in the prenatal, labor and delivery, postpartal, and noenatal periods. Additional chapters focus on special topics such as ethical, legal and cultural considerations; reproduction, fertility and infertility; family planning and contraception; fetal development; and laboratory and diagnostic testing. The final chapter includes issues of loss and grief in childbearing. The term *parent* or *parents* has been used in the book to indicate the primary caretaker(s) for the newborn. The authors understand and appreciate that there are a variety of family configurations in which a child can grow and thrive.

## ACKNOWLEDGMENTS

This book is a monumental effort of collaboration. Without the contributions of many individuals, this first edition of *Maternal-Newborn Nursing: Reviews and Rationales* would not have been possible. We gratefully acknowledge all the contributors who devoted their time and talents to this book. Their chapters will surely assist both students and practicing nurses alike to extend their knowledge in the area of maternal and newborn health.

We owe a special debt of gratitude to the wonderful team at Prentice Hall Health for their enthusiasm for this project, as well as their good humor, expertise, and encouragement as the series developed. Maura Connor, Executive Editor for Nursing, was unending in her creativity, support, encouragement, and belief in the need for this series. Marilyn Meserve, Senior Managing Editor for Nursing, devoted many long hours to coordinating different facets of this project, and tirelessly and cheerfully encouraged our efforts as well. Her high standards and attention to detail contributed greatly to the final "look" of this series. Jeanne Allison, Developmental Editor, actively kept in communication with the different writers in this book and also facilitated getting the book itself into production. Editorial assistants, including Beth Ann Romph, Sladjana Repic, and others, helped to keep the project moving forward on a day-to-day basis, and we are grateful for their efforts as well. A very special thank you goes to the designers of the book and the production team, led by Danielle Newhouse, who brought our ideas and manuscript into final form.

Thank you to the team at Pine Tree Composition, led by Project Coordinator Jessica Balch, for the detail-oriented work of creating this book. We greatly appreciate their hard work, attention to detail, and spirit of collaboration. A special thanks also goes to Yesenia Kopperman, Assistant Editor for Nursing at Prentice Hall, and to Carlos Cooper, Lisa Donovan, and staff at the Pearson Education Development Group for designing and producing the *Nursing Notes* clinical reference card that accompanies this book.

Finally, both Rita Glazebrook and Mary Ann Hogan acknowledge and gratefully thank our families, who sacrificed hours of time that would have been spent with them, to bring this book to publication. Their love and support kept us energized, motivated, and at times, even sane. We love you!

*Reference: National Council of State Boards of Nursing, Inc. *NCLEX Examination Test Plan for National Council Licensure Examination for Registered Nurses.* Effective April, 2001. Retrieved from the World Wide Web September 5, 2001 at http://www.ncsbn.org/public/resources/res/NCSBNRNTestPlan Booklet.pdf.

# Contributors

**Deb Bartnick, RN, MSN**
Instructor of Nursing
Indiana State University
Terre Haute, Indiana
*Chapter 10, Chapter 13, & Chapter 14*

**Rita S. Glazebrook, RN, CNP, PhD, MS BSN**
Associate Professor of Nursing
St. Olaf College
Northfield, Minnesota
*Chapter 3*

**Pamela Hamre, MS, RN, CNM**
Assistant Professor of Nursing
College of St. Catherine
St. Paul, Minnesota
*Chapter 2, Chapter 8, & Chapter 14*

**A. Jenny Harkey, RNC, MSN, ACCE**
Assistant Professor of Nursing
Southeast Missouri State University
Cape Girardeau, Missouri
*Chapter 11*

**Anita Kyle, MS, CNS-MCH, RNC**
Assistant Clinical Professor
Texas Woman's University
Houston, Texas
*Chapter 12*

**Karla Luxner, RNC, MSN**
Instructor of Nursing
Millikin University
Decatur, Illinois
*Chapter 7*

**Molly Meighan, RNC, PhD**
Assistant Professor of Nursing
Carson-Newman College
Jefferson City, Tennessee
*Chapter 9*

**Barbara Morrison, PhD, RN, FNP, CNM**
Associate Professor of Nursing
Millikin University
Decatur, Illinois
*Chapter 1*

**Patricia Posey-Goodwin, MN, RN**
Associate Professor of Nursing
Pensacola Junior College
Pensacola, Florida
*Chapter 3*

**Pamela Pranke, MSN, RNC**
Associate Professor of Nursing
Jamestown College
Jamestown, North Dakota
*Chapter 4*

**Angela Wood, PhD, RN-C**
Assistant Professor of Nursing
Carson-Newman College
Jefferson City, Tennessee
*Chapter 3, Chapter 5, & Chapter 6*

# Reviewers

**Judy F. Barnes, RN, MSN**
Assistant Professor
East Carolina University, School of Nursing
Kinston, North Carolina

**Irene Gonzales, PhD, RN, CNP, CLNC**
Nurse Practitioner and Assistant Professor
San Francisco State University, School of
    Nursing
San Francisco, California

**Judith Johnson Hilton, MSN, RNC**
Assistant Professor of Nursing
Lenoir-Rhyne College
Hickory, North Carolina

**Katherine A. Howe, RNC, MSN, MEd,
    WHNP**
Instructor, Nursing
Henry Ford Community College
Dearborn, Michigan

**Janet T. Ihlenfeld, RN, BSN, MSN, PhD**
Professor, Nursing
D'Youville College, Department of Nursing
Buffalo, NY

**Anne Katz, RN, PhD**
Assistant Professor
University of Manitoba, Helen Glass Centre for
    Nursing
Winnepeg, Canada

**Patricia A. Mynaugh, PhD, RN**
Associate Professor
Villanova University, College of Nursing
Villanova, Pennsylvania

**Carol S. Roane, RNC, MS**
Associate Professor of Nursing
Cecil Community College, Department of
    Nursing
North East, Maryland

**Stephanie Stewart, RN, PhD**
Undergraduate Program Director
University of Wisconsin-Oshkosh, College of
    Nursing
Oshkosh, Wisconsin

**Marcie Weissner, MSN, RNC**
Assistant Professor
University of Saint Francis
Fort Wayne, Indiana

**Susan Wilhelm, RNC, PhD**
Assistant Professor
UNMC College of Nursing, West Nebraska
    Division
Scottsbluff, Nebraska

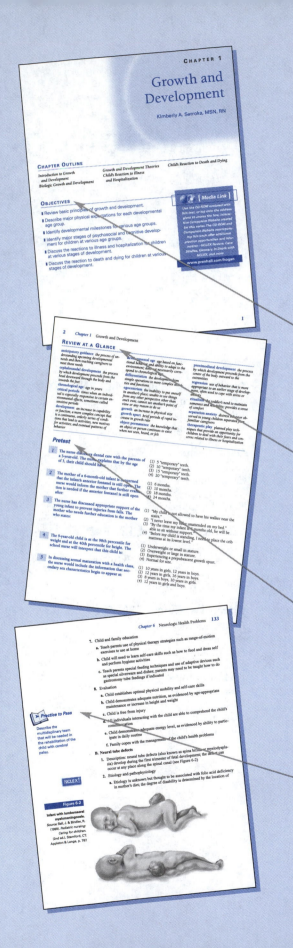

# A Guide To
## *Prentice Hall's Reviews and Rationales Series*

Each chapter has the following **feature elements** to guide you during review and study.

Chapter **Objectives** describe what you will be able to know or do after learning the material covered in the chapter.

**Review at a Glance** contains a glossary of key terms used in the chapter, with definitions provided up-front and available at your fingertips, to help you stay focused and make the best use of your study time.

The **Pretest** is a 10-question multiple choice test providing a sample overview of content covered in the chapter and helps you decide what areas need the most – or the least – review.

The **Practice to Pass** questions are open-ended questions that stimulate critical thinking and reinforce mastery of the chapter content.

**NCLEX** The NCLEX icon identifies information or concepts that are likely to be tested on the NCLEX licensing examination.

A detailed **Outline Review** of core content is given to provide both a comprehensive overview and review.

The **Case Study**, found at the end of the chapter, provides an opportunity for you to use your critical thinking and clinical reasoning skills to "put it all together." It describes a true-to-life client case situation and asks you open-ended questions about how you would provide care for that client and/or family.

The **Posttest** is a 10-question multiple-choice test at the end of the chapter providing new questions that are representative of chapter content. This posttest provides you with feedback about mastery of that content following review and study.

**Answers and Rationales** For all questions, answers and rationales for each correct answer are provided.

## CHAPTER 1

# Introduction to Maternity Nursing

Barbara Morrison, PhD, RN, FNP, CNM

## CHAPTER OUTLINE

*Legal Considerations*

*Ethical Issues*

*Cultural Health Beliefs and Cultural Competence*

*Family-Centered Maternity Care*

## OBJECTIVES

▮ Discuss legal considerations related to maternity nursing.

▮ Delineate ethical issues that influence maternal-newborn nursing practice.

▮ Identify culturally diverse health beliefs that impact the maternity cycle.

▮ Describe a philosophy of care that maintains maternal-newborn safety and fosters family unity.

[ *Media Link* ]

*Use the CD-ROM enclosed with this text, or log onto the address given to access the free, interactive Companion Website created for this series. The CD-ROM and Companion Website accompanying this book offer additional practice opportunities and information—NCLEX Review, Case Studies, Glossary, In Depth with NCLEX, and more.*

**www.prenhall.com/hogan**

## REVIEW AT A GLANCE

**belief** *something accepted as true, especially as a tenet or a body of tenets accepted by an ethnocultural group*

**cultural competency** *the awareness, knowledge and skills necessary to appreciate, understand and communicate with people of diverse cultural backgrounds*

**cultural imposition** *imposition of one's own values, beliefs, and practices on the client, family, or community in the belief that one's own lifeways are "best" and from ignorance of others' cultural practices*

**diversity** *differences in race, ethnicity, national origin, religion, age, gender, sexual orientation, ability/disability, social and economic status or class, education, and related attributes of groups of people in society*

**ethnocentrism** *assumption that one's own beliefs and ways of doing things are best or superior*

**family** *a group of individuals related by blood, marriage, or mutual goals*

**family-centered maternity care** *maternity care that is family oriented and views childbirth as a vital, natural life event rather than an illness*

**infant mortality rate** *the number of deaths of infants under one year of age per 1,000 live births in a given population*

**malpractice** *the failure of a professional person to act in accordance with the prevailing professional standards or failure to foresee consequences that a professional person, having the necessary skill and education, should foresee*

**maternity care** *health care provided to the childbearing family which involves physiologic, psychosocial, and cultural aspects of care*

**negligence** *omitting or committing an act that a reasonable prudent person would not omit or commit under the same or similar circumstances*

**scope of practice** *legally refers to permissible boundaries of practice for nurses and is defined by statute (written law), rules and regulations, or a combination of the two*

**standards of care** *documents describing the minimal requirements that define an acceptable level of care, which is to exercise ordinary and reasonable care to see that no unnecessary harm comes to the client*

**unlicensed assistive personnel** *health care workers who have no defined body of knowledge or educational preparation upon which to base their practice and who are uncredentialed*

## Pretest

**1**  A nurse admitted a client in her 38th week of pregnancy and complaining of severe upper-abdominal pain, nausea, and a persistent headache to the labor and delivery unit. The client's blood pressure (BP) was elevated on two different readings 20 minutes apart. The prenatal record indicated a history of elevated BP and protein in her urine. When the nurse notified the physician 20 minutes after the second elevated BP reading, she reported the elevated BPs, the abdominal pain and nausea, and the client's inability to void. The nurse did not report information about the client's headache, so the physician concluded the client had gastric disturbance from the flu. Later, the client had a grand mal seizure. Why would the nurse be considered negligent in this situation?

(1) The nurse did not maintain clear, concise, and accurate documentation of the client's condition.
(2) The nurse was not thorough in reporting assessment data to the physician.
(3) The nurse did not develop a positive empowering relationship with the client.
(4) The nurse told another nurse of not knowing that a headache was a symptom of preeclampsia.

**2**  Nurses often face dilemmas that have both legal and ethical implications. A legal implication is influenced by:

(1) Values and beliefs.
(2) Motives, attitudes, and culture.
(3) What is good for the individual.
(4) Rules and regulations.

**3** When a nurse signs an informed consent as a witness, what is the nurse affirming?

(1) That the client agreeing to the procedure was the person who signed the consent
(2) That the client understood the information about the procedure before making a decision
(3) That the physician explained all components of the informed consent
(4) That the nurse explained all the components of the informed consent

**4** As the nurse picks up the dinner tray, the nurse notices that a Vietnamese client did not eat any roast beef or mashed potatoes. Later her family members brought in some steamed fish and vegetables with rice, which she ate completely. Why did she prefer the food the family brought in?

(1) The client is acculturated to American foods and prefers hamburgers and french fries.
(2) Eating culturally desired foods is preferable to eating strange or taboo foods.
(3) The foods on the dinner tray are considered hot foods and should be avoided.
(4) The client's appetite was decreased because of her recent delivery.

**5** During the past 20 years, maternity care has changed dramatically. Which of the following changes has increased families' satisfaction with the birth experience?

(1) The expectant mother is transferred to multiple rooms during the birth process.
(2) The father of the baby is allowed to be present for the delivery.
(3) The infant will remain in the room with the family as long as it is well.
(4) Newborns are routinely separated from their parents immediate after birth.

**6** A client asks the nurse to explain the historical difference between midwifery and obstetrics. What should the nurse tell the client?

(1) Midwifery and obstetrics have always been practiced simultaneously.
(2) Midwifery is practiced in the home, while obstetrics is practiced in the hospital.
(3) The focus of midwifery is being with women and assisting the family in childbirth.
(4) The primary focus of obstetrics is the management of low-risk pregnancies.

**7** Several ethnic groups advise expectant mothers not to reach over their head because the cord will wrap around the infant's neck. What type of belief is this?

(1) Health-promotion belief
(2) Prescriptive belief
(3) Restrictive belief
(4) Taboo belief

**8** As the intake nurse at a prenatal clinic, you just completed the initial history for a 26-year-old client who is pregnant for the first time. The client is low-risk and very interested in being involved with the decisions regarding her care and learning all she possibly can about pregnancy and childbirth. Who would you recommend she see for prenatal care and birth?

(1) An obstetrician
(2) A family practice resident
(3) A physician's assistant
(4) A certified nurse-midwife

**9** The nurse manager of the maternal-child unit is evaluating how well the unit met the ACOG (American College of Obstetrics and Gynecology) standard of starting a cesarean section within 30 minutes of the decision for surgery. What is the best way for the nurse manager to assess if the standard is met?

(1) Do a chart review for documentation of time of decision and time surgery began and compare to the national standard.
(2) Interview the nurses involved in the case as to how long it took from decision to surgery.
(3) Assume that all emergency cesarean sections are done within the recommended 30 minutes.
(4) Ask the obstetricians how long it took from the time they ordered the surgery until they made the first cut.

**10** The nurse noticed that a fetus, who was a footing breech, was showing signs of fetal distress. The nurse notified the obstetrician and expressed concern about the fetus's well-being. The obstetrician did not take any action. What should the nurse have done next to remain legally accountable?

(1) Rely on the obstetrician's judgement and remain with the client until delivery.
(2) Ask another physician to review the fetal heart monitor strip.
(3) Notify the nursing supervisor promptly about the nurse's concern and the obstetrician's inaction.
(4) Tell the client that lack of action by the obstetrician warrants legal action.

*See pages 30–31 for Answers and Rationales.*

## I. Legal Considerations

### A. Two arenas for consideration of legal implications

1. Personal professional practice

2. Client care and advocacy

### B. Legal considerations in personal professional practice

1. **Scope of practice:** The Nurse Practice Act

    a. Broad definition of permissible boundaries of practice within a state

    b. Distinguishes nursing practice from practice of other health professionals

    c. Excludes untrained or unlicensed individuals from practicing nursing

    d. Rules and regulations promulgated by state boards of nursing provide official interpretation of nurse practice acts

    e. Correct interpretation and understanding of state practice acts enables the nurse

        1) To provide safe care within the limits of nursing practice

        2) To avoid the risk of being accused of practicing medicine without a license

2. **Standards of care**

    a. Definition

        1) Minimum criteria for competent, proficient delivery of nursing care

        2) Used to evaluate the quality of care provided

        3) Formulated from the skills and knowledge commonly possessed by members of a profession

4) Identify health, demographic, environmental, and psychosocial parameters of care

5) Reflect current knowledge in the field and, therefore, are dynamic and subject to change

  **b.** Uses of standards of care

1) Criterion for determining if a nurse has violated the state Nurse Practice Act

2) Criterion for determining if a nurse has violated state or city criminal codes

3) Criterion for elevating nursing practice to a professional level

  **c.** Internal standards of care: individual and institutional

1) Set by role and education of the nurse: job description, education, and expertise

2) Set by individual institutions: policies and procedures

  **d.** External or national standards of care

1) External because they supercede individual practitioners and single institutions

2) Broader than *locality rules:* standards of care viewed from the perspective of care within a geographic area

3) Based on reasonableness and average degree of skill, care, and diligence practiced by members of the profession across the nation

4) Nurses in a variety of settings and locals must meet the same standards

    a) Apply to homes, alternative birthing centers, hospitals, and ambulatory-care settings

    b) Apply equally in urban, suburban, and rural localities

5) Standards established by

    a) State boards of nursing through nurse practice acts or promulgated rules and regulations

    b) Professional organizations: e.g., American Nurses Association (ANA), Congress for Nursing Practice, International Council of Nursing (ICN)

    c) Specialty nursing organizations: e.g., Association of Women's Health, Obstetric, and Neonatal Nurses (AWHONN), National Association of Neonatal Nurses (NANN), American College of Nurse-Midwives (ACNM)

    d) Federal organizations and guidelines: e.g., Joint Commission on Accreditation of Healthcare Organizations (JCAHO)

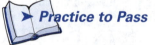

### ➤ Practice to Pass

A nurse waited until the end of the shift to chart the medications given while on duty. The nurse also gave pain medications based on her knowledge of the physician's routine orders without looking at the medication record, relying on information passed on during shift report. Inadvertently the nurse gave a pain medication an hour after the previous dose had been given. Discuss why the nurse should or should not be terminated by the employer.

e. Standards of care and negligence and malpractice

1) **Negligence** is omitting an act or deviation from the standard of care that a reasonably prudent person would not omit or commit under similar circumstances

a) Examples of omission: failing to give a medication, failing to assess properly, failing to notify a physician of a change in a client's condition

b) Examples of commission: giving medication to the wrong patient, placing an infant in the wrong crib

2) Elements of negligence

a) There was a duty to provide care

b) The duty was breached

c) Injury occurred

d) The breach of duty caused injury

3) **Malpractice:** negligent action of a professional person

4) Nurses not meeting appropriate standards of care could be subject to allegations of negligence or malpractice

f. Nurse's responsibility in preventing negligence and malpractice

1) Obtain and maintain current information regarding the state Nurse Practice Act

2) Obtain and maintain current information on internal and external standards of practice

3) Seek continuing education to remain current in specialty area

4) Develop a positive, empowering relationship with clients; see clients as important members of the healthcare team

5) Be thorough in completing and reporting assessments and implementing care

6) Maintain clear, concise, accurate, and complete documentation

7) Question appropriateness of care when harm to a client may occur

C. **Legal considerations for client care**

1. Healthcare reform

a. The United States leads the world in healthcare spending, yet has one of the highest **infant mortality rates** among all industrialized countries

b. One of the primary factors related to infant mortality, deaths under one year of age per 1,000 live births, is an increase in the delivery of low birthweight infants, which is linked to the lack of prenatal care

c. Barriers to access to prenatal care

1) Costs of health care, which are out of control

2) Limited financial resources

3) Uncoordinated service systems

4) Individual behaviors and beliefs concerning health care

5) Bureaucratic obstacles, such as complicated, lengthy application forms for Medicaid

6) Unavailability of maternal services in certain parts of the country

7) Underfunded and overcrowded publicly supervised clinics

8) Difficulty in recruiting and retaining healthcare providers in publicly subsidized clinics

9) Lack of coordinated services for needy individuals

10) Inaccessibility to prenatal services because of transportation, location, and lack of child care facilities

d. Federal and state governments, through policies and legislation, have begun to implement strategies to resolve these barriers by:

1) Broadening health insurance coverage for childbearing women and infants

2) Improving coordination and funding of public programs

3) Simplifying bureaucratic procedures

4) Increasing the number of maternity care providers

5) Establishing a national council on children and health

6) Raising public awareness throughout the country

e. Need to continue to seek reform to further control costs, improve access to care, and improve quality of health care

1) Develop a new way of thinking about and providing healthcare services with primary healthcare services as the foundation upon which all other secondary and tertiary services are built

2) Primary health care, provided to all segments of the population, focusing on:

a) Health promotion

b) Prevention

c) Individual responsibility for one's own health

2. Managed care: Private sector solution for decreasing health care costs

a. Health insurance plans that combine

1) Delivery of healthcare services

2) Financing of those services

3) Controlling the use of services

b. Philosophy of managed care organizations includes

1) Health promotion and disease prevention

2) Desire to avoid serious disease and costly treatment services

      **c.** To meet expenses and make reasonable profits, companies are providing providers with less money per client served while increasing case loads

      **d.** Creates a climate in which providers have

          1) Little time and few resources with which to provide care

          2) Financial disincentives for providers to give adequate services to their clients

      **e.** Consequences

          1) Fewer expensive tests or costly procedures performed, even if provider believes they are justified

          2) Shortened hospital stays

          3) Increased use of unlicensed unlicensed healthcare workers

**3.** Shortened hospital stays

      **a.** During the early to mid-1990s hospital stays after birth were shortened to 24 hours or less

      **b.** Consequently, there is not enough time for maternal and parental teaching regarding self and infant care

          1) Cases of infant dehydration with harmful consequences reported

          2) First-time mothers unable to master breast-feeding before discharge

          3) Some mothers not able to recognize signs of jaundice that may lead to brain damage

      **c.** Several states passed laws requiring longer stays

      **d.** U.S. Congress passed Senate Bill 969, the Newborns' and Mothers' Health Protection Act of 1996

          1) Set a national standard requiring health insurance and employer-provided benefit plans to cover minimum hospital stays of:

             a) 48 hours after a vaginal delivery

             b) 96 hours after delivery by cesarean section

             c) Physicians can write an early discharge order after consulting with the mother and if the health plan provides post-delivery follow-up care, including home care, within 24 to 72 hours of discharge

          2) Even with federal law mandating a longer postpartum stay, nurses are still responsible for:

             a) Verbal and written instructions about infant and self-care, and signs and symptoms indicating a problem

             b) Evaluation of parents' learning

             c) Recommending timely follow-up care, including a home visit, when mother seems at risk after a longer stay

4. **Unlicensed assistive personnel (UAP)**

   a. UAPs are healthcare workers who have no defined body of knowledge or educational preparation upon which to base their practice

      1) Uncredentialed

      2) No state or federal regulatory body to validate their competence

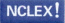

   b. Nurses are responsible for the delegation of tasks to UAPs

      1) UAPs can perform repetitive tasks, which are clearly defined and for which they have been trained

      2) Nurses should obtain information on UAPs' training and skills prior to delegating tasks

      3) Inappropriate delegation to UAPs increases the nurse's liability and may jeopardize the nurse's license

   c. What cannot be delegated to UAPs

      1) Essential nursing processes of assessing, diagnosing of a problem, planning client care, implementing that care, and evaluating the outcomes

      2) Judgements about client status

5. Nurse's role as client advocate

   a. Maintain current information about issues critical to client care

   b. Educate clients and other significant persons about such issues

   c. Become involved in the political process as an advocate for quality healthcare for all healthcare recipients

## II. Ethical Issues

### A. Ethics and legal issues are interrelated as shown in Table 1-1

1. Law is based on a rights model establishing rules of conduct to define:

   a. Relationships among individuals

   b. Relationships to impersonal entities like agencies or hospitals

   c. Formal and binding relationships

2. Ethics is based on a responsibility or duty model examining what our behavior ought to be in relation to ourselves, other human beings, and the environment

   a. Incorporates factors such as:

      1) Risks

      2) Benefits

      3) Other relationships

      4) Concerns

      5) The needs and abilities of persons affected by and affecting decisions

   b. Subject to philosophical, moral, and individual interpretations

| Table 1-1 | | Law | Ethics |
|---|---|---|---|
| **Differences between Law and Ethics** | **Origin** | Social rules and regulations, external to the individual | Individual values, beliefs, and interpretations; internal to the individual |
| | **Focus** | Society as a whole, behavior of individuals; acts committed or omitted | Individual in society; relationship of attitudes and motives to behavior; desired behavior to achieve goodness |
| | **Regulation** | Boards of nursing, statutes, courts | Professional organizations, ethics committees |

**B. Some ethical principles used in clinical practice**

1. Respect: recognition of the dignity of each person, of their right to make decisions and to live or die by those decisions

2. Autonomy: recognition of an individual's personal freedom and self-determination; the right to choose what will happen to one's own person

3. Beneficence: duty to do good

4. Nonmaleficence: duty to do no harm

5. Veracity: duty to tell the truth

6. Fidelity: duty to keep one's promise or word

7. Justice: equitable distribution of risks and benefits, obligation to be fair to everyone

8. Confidentiality: holding information entrusted in the context of special relationships as private or protection of the individual's right to privacy

9. Informed consent: contains four elements—disclosure or information, comprehension, voluntary agreement, competency to make decisions

10. Universality: same principle must apply for everyone regardless of time, place, or person involved

**C. Ethical decision-making framework (similar to the nursing process); use acronym MORAL**

1. M: Massage the dilemma

   a. Identify and define issues in the dilemma

   b. Determine who owns the problem, the information, the decision, and the consequences of it

   c. Establish the facts as best possible

   d. Consider the opinions, values, and moral position of the major players

   e. Identify value conflicts

2. O: Outline the options

   a. Examine all options fully, including the less realistic and conflicting ones

   b. Identify pros and cons of all the options

   c. Fully comprehend the options and alternatives available

3. R: Resolve the dilemma

   a. Review the issues and options

   b. Apply ethical principles to each option

   c. Decide the best option for action based on the views of all those concerned

4. A: Act by applying the chosen option

5. L: Look back and evaluate the entire process, including the implementation

   a. Ensure that all those involved are able to follow through on the final option

   b. Revise the decision as indicated, starting the process with the initial step

**D. Ways nurses can maintain legal rights within ethical dilemmas**

1. Recognize the difference between legal rights and ethical views; legal rights must be provided to the client

2. Realize that personal ethical views and values may differ greatly from the client's value system

   a. Understanding personal views and values allows objectivity when caring for clients and when serving as a consultant for decision making by the client

   b. Diminishes judgemental actions

3. Remain current about recent judicial decisions in the jurisdiction and incorporate these standards and rights into nursing care

4. If a legal standard does not exist for a particular ethical issue, practice is guided by the ethics of the profession and by personal moral values

5. Remove self from client's nursing care if values come into major conflict

6. Established legal principles should be followed first when conflict occurs

**E. "Clients' rights" intersect law and ethics in maternity nursing practice**

1. Informed consent

   a. Designed to allow clients to make intelligent decisions regarding their own health care

   b. Information to be provided by the individual who is ultimately responsible for the treatment or procedure, generally the physician

   c. The information must be clearly and concisely presented in a manner understandable to the client

   d. Components of informed consent

      1) Nature and purpose of the treatment or procedure

      2) Risks and benefits

      3) Significant treatment alternatives

      4) Probabilities of success

      5) Consequences of receiving no treatment or procedure

      6) Right to refuse a specific treatment or procedure and that refusing the specific treatment will not result in the withdrawal of all support or care

     **e.** Nurse's role in obtaining informed consent

       1) Preferably, be present during the physician's conversation with the client about informed consent

       2) Clarify information the physician provides

       3) Determine that the client understands the information prior to making a decision

       4) Sign the consent form as witness to the client's signature, attesting that the client agreeing to the treatment or procedure was the person who signed the informed consent form

       5) Client may need to sign a form to release the physician and agency from liability when treatment, medication, or procedure is refused after appropriate information has been provided

**2.** Right to privacy

     **a.** The right of clients to keep their person and property free from public scrutiny

     **b.** Only the health professional responsible for a client's care should examine the client and share information about the client's treatment, condition, and prognosis

     **c.** If information needs to be shared with others, such as insurance companies or referral healthcare professionals, an authorization for the release of client information should be obtained from competent clients or their surrogate decision maker

     **d.** Whatever the situation requiring release of information, the client should be consulted regarding what information may be released and to whom

**3.** Confidentiality

     **a.** Maintaining confidentiality is crucial for the development of a trusting relationship between client and provider

       1) Information requested of clients is highly personal and intimate

       2) Considered privileged conversation

     **b.** Right to confidentiality of medical records may be waived by action or word when:

       1) Lawsuit is pursued, records a source of evidence

       2) Consent is given for information to be released to insurance companies or employers

       3) Public good takes precedence and providers are required by law to report some findings, e.g., child abuse, gunshot wounds, some communicable diseases

**F. Ethical considerations in maternity nursing**

    **1.** Assisted reproduction

      **a.** Artificial insemination

      **b.** In vitro fertilization and embryo transfer

      **c.** Gamete intrafallopian transfer

      **d.** Surrogate childbearing

  **2.** Amniocentesis and chorionic villus sampling

  **3.** Abortion

  **4.** Fetal or embryo research

  **5.** Cord blood banking

  **6.** The Human Genome Project and genetic counseling

  **7.** Fetal rights versus maternal rights

      **a.** Fetus is not viewed as a person by U.S. Supreme Court even if "viable"

      **b.** Advances in technology have enabled monitoring and treatment of the fetus

      **c.** Fetus is given consideration as a client separate from the mother

         1) Treatment of the fetus involves the mother

         2) Leads to contradictory moral claims on the ethical obligation to do good and avoid harm

         3) Fundamental right of expectant mothers to make informed, uncoerced decisions regarding medical intervention to themselves and the fetus

         4) When maternal-fetal conflict occurs, it involves two clients, both of whom deserve respect and treatment

         5) Cases are best resolved through internal hospital mechanisms such as counseling, interventions of specialists, or ethics committees

         6) Judicial intervention should be a last resort

**G. Nurses' responsibilities when preparing for ethical decision making in maternity nursing**

  **1.** Learn to anticipate ethical dilemmas

  **2.** Identify attitudes, values, and beliefs about ethical dilemmas taking into consideration the influence of cultural, religious, and social factors on the development of values

  **3.** Recognize the influence personal values have on care provided for clients by engaging in self-values clarification activities

  **4.** Review and update theoretical bases

      **a.** Gather current information on technologic advances and changing trends in maternity nursing

      **b.** Review ethical principles and practice codes in regard to new technology and trends

      **c.** Become familiar with the client's knowledge base by reading lay literature related to maternity advances

5. Attend continuing education programs related to ethical issues and decision making

  a. Participate in ethics committees with other healthcare professionals

  b. Inservice peers on ethical issues and decision making

6. Review research journals regarding current trends in ethical decision making, comparing and contrasting the results with what is occurring in clinical practice

7. Evaluate current social norms by following social, legal, religious, and political debates that may influence clinical decision making and quality care for clients experiencing dilemmas

8. Avoid judgements about the life decisions of others

  a. Aim to accept the values of others and their decisions regarding issues and provisions of care

  b. Do not allow personal beliefs and values to interfere with the provision of quality care

9. Understand the legal implications of the issues

10. Develop appropriate strategies for ethical decision making

### III. Cultural Health Beliefs and Cultural Competence

A. **Beliefs about pregnancy and childbearing:** significantly influenced by the culture or cultures in which the expectant family was raised and is now living

  1. Ideas about conception, pregnancy, and childbearing practices are passed down from generation to generation

  2. Beliefs are acculturated into the society without validation or being completely understood

  3. Many societies do not consider pregnancy an illness

    a. May not seek advice from healthcare professionals or prenatal care

    b. May seek and follow advice from elders and family members

B. **National and global populations:** characterized by increasing diversity

C. *Diversity:* differences in race, ethnicity, national origin, religion, age, gender, sexual orientation, ability/disability, social and economic status or class, education, and related attributes of groups of people in society

D. **Every human being is** *ethnocentric*

  1. Subconsciously view other people by using our own group of customs as the standard for all judgements

  2. View others' ways as inferior to personal ways

  3. Need to avoid **cultural imposition:** imposing personal cultural beliefs and practices on clients while trivializing or disregarding theirs

E. **Developing** *cultural competency*

  1. The concept of cultural competency

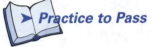

**Practice to Pass**

The recommended lifesaving treatment for a newborn's congenital anomaly is surgery. The parents refuse surgery for their newborn. When exploring the reasons for their refusal, the nurse finds the parents have strong beliefs that intentional cutting of the body will result in spiritual death. How can the nurse help resolve the conflict between the parents' convictions and the recommended medical treatment?

NCLEX!

a. The complex integration of knowledge, attitudes, and skills that enhance cross-cultural communication and appropriate, effective interaction with others

b. A process in which one continuously strives to effectively work within the cultural context of an individual, family, or community from a diverse cultural background

2. Components of cultural competency

   a. Cultural awareness

   b. Cultural knowledge

   c. Cultural skill

   d. Cultural encounter

3. To become culturally competent the nurse should:

   a. Critically examine one's own cultural beliefs

   b. Identify personal biases, attitudes, stereotypes, and prejudices

   c. Make a conscious decision to respect the values and beliefs of others

   d. Use sensitive, current language when describing the client's culture

   e. Learn the ritual, customs, practices, values, and beliefs for the major cultural and ethnic groups with whom one has contact

   f. Include cultural assessment and assessment of the family's expectations of the healthcare system as a routine part of perinatal nursing care

   g. Incorporate the family's cultural practices into perinatal care as much as possible

   h. Foster an attitude of respect for and cooperation with alternative healers and caregivers whenever possible

   i. Provide for the services of an interpreter if language barriers exist

   j. Learn the language (or at least key phrases) of at least one of the cultural groups with whom one interacts

   k. Recognize that ultimately it is the expectant mother's right to make her own healthcare choices

   l. Evaluate whether the client's health beliefs have any potential negative consequences for the client's health

**F. Incorporating cultural assessment and planning into perinatal care**

1. Cultural assessment

   a. Identify main beliefs, values, and behaviors that relate to pregnancy and childbearing

     1) Ethnic background

     2) Amount of affiliation with the ethnic group

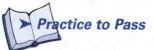

**► Practice to Pass**

As a new manager on the obstetric unit, the nurse quickly realized that there were cultural conflicts between the nursery nurses, who were Filipino, and the new mothers, most of whom were African-American or Latino and of low socioeconomic status. How can the nurse manager help to improve communication and cultural sensitivity between the nursery nurses and the new mothers?

3) Patterns of decision making

4) Religious preferences

5) Language

6) Communication style

7) Common etiquette practices

   **b.** Explore expectant mother's and family's expectation of the healthcare system

2. Planning to meet cultural beliefs

   **a.** Consider the extent to which the expectant mother's personal values, beliefs, and customs agree with

     1) The expectant family's identified cultural group

     2) The nurse providing care

     3) The health care agency

   **b.** If there are discrepancies, is the expectant family's system supportive, neutral, or harmful in relation to possible interventions?

   **c.** If supportive or neutral, incorporate cultural practices into the plan of care

   **d.** If cultural practices might pose a threat to the health of the expectant mother or fetus:

     1) Discuss with client and understand the reasons for refusal

     2) Identify ways to persuade the expectant mother to accept the proposed interventions

     3) Accept the expectant mother's decision to refuse the intervention if the client is not willing to adapt her belief system

     4) Explain alternative therapies that might be acceptable to the expectant mother within her cultural beliefs

**G. Cultural variation during pregnancy, labor, birth, and the postpartum**

1. Support system

   **a.** Formalized assistance from healthcare providers

     1) Western medicine perceived as having curative rather than preventive focus, pregnancy a physiologic state that will become pathologic

     2) Subcultures view pregnancy as a normal physiologic process, not an illness or condition requiring curative services of a doctor, which may result in delay or neglect in seeking prenatal care

   **b.** Nontraditional support systems

     1) Traditionally, emphasis on female support and guidance

     2) Some ethnic/cultural groups, such as Orthodox Jews, Muslims, Chinese, or Asian Indians, have strict religious and cultural prohibitions against husbands or any man viewing a woman's body during labor and birth

        3) Family and social network, especially grandmother or other maternal relatives, are of primary importance in advising and supporting the expectant mother

        4) Traditional healers

**2.** Prescriptive, restrictive, and taboo beliefs and practices

    **a.** Prescriptive beliefs and practices: describe expectancies of behavior, those things that an expectant mother should do to have a healthy pregnancy and baby, phrased positively

    **b.** Restrictive beliefs and practices: limit choices and behaviors, those things that the mother should not do to have a positive outcome, phrased negatively

    **c.** Taboo beliefs and practices: restrictions with supernatural consequences, those things that are likely to harm the mother or baby

    **d.** Box 1-1 provides examples of prescriptive, restrictive, and taboo beliefs and practices

**3.** Expressions of labor pain

    **a.** Factors interacting to influence labor and the perception of pain

        1) Cultural attitude toward the normalcy and conduct of birth

        2) Expectations of how a woman should act in labor

        3) Role of significant others

        4) The physiologic processes involved

    **b.** Examples of responses to labor by many women of a cultural group

        1) Filipino women feel it is best to lie quietly

        2) Middle Eastern women are verbally expressive, sometimes crying and screaming loudly while refusing pain medication

        3) Samoan women believe that no verbal expressions of pain are permissible and only "spoiled" Caucasian women need any analgesia

        4) Hispanic women are instructed by their *parteras* to endure the pain with patience and close the mouth, for opening it to cry out would cause the uterus to rise

        5) Japanese, Chinese, Vietnamese, Laotian, and others of Asian descent maintain that screaming or crying out during labor or birth is shameful; birth is believed to be painful but something to be endured

    **c.** Culturally appropriate ways of preparing for labor and birth

        1) Assisting with or participating in birth from the time of adolescence

        2) Listening to birth and baby stories told by respected elderly women

        3) Following special dietary and activity prescriptions in the antepartal period

        4) Learning formal breathing and relaxation techniques

## Box 1-1

**Examples of Prescriptive, Restrictive, and Taboo Practices During Pregnancy, Labor, Birth, and the Postpartum for a Variety of Cultural Groups**

*Prescriptive Practices*

**Navajo:** During labor, wear a necklace made of juniper seeds and beads to assist with a safe birth; bury the placenta after birth to symbolize child being tied to the land; feed the baby a mixture with juniper to cleanse the baby's insides and rid it of mucus

**Crow Indian:** Remain active during pregnancy to aid baby's circulation

**Polish-Americans:** To have a healthy pregnancy and baby, pregnant mothers are expected to seek preventive care, eat well, and get adequate rest

**Latino:** Wear a *muneco* (special article of clothing) to ensure a safe delivery and prevent morning sickness

**Chinese:** Add more meat to the diet to makes the blood stronger for the fetus

**Mexican:** Keep active during pregnancy to ensures a small baby and easy delivery

**Filipino:** Continue daily baths and frequent shampoos during pregnancy to produces a clean baby

**Haitian, Mexican:** Continue sexual intercourse to lubricates the birth canal and prevent a dry labor

**Hispanic:** Bury the placenta to prevent the mother from having afterbirth pains

*Restrictive Practices*

**Egyptian:** Don't bathe during the postpartum period as it could expose the mother to colds and chills

**Navajo:** Clothes should not be purchased for the infant before birth as preparing for the infant is forbidden by Indian tradition and the newborn may not survive; do not tie knots or braids or allow the baby's father to do so as it will cause difficult labor

**African-American, Latino, white, Asian:** Do not reach over your head as the cord will wrap around the baby's neck

**Vietnamese:** Avoid weddings and funerals or bad fortune will come to the baby

**Vietnamese, Filipino, Samoan:** Do not continue sexual intercourse; harm will come to the expectant mother and baby

**Latino:** Fathers are not allowed in the delivery room or to see the mother or baby before they have been cleaned as this can cause harm to the baby

*Taboo Practices*

**Navajo:** Do not have a weaving comb (rug) with more than five points or the baby will have extra fingers; do not jump around or ride a horse if you are pregnant or it will induce labor; do not cut a baby's hair when it is small or it won't think right when it is older

**Mexican:** Avoid lunar eclipses and moonlight or the baby may be born with a deformity

**Haitian:** Do not get involved with persons who cast spells or the baby will be eaten in the womb

**Orthodox Jewish:** Do not say the baby's name before the naming ceremony or harm might come to the baby

**African-American:** Do not have your picture taken during pregnancy or it might cause stillbirth

**Korean:** Do not eat chicken, duck, rabbit, goat, crab, sparrow, pork, or blemished fruit to guard the child from unwanted physical characteristics (chicken may cause bumpy skin, blemished fruit may cause an unpleasant child)

4. Postpartum

   a. Pregnancy and birth considered most dangerous and vulnerable by Western medicine

   b. For many other cultures the postpartal period is the time of vulnerability for the mother and newborn and require special practices which:

      1) Serve to mobilize support for the new mother

      2) May involve restrictive dietary customs, activity level, taboos, and rituals associated with purification and seclusion which positively influence the mother's mental health after delivery

   c. Concept of postpartum vulnerability is based on beliefs related to imbalance or pollution

      1) Imbalance: disharmony caused by the processes of pregnancy and birth

      2) Pollution: caused by the *unclean* bleeding associated with birth and the postpartum period

      3) Ritual seclusion and activity restrictions may reduce the risk of increasing personal vulnerability to spirit influence or of spreading evil and misfortune

      4) Restitution of physical balance and purification occur through mechanisms such as dietary restrictions, ritual baths, seclusion, restriction of activity, and other ceremonial events

5. Hot and cold theory: humoral balance and imbalance

   a. Health is a state of balance among the body humors or body fluids (blood, phlegm, black bile, and yellow bile) that manifests itself in a somewhat wet, warm body

   b. Illness results from a humoral imbalance causing the body to become excessively dry, cold, hot, wet, or a combination of these states

   c. Natural balance can be restored by the therapeutic use of food, herbs, and medications, which are also classified as wet or dry, hot or cold

   d. To achieve balance, illnesses are treated with substances having the opposite property of the illness

   e. Pregnancy is a "hot" state and a great deal of heat is thought to be lost during the birth process

   f. Postpartum practices focus on restoring the balance between hot and cold

      1) Avoidance of cold: air or food

      2) Example: Haitians believe that exposure to cold air may cause a uterine cold, use of sanitary napkin is thought to prevent air from entering into the vagina

      3) Fruits and vegetables, milk products, and foods that are sour to taste may be considered "cold" foods; animal products, chilies, spices and ginger may be considered hot foods

**H. An example of cultural influences on an expectant family:** the African-American family

1. Variations in African-American families

    a. Influenced by geographic location, level of acculturation, religious background, and socioeconomic status

    b. Socioeconomic status very significant to consider as persons of different cultural backgrounds who live in poverty share similar social problems

2. Adaptive strengths of the African-American family that help bring about positive pregnancy outcomes

    a. Kinship bonds

        1) Kinship network important source of support

        2) Not always along "bloodlines"

        3) Based on complex patterns of co-residence and kinship-based exchange networks linking various domestic units

        4) Family units have broad household boundaries with strong bonds to three generations of households

        5) Individuals within the network are involved in cooperative domestic exchanges

        6) May include a large number of people inside and outside the nuclear family creating a complex family network: partner, parents, children, uncles, aunts, preachers, friends, siblings, cousins

        7) Networks are often well-organized and provide lifelong relationships that offer stability

    b. Family roles

        1) Role of men is difficult, but many men have a great investment in the family

        2) Women and men may have significant role flexibility, especially in care of children, childrearing, and household responsibilities

        3) Members of the kinship network may take on roles usually assumed by nuclear family members

            a) Maternal or paternal aunt or grandmother may share or assume responsibility for child care

            b) Infant may be adopted informally and reared by extended family members who have resources not available to the child's parents

    c. Religion and the church

        1) Religious system provides support in pastors, deacons, deaconesses, and other church members

        2) Spirituality influences health and well-being

        3) Religious beliefs provide spiritual comfort and support

        4) Church activities may provide a social life for members of the whole family

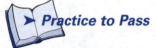

**► Practice to Pass**

A nurse was caring for a 15-year-old African-American client on the day of discharge after the birth of her first infant. When the nurse entered the room, both the maternal and paternal grandmothers were present and continually made comments about the care and teaching the nurse was providing the client. How should the nurse handle the situation so the provision of care and education of the new mother can continue?

5) During pregnancy, church family may promote physical health of the expectant mother by encouraging early prenatal care and maintaining a lifestyle that fosters healthy pregnancy outcomes

## IV. Family-Centered Maternity Care

**NCLEX!**

### A. What is a *family*?

1. A group of individuals related by blood, marriage, or mutual goals

2. A group of individuals who are bound by strong emotional ties, a sense of belonging, and a passion for being involved in one another's lives

3. Critical attributes of family

   a. The family is a system or unit

   b. Its members may or may not be related and may or may not live together

   c. The unit may or may not contain children

   d. There is a commitment and attachment among unit members that include future obligation

   e. The unit caregiving functions consist of protection, nourishment, and socialization of its members

4. Types of families

   a. Traditional forms

   1) Nuclear family: father, mother, and child living together but apart from both sets of grandparents

   2) Extended family: three generations, including married brothers and sisters and their families

   b. Nontraditional forms

   1) Single-parent family: divorced, never married, separated, or widowed man or women and at least one child

   2) Three-generational family: any combination of first-, second-, and third-generation members living within a household

   3) Dyad family: husband and wife or other couple living alone without children

   4) Stepparent family: one or both spouses have been divorced or widowed and have remarried into a family with at least one child

   5) Blended or reconstituted family: a combination of two families with children from one or both families and sometimes children of the newly married couple

   6) Cohabiting family: An unmarried couple living together

   7) Gay or lesbian family: A homosexual couple living together with or without children; children may be adopted, from previous relationships, or artificially conceived

   8) Adoptive family: single persons or couples who have at least one child who is not biologically related to them and to whom they have legally become parents

5. Family is a system nested within and influenced by broader systems such as neighborhood, class, region, and country

6. These broader systems are the context which permeates and circumscribes individuals and their family, and include:

   a. Ethnicity

   b. Race

   c. Social class

   d. Religion and spirituality

   e. Environment

B. **The family development theory of the family life:** eight stages in family development from leaving home as single young adult to aging families accepting shifting generational roles

   1. Family stage identified by age of the oldest child

   2. Theories initially developed to describe middle-class North American family life

   3. Developmental tasks for the family during childbearing years

      a. The joining of families: couples without children

         1) Finding, furnishing, and maintaining a first home

         2) Establishing mutually satisfactory means of support

         3) Allocating responsibilities

         4) Establishing mutually acceptable personal, emotional, and sexual roles

         5) Interacting with in-laws, relatives, friends, and community

         6) Planning for children or no children

         7) Maintaining couple motivation and morale

      b. Families with young children: childbearing with oldest child under 30 months

         1) Arranging space (territory) for child

         2) Financing childbearing and childrearing

         3) Assuming mutual responsibility for child care and nurturing

         4) Facilitating role learning of family members or defining and assuming maternal and paternal roles

         5) Adjusting to changed communication patterns to accommodate a newborn and young child

         6) Planning for subsequent children

         7) Realigning intergenerational patterns to establish grandparent roles and grandparent-grandchild subsystems

         8) Maintaining family members' motivation and morale

         9) Establishing family rituals and routines

4. Theory has been adapted and modified to describe a variety of family life-cycles including divorced families, remarried families, economically disadvantaged families, and adoptive families

C. **The childbearing family:** a family in crisis

1. Childbearing is a developmental crisis

   a. Normal and routinely experienced in the process of growth and development

   b. Periods of marked physical, psychological, and social change characterized by disturbances in life's patterns or a sense of disorganization

   c. Certain tasks must be faced and mastered by individual or family to achieve next maturational stage and be ready for further growth and development

2. Situational crises are unexpected, stressful external events that may or may not coincide with a developmental crisis, such as a high risk pregnancy

D. **Historical trends in moving toward family-centered maternity care**

1. Midwifery, originally the branch of medicine that dealt with the practice of assisting in childbirth, has been practiced since the earliest of times

   a. Midwives mentioned in the Bible

   b. The midwife, meaning "with women," was responsible for the delivery of infants

2. Obstetrics, as a branch of medicine, was introduced in the late-19th century

   a. Branch of medicine that deals with the phenomena and management of pregnancy, labor, and the postpartum in low- and high-risk circumstances

   b. Midwifery is now used to delineate the practice of nurses who are responsible for the management of childbearing women and neonates in collaboration with other providers

3. During the 1920s and 1930s, childbirth moved from the home to the hospital

   a. Advances in medical services introduced various drugs and obstetric procedures to control pain and combat infection; provided by hospitals and superceded giving birth in the home environment

   b. Mobility and urbanization minimized the social network of female support for childbearing women

   c. Childbirth viewed as a pathophysiologic, physician-centered process

   d. Traditional maternity care reorganized into subspecialities

   e. Intrapartum care based on a surgical, multitransfer system

      1) Mothers labored in one room, delivered in another, recovered in a third room, spent the remainder of their hospital stay on a postpartum unit

      2) Newborns were immediately separated from their mothers and kept in a separate nursery to be transported to their mothers for feedings on a predetermined schedule

**f.** After World War II, the focus of care shifted from the provider of care to the recipient of care to a broader focus involving psychosocial, cultural, and physiologic aspects of the woman

**g.** By 1960s, professionals and consumers were concerned with the continuing assumption that every woman was a disaster waiting to happen

1) Traditional hospital care detracted from biophysical development of the new family

2) Consumers sought to understand technology and to take interest in their own health and basic self-care skills, assuming many primary care functions

3) Focus of care needed to shift to promote health and well-being with the family unit the recipient of care

4) Nurses have become significant members of the health care team

   a) Foster self-care by readily providing information

   b) Acknowledge family members' right to ask questions and become actively involved in their own care

   c) Encourage family members to speak up for preferences in dealing with healthcare providers

**E. Philosophy of family-centered maternity care:** childbirth is a natural event

**1.** Components of the family-centered maternity care philosophy

**a.** Childbearing is a family affair

1) Family members need to be included in all aspects of care

2) Family members are capable of making decisions about childbearing care when provided education, support, and advocacy

**b.** The reproductive health of the total family is important to the health of society

**c.** Childbirth is a normal physiologic process that generally requires few medical interventions, a natural life event rather than an illness

1) Childbirth is generally an uncomplicated, joyful event for families

2) Understanding the social and psychological factors related to childbirth improves family satisfaction and provision of meaningful care

**d.** Parenting is learned

1) Many physical, psychological, and social changes to be navigated during the transition to parenthood

2) Nurses and healthcare professionals can help expectant families develop appropriate expectations, knowledge, and skills for good parenting

**2.** Goals of care

**a.** To assist the expectant parents to make informed decisions about their own health care

**b.** To foster family unity while providing safe, quality, cost-effective care

**3.** Components of care

   **a.** Collaboration with parents, siblings, and extended family members during the entire childbearing experience

   **b.** Childbirth preparation of both parents, siblings, and others as designated by the mother

   **c.** Involvement of the father in the entire birthing process

   **d.** Choice of birthing environment when possible

   **e.** Sibling visitation

   **f.** Early discharge programs for mother and infants

   **g.** Strategies to foster family members' attachment to the newborn

   **h.** Parental leave options for both parents

   **i.** Nursing management for families throughout the childbearing cycle

**F. Prenatal care providers and expertise are presented in Table 1-2**

   **1.** Maternity health care providers differ in their philosophical approach to care

   **2.** Expectant women and their families need to know their options and choose the provider with whom they are most comfortable

| Table 1-2 | Levels of Prenatal Care | Types of Care Provider | Prenatal Care Expertise |
|---|---|---|---|
| **Prenatal Care Providers and Expertise** | Low-risk pregnancy (basic care) | Family physician<br>Nurse practitioner<br>Certified nurse-midwife<br>Obstetrician | Initial and ongoing risk assessment; routine physical and laboratory assessment; monitoring normal pregnancy progress; psychosocial support; childborth education; consultation and referral |
| | Moderate-risk pregnancy (specialty care | Family physician<br>Obstetrician | Basic care; basic fetal diagnostic testing (ultrasound, biophysical profile, amniotic fluid analysis); management of medical and obstetric complications; consultation and referral |
| | High-risk pregnancy (sub-specialty care) | Maternal-Fetal medicine specialist<br>Geneticist | Basic and specialty care; advanced fetal diagnostic testing (targeted ultrasound, echocardiogram); advanced fetal treatment (intrauterine transfusion, cardiac arrhythmia management); medical, surgical, and genetic consultation; management of severe obstetric complications |

## G. Nursing members of the healthcare team

1. Professional nurses: the nurse generalists who have graduated from an accredited basic nursing program and have additional continuing education in the specialized area of maternity nursing

2. Nurse specialists or advanced practice nurses: professional nurses who have additional education preparation at least at the graduate level, expertise in a specific clinical area, and function in an expanded role

   a. Certified nurse-midwives (CNMs): individuals educated in the two disciplines of nursing and midwifery, and are certified by the American College of Nurse-Midwives (ACNM)

      1) Prepared to manage independently the care of women and families at low risk for complications during pregnancy and birth and the care of normal newborns

      2) Take a holistic approach to assessment and identification of needs of the expectant mother and her family

      3) Provide cost-effective care that achieves outcomes that are consistently better than national statistical averages

   b. Nurse practitioners (NPs): primary care providers focusing on physical and psychosocial assessments leading to clinical diagnosis and treatment while seeking physician consultation when necessary

   c. Clinical nurse specialists (CNSs): assume a leadership role within their specialty, focus on improving client care by evaluating nursing practice, recommending improvements, establishing standards of care, and conducting research studies

3. Unlicensed assistive personnel

## H. Environments for birth

1. Single-room maternity care (SRMC)

   a. Replaced multi-transfer system that characterized traditional childbirth care

   b. Labor/delivery/recovery and/or postpartum (LDR/LDRP) rooms

      1) Designed and equipped to accommodate entire birthing process, including complicated vaginal deliveries

      2) No screening criteria

      3) Equipment brought to expectant mother based on her individual needs and different stages of the childbearing process

      4) Newborns are not routinely separated from parents and family after birth

      5) Well infants may remain in room with family under care of maternity nurses who are proficient in both maternal and neonatal nursing

      6) Cesarean births occur in delivery/operating rooms

      7) Preterm and ill newborns are cared for in high-risk nurseries

> **▶ Practice to Pass**
>
> Your best friend just discovered she is pregnant. She asks you, a nurse, who she should go to for prenatal care. How will you respond?

**c.** Advantages of single-room maternity care

1) Clinical safety

a) Increased effectiveness in responding to emergencies

b) Improved communication and continuity of care

c) Decreased risk of client exposure to many different areas and departmental staff

2) Marketability

a) Non-institutional environment increases market share by attracting parents-to-be and promotes their using the facility for future family needs

b) Continuity of care and comprehensive cross-training promote recruitment and retention of staff

3) Cost efficiency

a) Space is more efficient since SRMC eliminates need for duplication of support area (i.e., utility and linen rooms)

b) Staffing for one area rather than three combined with increased flexibility of staff through cross-training reduces personnel costs

c) Non-transfer of care and smaller space decreases cleaning and maintenance

d) Combined practices of physiologic management with mother-baby nursing help to decrease use of technology and provide support needed for early discharge, thereby reducing operational costs

**d.** Risk to implementing SRMC: inability to change culture, staff attrition, and loss of commitment

**2.** Birth centers

**a.** Maternity unit that provides low-technology care in a homelike setting, families generally return home shortly after giving birth

**b.** Types of birth centers

1) Freestanding

a) Separate from acute care hospital setting

b) Has more autonomy in formulating policies and procedures for center operations and programs of care for clients

c) Provide comprehensive maternity services including prenatal care, education and counseling, intrapartum, and postpartum care with home visiting and family planning

2) In-hospital birth centers

a) Located on hospital grounds or inside a hospital

b) Generally provide only intrapartum and early postpartum care

       3) Commonalties

         a) Both types of centers have capabilities of initiating emergency procedures

         b) Have contingency plans for in-hospital obstetric and newborn services

         c) Caregivers: nurse midwives, obstetricians, pediatricians, professional nurses

  **3.** Home births

    **a.** Some families choose to give birth at home as a rejection of physician-directed and hospital-based rituals

      1) Many of these expectant mothers are well-educated, especially related to childbearing, and are middle-to upper-middle-class

      2) Low-risk, healthy clients motivated to actively participate in the whole childbearing process

    **b.** Some women give birth at home through lack of choice or access to the health care system

---

## Case Study

During the pregnancy with their second child, an Asian-Indian Hindu couple discovered their son had Wiskott-Aldrich syndrome. This syndrome is an X-linked recessive disorder that leads to an early death from a super infection. At the birth of their daughter, the stem cells were harvested from the umbilical cord for a bone marrow transplant to their son.

❶ What are the ethical issues involved in using stem cells from one child to improve the health and well-being of another?

❷ Are there any cultural conflicts in harvesting stem cells for Hindus or Asian Indians?

❸ What is the significance of having a son or daughter for an Asian Indian family?

❹ Who might be available to support the family as they adapt to a new child and await the results of the compatibility test on the stem cells?

❺ What steps should the nurses take to be able to support the family and give appropriate guidance in this situation?

*For suggested responses, see page 336.*

## Posttest

**1** A client who is a brittle diabetic is seeking to get pregnant. Who should she choose as a care provider?

(1) A certified nurse-midwife
(2) A family nurse practitioner
(3) An obstetrician
(4) A maternal-fetal medicine specialist

**2** The nursery nurses routinely keep the newborns in the nursery except for feeding times. They justify this action by saying that the infants need to be available for the pediatricians when ever they might make rounds. The nurses also feel that they can monitor the newborns better if they are in the nursery. What type of views are the nursery nurses expressing?

(1) Ethnocentric views
(2) Culturally aware views
(3) Culturally sensitive views
(4) Culturally diverse views

**3** A client, who is a gravida 14, para 10-3-0-16, gave birth to all her children vaginally. She presents in labor and upon vaginal examination the obstetrician discovers the infant is in footling breech position. The obstetrician plans to do a cesarean section immediately but the patient adamantly refuses. How can the nurse help resolve the dilemma?

(1) Follow the physicians orders and prepare the client for surgery.
(2) Help identify all the options, taking action on the best option for all concerned.
(3) Side with the client and refuse to prepare her for surgery.
(4) Call the supervisor so she can mediate the dispute.

**4** A 16-year-old client, who lives in a state without an emancipated minor law, needs to have a dilatation and curettage (D&C) after the manual delivery of the placenta. Who can legally give informed consent for the client to have this procedure?

(1) The client
(2) The client's physician
(3) The client's mother
(4) The client's best friend

**5** The young children of a client call the woman who stays in their home three days a week "Auntie." Why might she be considered part of the family unit?

(1) She is the client's closest colleague.
(2) She lives in another city four days a week.
(3) She has no children of her own.
(4) She has strong emotional ties with the children.

**6** Childbearing is considered a developmental crisis for a family because:

(1) It is an abnormal experience in the process of growth and development.
(2) It is a period of physical, psychological, and social change causing a sense of disorganization.
(3) It is a stressful, unexpected event caused by external factors.
(4) The family has already mastered the tasks of this maturational stage.

**7** A nurse is the defendant in a suit brought by a client who had a postpartum hemorrhage requiring transfusion of 20 units of blood and a hysterectomy after the delivery of her third child. The client had an epidural before delivery and immediately after delivery of the placenta the client had persistent uterine atony with heavy bleeding. In the immediate postpartum, the client's uterus continued to get boggy and the client had a heavy, bright rubra lochial flow. The nurse is being sued for not providing appropriate care. Which of the following would be the standard of care for a client experiencing a postpartum hemorrhage?

(1) Palpate the fundus every 10 to 15 minutes and if boggy, massage to expel clots.
(2) Have the client empty her bladder only when she has the urge to void.
(3) Discontinue the pitocin IV when the uterus is firm and 4 centimeters above the umbilicus.
(4) Do assessments every 30 minutes as indicated on the postpartum flow sheet.

**8** During labor the nurse notices that the husband of a Ukrainian client just sits beside the bed and is not actively involved with the client. While the nurse interprets this as not being very supportive, how might the client interpret her husband's actions?

(1) The client would prefer more active involvement in coaching from her husband.
(2) The client interprets her husband's presence in the labor room as caring.
(3) The client would like him to leave the room so her mother could be there instead.
(4) The client wants to labor alone with only the hospital staff present.

**9** The United States has one of the highest infant mortality rates among all industrialized nations. Preterm labor and delivery of low birth-weight infants are several of the primary factors related to infant mortality and can be linked to the lack of prenatal care. Why are many client's unable to obtain prenatal care?

(1) Health care and other services are well-coordinated for needy clients.
(2) All uninsured pregnant women are eligible for Medicaid.
(3) Prenatal care services and providers are not available in certain areas.
(4) Many healthcare providers are willing to provide care in subsidized clinics.

**10** A client from the Gusii tribe in Kenya presents in active labor. As the nurse does a vaginal exam she realizes that the client has been circumcised and the vaginal opening is not large enough to admit two fingers. The nurse believes female circumcision is a type of mutilation. What should the nurse do so she can continue to give appropriate, supportive care?

(1) Recognize that her personal beliefs and values differ from those of the client.
(2) Report the finding of the circumcision to the primary care provider.
(3) Avoid entering the client's room and making further assessments.
(4) Accept that personal values and beliefs will interfere with the provision of care.

*See pages 31–32 for Answers and Rationales.*

## Answers and Rationales

### Pretest

**1** **Answer: 2** *Rationale:* Reporting all information gathered, such as the headache, may have heightened the physician's concern about progressing preeclampsia. It is the nurse's responsibility to report all information from an assessment. The nurse furthered her negligence by not recognizing all the signs of preeclampsia, an accepted standard of maternal-newborn practice, but the immediate concern of this case study was not reporting all information to the physician.
*Cognitive Level:* Analysis
*Nursing Process:* Assessment; *Test Plan:* PHYS

**2** **Answer: 4** *Rationale:* The legal system is founded on rules and regulations that are external to oneself and that guide society in a formal and binding

manner. Ethical issues are subject to an individual's values, beliefs, culture, and interpretation.
*Cognitive Level:* Analysis
*Nursing Process:* Assessment; *Test Plan:* HPM

**3** **Answer: 1** *Rationale:* A nurse signs the consent form as witness to the client's signature.
*Cognitive Level:* Application
*Nursing Process:* Implementation; *Test Plan:* PSYC

**4** **Answer: 2** *Rationale:* When clients can eat the foods they prefer, they are more satisfied and recover more quickly. Foods that are provided by the hospital kitchen might be unknown to the client. When one is under stress or ill, there is a longing for foods that are known and liked.
*Cognitive Level:* Analysis
*Nursing Process:* Analysis; *Test Plan:* HPM

**5** **Answer: 3** *Rationale:* As maternity care has become more family-centered efforts are made to keep the family together all the time. This is done by providing single-room maternity care, letting the client define her family and designate who she wants to have present at the birth, and encouraging the family to keep the infant with them in the room so they have more opportunity for bonding and learning about each other.
*Cognitive Level:* Analysis
*Nursing Process:* Evaluation; *Test Plan:* PSYC

**6** **Answer: 3** *Rationale:* Midwifery is the branch of nursing that deals with the practice of assisting women and their families in childbirth. It has been practiced since very early times. Obstetrics was not introduced to medicine until the late 1800s and primarily focuses on high-risk circumstances in pregnancy, labor, and the postpartum. Only a small percentage of nurse-midwives currently practice in the home.
*Cognitive Level:* Application
*Nursing Process:* Planning; *Test Plan:* SECE

**7** **Answer: 3** *Rationale:* Restrictive beliefs and practices are those things an expectant mother should not do or avoid so that she will have a positive pregnancy outcome.
*Cognitive Level:* Analysis
*Nursing Process:* Analysis; *Test Plan:* PSYC

**8** **Answer: 4** *Rationale:* Certified nurse-midwives are prepared to manage independently the care of women and their families who are at low-risk for complications during pregnancy and birth. They take a holistic approach to assessment and identification of needs,

providing education and information to empower the expectant mother and her family for active involvement during the reproductive years.
*Cognitive Level:* Application
*Nursing Process:* Planning; *Test Plan:* HPM

**9** **Answer: 1** *Rationale:* Documentation needs to reflect the standards of care. If the nurses routinely chart time of the decision and time surgery began, data can be collected to compare the unit's practice with national standards.
*Cognitive Level:* Analysis
*Nursing Process:* Evaluation; *Test Plan:* SECE

**10** **Answer: 3** *Rationale:* It is the nurse's responsibility to report the situation to the nurse's supervisor when the physician does not act on information from the nurse regarding concerns about client safety. The nurse also needs to document that the obstetrician was notified, the obstetrician's response, and the nurse's further actions in reporting to the supervisor.
*Cognitive Level:* Application
*Nursing Process:* Implementation; *Test Plan:* HPM

**Posttest**

**1** **Answer: 4** *Rationale:* A person who is a brittle diabetic is considered high-risk and will need to be monitored closely. Many obstetricians have expertise in management of medical complications and will recognize situations when the client needs referral to a maternal-fetal medicine specialist.
*Cognitive Level:* Application
*Nursing Process:* Planning; *Test Plan:* PHYS

**2** **Answer: 1** *Rationale:* The views of the nursery nurses are ethnocentric and based on the culture of the Western health care system where convenience for the pediatricians is of primary importance and only the nurses can adequately monitor the clients.
*Cognitive Level:* Analysis
*Nursing Process:* Assessment; *Test Plan:* SECE

**3** **Answer: 2** *Rationale:* One of the steps in an ethical decision-making framework is to identify the options. The next step is to resolve the dilemma by deciding on the best option for action based on the views of all concerned. Since this client has successfully delivered vaginally numerous times, there are several options available to the client. Using an ethical decision-making framework is a good way to resolve the dilemma.
*Cognitive Level:* Application
*Nursing Process:* Implementation; *Test Plan:* PHYS

**4**    **Answer: 3** *Rationale:* In a state with no emancipated minor law, the client's parents are granted the authority and responsibility to give consent for their minor children.
*Cognitive Level:* Application
*Nursing Process:* Implementation; *Test Plan:* SECE

**5**    **Answer: 4** *Rationale:* A family can be defined as a group of individuals who are bound by strong emotional ties, a sense of belonging, and a passion for being involved in one another's lives. They may or may not be related or live together on a permanent basis.
*Cognitive Level:* Analysis
*Nursing Process:* Assessment; *Test Plan:* PSYC

**6**    **Answer: 2** *Rationale:* Childbearing is a developmental crisis because it is a normal period of growth and development. As new roles are learned and assumed, the changes may cause disturbances in life's patterns and a sense of disorganization.
*Cognitive Level:* Analysis
*Nursing Process:* Evaluation; *Test Plan:* PSYC

**7**    **Answer: 1** *Rationale:* Standard of care for clients experiencing a postpartum hemorrhage requires frequent, every 10 to 15 minutes, assessments of vital signs, uterine tone and placement, characteristics and amount of lochia, condition of the perineum, urinary elimination, and level of pain. Massaging the uterus helps to assure that the uterus stays firm, empty, and involutes toward the umbilicus. Right after delivery

the client might not have an urge to void and needs to be encouraged to do so, especially when the uterus is rising above the umbilicus. The IV should be maintained until there is no further risk of postpartum hemorrhage.
*Cognitive Level:* Application
*Nursing Process:* Analysis; *Test Plan:* PHYS

**8**    **Answer: 2** *Rationale:* As Ukrainian men become more acculturated they are learning to be supportive of and involved with their wives during pregnancy and labor. The women interpret the presence of their spouses as an indication of care.
*Cognitive Level:* Analysis
*Nursing Process:* Evaluation; *Test Plan:* PSYC

**9**    **Answer: 3** *Rationale:* Many barriers to prenatal care have been identified including the lack of available prenatal care services and providers in many areas of the country.
*Cognitive Level:* Application
*Nursing Process:* Assessment; *Test Plan:* SECE

**10**    **Answer: 1** *Rationale:* Personal values and beliefs clarification is the first step in appreciating that personal ethical views may differ greatly from the client's value system. Understanding the differences allows the nurse to remain objective when providing care and when serving as a consultant for decision making by the client.
*Cognitive Level:* Analysis
*Nursing Process:* Assessment; *Test Plan:* SECE

# References

Andrews, M. M. (1999). Theoretical foundations of transcultural nursing. In M. M. Andrew & J. S. Boyle (Eds.), *Transcultural concepts in nursing care* (3rd ed.). Philadelphia: Lippincott, pp. 3–22.

Andrews, M. M. & Boyle, J. S. (1999). *Transcultural concepts in nursing care* (3rd ed.). Philadelphia: Lippincott.

Andrews, M. M. & Hanson, P. A. (1999). Religion, culture, and nursing. In M. M. Andrew & J. S. Boyle (Eds.), *Transcultural concepts in nursing care* (3rd ed.). Philadelphia: Lippincott, pp. 378–443.

Bohay, I. Z. (2001). Culture care meanings and experiences of pregnancy and childbirth of Ukrainians. In M. M. Leininger (Ed.) *Culture care diversity & universality: A theory of nursing.* Boston: Jones and Bartlett, pp. 203–229.

Driscol, K. M. & Nichols, F. H. (1997). Legal aspects of maternal-newborn nursing. In F. H. Nichols & E. Zwelling (Eds.), *Maternal-newborn nursing Theory and practice.* Philadelphia: W. B. Saunders Company, pp. 138–153.

Gardner, S. L., & Enzman Hagedorn, M. I. (1997). *Legal aspects of maternal child nursing practice: Concepts and strategies in risk management.* Menlo Park, CA: Addison-Wesley, 102–107.

Goodwin, L. & Nichols, F. H. (1997). Roles of the maternal-newborn nurse. In F. H. Nichols & E. Zwelling (Eds.), *Maternal-newborn nursing Theory and practice.* Philadelphia: W. B. Saunders Company, pp. 49–56.

Guido, G. W. (2001). *Legal and ethical issues in nursing* (3rd ed.). Upper Saddle River, NJ: Prentice Hall, pp. 52–58.

Jones, L. C. & Maestri, B. O. (1997). Maternal-newborn nursing practice. In F. H. Nichols & E. Zwelling (Eds.), *Maternal-newborn nursing: Theory and practice.* Philadelphia, PA: W. B. Saunders Company, pp. 20–48.

Kruger, S. F., & Nichols, F. H. (1997). Family dynamics. In F. H. Nichols & E. Zwelling (Eds.), *Maternal-newborn nursing: Theory and practice.* Philadelphia: W. B. Saunders Company, pp. 57–86.

Lauderdale, J. (1999) Childbearing and transcultural nursing care issues. In M. M. Andrews & J. S. Boyle, *Transcultural concepts in nursing care* (3rd ed.). Philadelphia: Lippincott, pp. 36–37, 81–106.

Leininger, M. (1995). *Transcultural nursing: Concepts, theories, research & practices* (2nd ed.). New York: McGraw-Hill, p. 199.

Nichols, F. H., & Zwelling, E. (1997). *Maternal-newborn nursing: Theory and practice.* Philadelphia: W. B. Saunders Company.

Norton, M. E. (1999). Ethics and culture: Contemporary challenges. In M. M. Andrews & J. S. Boyle, *Transcultural concepts in nursing care* (3rd ed.). Philadelphia: Lippincott, pp. 444–470.

Olds, S. B., London, M. L., & Ladewig, P. A. (2000). *Maternal-newborn nursing: A family and community-based approach.* (6th ed.). Upper Saddle River, NJ: Prentice-Hall, Inc., pp. 6, 10.

Purnell, L. D. & Paulanka, B. J. (1998). *Transcultural health care: A culturally competent approach.* Philadelphia: F. A. Davis Company.

Satyshur, R. D. & Nichols, F. H. (1997). Ethical issues in maternal-newborn nursing. In F. H. Nichols & E. Zwelling (Eds.), *Maternal-newborn nursing: Theory and practice.* Philadelphia: W. B. Saunders Company, pp. 154–167.

Sherwen, L. N., Scoloveno, M. A., & Weingarten, C. T. (1999). *Maternity nursing: Care of the childbearing family* (3rd ed.). Stamford, CT: Appleton & Lange, pp. 4, 8, 36, 59, 250–251.

Spector, R. E. (2000). *Cultural diversity in health & illness* (4th ed.). Upper Saddle River, NJ: Prentice-Hall, Inc.

Wright, L. M., & Leahey, M. (2000). *Nurses and families: A guide to family assessment and intervention* (3rd ed.). Philadelphia: F. A. Davis Company, p. 69.

Zwelling, E. (1997). Sociocultural aspects of pregnancy. In F. H. Nichols & E. Zwelling (Eds.). *Maternal-newborn nursing: Theory and practice.* Philadelphia: W. B. Saunders Company. pp. 474–489.

## CHAPTER 2

# Reproduction, Fertility, and Infertility

Pamela Hamre, MS, RN, CNM

## CHAPTER OUTLINE

## OBJECTIVES

- Describe the structure and function of the female and male reproductive systems.
- Summarize the components essential for fertility.
- Discuss possible psychological reactions of an infertile couple.
- Describe common diagnostic studies used to evaluate fertility.
- Describe nursing care of clients receiving treatment for infertility.

[ *Media Link* ]

*Use the CD-ROM enclosed with this text, or log onto the address given to access the free, interactive Companion Website created for this series. The CD-ROM and Companion Website accompanying this book offer additional practice opportunities and information—NCLEX Review, Case Studies, Glossary, In Depth with NCLEX, and more.*

**www.prenhall.com/hogan**

## REVIEW AT A GLANCE

**artificial insemination**  *treatment of infertility where sperm are directly inserted into the uterus*

**anovulatory menstrual cycles**  *menstrual cycles that are not preceded by ovulation*

**basal body temperature (BBT)**  *the resting body temperature, taken daily prior to arising from bed; when graphed will detect ovulation*

**endometrial biopsy**  *a diagnostic test whereby the endometrium is sampled via a catheter inserted through the cervix and into the body of the uterus, and a small amount of the endometrium is suctioned and sent to a laboratory for analysis*

**fertility awareness**  *the use of BBT graphing and daily cervical mucous examination to detect ovulation, and therefore determine the optimal day to have intercourse to achieve pregnancy*

**gamete intrafallopian transfer (GIFT)**  *multiple ova are harvested via large-bore needle under ultrasound guidance and are*

*inserted via a large-bore needle under ultrasound guidance into the fallopian tube; spermatozoa that have been collected via masturbation are also inserted via a large-bore needle under ultrasound guidance into the fallopian tube; fertilization occurs in the fallopian tube*

**hysterosalpingogram (HSG)**  *a diagnostic test in which radio-opaque dye is instilled into the uterus and fallopian tubes via a catheter inserted through the cervix; used to detect uterine or tubal anomalies*

**in vitro fertilization (IVF)**  *Multiple ova are harvested via large-bore needle under ultrasound guidance and mixed with sperm in the laboratory; the gametes or embryos are either reinserted into the fallopian tubes or uterus, or frozen for later use.*

**pelvic inflammatory disease (PID)**  *Inflammation of the uterus and fallopian tubes, usually caused by an infectious agent such as* Chlamydia trachomatis *or* Gonorrhea neisseria

**postcoital exam**  *the couple is asked to have intercourse 8 to 12 hours prior to the exam, which should be scheduled 1 to 2 days before expected ovulation; mucus from the endocervical canal is aspirated into a catheter and examined microscopically for infection, consistency and ferning of the cervical mucus, and number and type of active and non-motile sperm*

**tubal embryo transfer (TET)**  *multiple ova are harvested via large-bore needle under ultrasound guidance and fertilized in vitro (in the laboratory); up to four of the subsequent embryos are reinserted into the fallopian tube*

**zygote intrafallopian transfer (ZIFT)**  *multiple ova are harvested via large-bore needle under ultrasound guidance and fertilized in vitro (in the laboratory); up to four of the subsequent fertilized ova (zygotes) are reinserted into the fallopian tube*

## Pretest

1  A client's basal body temperature (BBT) graph shows a nearly straight line. Which of the following describes the etiology of what the graph means?

(1) The client is not ovulating.
(2) The client is not having intercourse.
(3) The client is ovulating late in her menstrual cycle.
(4) The client is not taking her temperature correctly.

2  A client who has had pelvic inflammatory disease (PID) caused by *Chlamydia trachomatis* is at risk for which of the following?

(1) Anovulatory menstrual cycles
(2) Ectopic pregnancy
(3) Multifetal pregnancy
(4) Cervical dysplasia

3  The nurse explains to a male client with vas deferens blockage to expect which of the following problems?

(1) Frequent urination
(2) Oligospermia
(3) Impotence
(4) Decreased libido

4  Which of the following statements tells you that a client needs further teaching? "To become pregnant, we should:

(1) Have intercourse on the fourteenth day of my menstrual cycle."
(2) Have intercourse when my basal body temperature rises."
(3) Have intercourse every other day during the week before and after ovulation."
(4) Abstain from intercourse for the month prior to the month we want to conceive."

**5** An infertile couple will likely have which of the following tests ordered?

(1) Semen analysis and hystersalpingogram
(2) Hysterosalpingogram and Pap smear
(3) Colposcopy with endocervical biopsy
(4) Sexually transmitted infection testing and artificial insemination

**6** Nursing care of the infertile couple would include which of the following?

(1) Assistance in dealing with feelings of guilt and shame
(2) Facilitation of verbalizing which partner is to blame
(3) History and vital sign analysis only
(4) Discussion of the advantages of adoption instead of infertility treatment

**7** A client with fallopian tube blockage would be a candidate for which of the following methods of achieving pregnancy?

(1) Natural family planning
(2) In vitro fertilization
(3) Tubal ligation
(4) Sperm washing

**8** The client has been scheduled to have a hysterosalpingogram. Which of the following questions does the nurse need to ask?

(1) "Do you have any metal implants?"
(2) "When was the last time you had intercourse?"
(3) "When was the first day of your last menstrual cycle?"
(4) "What was your age at menarche?"

**9** Which of the following statements made by the client scheduled for in vitro fertilization would indicate the need for additional teaching?

(1) "The egg retrieval procedure may be uncomfortable, but medication will be available for me."
(2) "The fertilized eggs will be implanted into my uterus 2 to 3 days after the egg retrieval."
(3) "I will need to limit my activities the day of the egg retrieval and the day of implantation."
(4) "I will have eight embryos implanted to maximize my chance of carrying a baby to term."

**10** The procedure of partner sperm intrauterine insemination is indicated for a couple when:

(1) The male partner has a varicocele.
(2) The female partner has irregular menses.
(3) The female produces anti-sperm antibodies.
(4) The male partner has human immunodeficiency virus.

*See pages 47–48 for Answers and Rationales.*

## I. The Reproductive System

### A. Female structures

1. External structures

   **a.** Labia majora: fleshy longitudinal folds of tissue that cover and protect underlying structures

   **b.** Labia minora: small, soft folds of tissue beneath the labia majora that directly cover the vaginal introitus

   **c.** Clitoris: small (6 mm × 6 mm) erectile tissue with rich blood and nerve supply covered by the labia minora

2. Internal structures (Figure 2-1)

   **a.** Vagina: muscular, membranous tube with side walls covered with rugae that connect the external genitalia with the cervix and uterus; also called

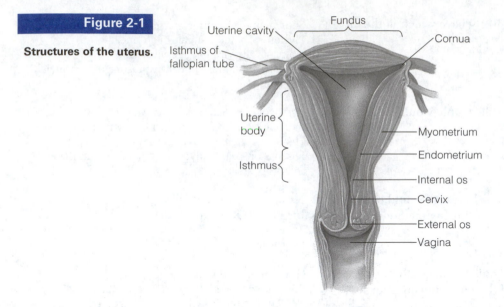

**Figure 2-1**

**Structures of the uterus.**

the birth canal; provides a passageway for sperm when attempting conception, menstrual flow during menstruation, and the fetus during childbirth

**b.** Cervix: neck of the uterus, extends down into the vagina; consists of fibrous tissue that distends during labor

**c.** Uterus: hollow muscular organ at the superior end of the vagina; also called the womb; sheds endometrium with menstrual cycles, and holds the fetus during pregnancy; superior portion known as the fundus; inferior portion ends in the cervix

**d.** Fallopian tubes: connect each ovary with the uterine body; ciliated to transport ovum or zygote; portion which attaches to the uterus is the isthmus; middle section is the ampulla; ends at the ovary in funnel-shaped infundibulum, which has finger-like fimbriae reaching towards the ovary

**e.** Ovaries: almond-sized endocrine functioning glands that secrete estrogen and progesterone; mature one follicle and ovum during each menstrual cycle from menarche to menopause, except during pregnancy

**B. Male structures**

 **1.** External

**a.** Foreskin: circular fold of skin that covers the glans, removed via circumcision

**b.** Penis: vascular shaft that contains urethra and erectile tissue which lengthens and elongates through stasis of blood in the vessels; the glans is the tip of the penis, and has the urethral meatus centered in it; the shaft is the midportion, and the base attaches to the scrotum and groin

**c.** Scrotum: rugated covering of the testes composed of muscle tissue that raises and lowers the testes to control their temperature for optimal sperm production

2. Internal

   a. Testes: two lobular oval glands located within the scrotum where spermatogenesis takes place via meiosis

   b. Epididymis: tube-like duct arising from the top of each testis and ending in the vas deferens

   c. Vas deferens: connects the epididymis to the prostate gland

   d. Prostate gland: encircles the urethra just below the bladder, producing alkaline fluid that is released during ejaculation

   e. Seminal vesicles: lobular glands located just superior to the prostate, produce seminal fluid that is secreted during ejaculation to support sperm metabolism and motility

   f. Urethra: tube that passes through the prostate gland and connects the bladder and the urethral meatus; also is passage for ejaculate

   g. Semen: male ejaculate comprised of spermatozoa and glandular secretions; milky white in color; average volume from 2 to 5 ml

**C. Functions of female structures**

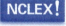

1. Oogenesis: all oocytes are present at birth; meiosis leads to maturation of an individual ovum under the influence of follicle stimulating hormone (FSH); luteinizing hormone (LH) transforms the follicle into the corpus luteum, which maintains the pregnancy through the production of progesterone; ovaries produce estrogen and progesterone in both the pregnant and nonpregnant state

2. Menstruation occurs if the ovum is not fertilized and the corpus luteum disintegrates; the endometrium becomes ischemic as progesterone and estrogen levels drop in the last week of the menstrual cycle, leading to sloughing of the myometrium

3. Conception occurs in the fallopian tube when a 23 chromosome-containing spermatozoon enters a 23 chromosome-containing ovum and produces a 23 chromosome pair-containing diploid zygote

4. Pregnancy: cleavage (rapid mitotic division of the zygote) creates a blastocyst, which in turn becomes a multicellular solid ball of 16 cells (morula); further division leads to trophoblast stage, when it implants within the endometrium

5. Secretion production: cervical secretions become stratified during ovulation to facilitate sperm transport towards the ovum; endometrial secretions are rich in glycogen to nourish the developing embryo until placental circulation is in place

**D. Age related changes of the female reproductive system**

1. Menses begin during puberty, stimulated by the release of estrogen and progesterone

2. Menopause is characterized by 1 year of amennorhea, and occurs on average at age 50; postmenopausal changes of the reproductive tract include thinning and atrophy of external and internal structures

### E. Functions of the male structures

1. Spermatogenesis takes place in the testes; the spermatozoa then proceed through the tubules of the epididymis where motility and fertility develop, finally being stored in the reservoir of the epididymis

2. Ejaculation is a series of muscular contractions that release spermatozoa and seminal fluid through the penis

3. Urination also takes place through the urethra in the penis

4. Secretion production: the prostate gland and seminal glands create a milky-white fluid that nourishes the spermatozoa during and after ejaculation

### E. Age related changes of the male reproductive system

1. Puberty is characterized by greatly increased serum levels of testosterone, which in turn stimulate elongation and thickening of the penile shaft, spermatozoa production, and enlargement of the testes and scrotum

2. Spermatozoa count, motility, and morphology begin to decrease in middle age

3. External organs atrophy in the elderly

## II. Fertility

### A. Female components

1. Primary infertility is that which occurs prior to ever having conceived; secondary infertility occurs after a pregnancy

2. Menstrual cycle: the follicular phase is days 1 to 14 of the cycle, incorporating the menstrual phase (menses) and proliferative phase (beginning of endometrial thickening); variations in the length of the menstrual cycle are caused by variations in the length of the follicular phase; the luteal phase is days 15 to 28 of the cycle, and includes the secretory phase (the plush endometrium secretes glycogen in preparation for implantation of a fertilized ovum) and the ischemic phase (beginning of the breakdown of the endometrium when fertilization has not occurred); the luteal phase is always 12 to 14 days in length

3. Ovulation: an ovum begins to mature during the follicular phase as a result of FSH production; at the onset of the luteal phase, a blister-like graafian follicle appears and enlarges on the surface of the ovary under the influence of FSH and LH; the ovum oozes out of the follicle at the time of ovulation; the ruptured follicle becomes the corpus luteum, which disintegrates if fertilization does not occur or creates progesterone if fertilization has occurred; a body fat percentage of 14 percent or more is needed to support ovulation (caused by estrogen being stored in body fat); lower than 14 percent body fat will result in irregular menses or amenorrhea

4. Cervical mucus: becomes more plentiful, a thinner and more stretchy consistency, and forms columns during ovulation to facilitate the transport of sperm into the uterus; cervical mucus production can be impeded by surgical treatments for abnormal Pap smears

5. Uterine structure: a septum (a fibrous, vertical, wall-like structure in the center of the uterine body), a unicornate uterus (one-sided, banana-shaped uterus) or a bicornate uterus (two banana-shaped uteri side by side, curving away

from each other; may end at one cervix, or have two cervices and vaginas) will have less normal myometrium and fewer healthy places for an embryo to implant successfully; a bicornate uterus may have one underdeveloped horn and ovary and be ovulating and fertile every other cycle; a complete bicornate uterus with double vagina may result in sperm being present in the horn of the uterus which is not ovulating or is underdeveloped (see Figure 2-2)

6. Hormones

   a. Estrogen: produced by ovaries, especially the ovarian follicle during ovulation; responsible for the development of secondary sex characteristics at puberty; peaks in the follicular phase of the menstrual cycle; inhibits FSH and LH production

   b. Progesterone: secreted by the corpus luteum; peaks during the luteal phase; stimulates FSH and LH secretion; responsible for endometrial thickening

   c. FSH: anterior pituitary hormone that matures one ovarian follicle each cycle

   d. LH: anterior pituitary hormone that completes maturation of the ovarian follicle; ovulation occurs 10 to 12 hours after LH peaks

7. Fallopian tube must be patent for sperm to reach the ovum and for the fertilized ovum to reach the uterus; scarring can occur from an infection, such as a ruptured appendix during adolescence or **pelvic inflammatory disease (PID),** an infection of the uterus and fallopian tubes; the cilia in the fallopian tubes, which propel the ovum toward the oncoming sperm, will have decreased motility in cigarette smokers, thereby decreasing fertility

**B. Male components**

**NCLEX!**

1. Sperm production

   a. Morphology: at least 50 percent of the sperm must have normal form to achieve optimal fertility

   b. Count: normal levels are > 20 million sperm per milliliter of ejaculate

   c. Motility: at least 50 percent of sperm should have normal motion patterns

   d. Decreased sperm count and motility can be caused by increased scrotal temperature resulting from frequent hot tub or sauna use, tight clothing, or varicocele; heavy alcohol, marijuana, or cocaine use; trauma to the scrotum; mumps during adulthood; developmental factors; and cigarette smoking

**Figure 2-2**

**Uterine structures.**

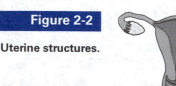 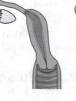 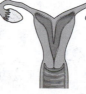 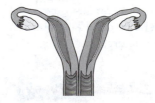 

**A** Normal          **B** Unicornate          **C** Septate          **D** Bicornate with double vagina

2. Testosterone is the primary hormone responsible for libido, sperm production, ability to have and maintain an erection, and ejaculation

3. Erections must be able to be maintained long enough for ejaculation to occur in the vagina and near the cervix for optimal fertility

4. Ejaculation must occur and contain sufficient numbers of normally formed and motile sperm to achieve fertility

## III. Nursing Care of the Infertile Couple

### A. Assessment

1. Common diagnostic studies to detect physiological factors associated with infertility

   **a.** Female

   1) **Basal body temperature (BBT),** or resting body temperature, is obtained by the woman taking her oral temperature each day prior to arising from bed and graphing the results on a month-long graph; a sudden dip occurs the day prior to ovulation and is followed by a rise of 0.5 to 1.0°F, which indicates ovulation; this rise will remain until menstruation begins; **fertility awareness** includes monitoring the BBT and cervical mucus changes to detect ovulation

   2) Serum hormone testing: venous blood is drawn to assess levels of FSH and LH in infertile women, which are indicators of ovarian function

   3) **Postcoital exam:** couple is instructed to have intercourse 8 to 12 hours prior to the exam, 1 or 2 days before expected ovulation; a 10-cc syringe with catheter attached is used to collect a specimen of secretions from the vagina; and the secretions are examined for signs of infection, number of active and non-motile spermatozoa, sperm-mucus interaction, and consistency of cervical mucus

   4) **Endometrial biopsy** (obtaining an endometrial tissue sample for examination) is achieved by positioning the client on the exam table with her feet in stirrups; the provider will then insert a vaginal speculum to visualize the cervix; a paracervical block is first administered to decrease cramping and pain; the sample of endometrium is obtained by inserting a sharp-tipped stiff catheter that is attached to a syringe for suction; the sample is then biopsied to check for a luteal phase defect (lack of progesterone); preprocedure care should include assisting the client (after undressing below the waist) onto the exam table with feet in stirrups and advising the client that she will feel crampy discomfort both during paracervical block administration and during the aspiration; postprocedure care should include providing sanitary napkins for the client as vaginal bleeding will occur and assessing the client for a vaso-vagal response (sudden fainting caused by hypotension induced by vagus nerve stimulation) prior to arising from the exam table

   5) **Hysterosalpingogram** (HSG) detects uterine anomalies, such as septate, unicornate, or bicornate structures, and tubal anomalies or blockage; after sedation or anesthesia is obtained, iodine-based radio-opaque dye is instilled through a catheter into the uterus and tubes to outline these structures and x-rays are taken to document the findings

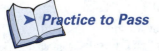

**Practice to Pass**

The client has been instructed to start taking her basal body temperature and graph the results. She tells you that she works the night shift. When is the best time for her to take her daily temperatures?

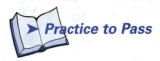

**Practice to Pass**

The client scheduled for a hysterosalpingogram reports an allergy to shellfish. What should the nurse do?

NCLEX!

6) Laparoscopy is carried out under general or epidural anesthesia; the abdomen is insufflated with carbon dioxide, one or more trochars are inserted into the peritoneum near the umbilicus and the symphysis pubis; the laparoscope is then used to visualize the structures in the pelvis or perform surgical procedures

b. Male: semen analysis: the client ejaculates into a specimen container, and the ejaculate is examined microscopically for the number, morphology, and motility of sperm; Table 2-1 presents the normal results of the semen analysis

c. Male and female partner: anti-sperm antibody evaluation of cervical mucus and ejaculate are tested for agglutination, an indication that secretory immunological reactions are occurring between cervical mucus and spermatozoa

2. Psychological factors associated with infertility: many couples will experience shame, guilt, blame, or the stages of grief when faced with a diagnosis of infertility as well as during treatment for infertility; the nurse should facilitate communication between the couple and provide information to the couple on resources for coping with infertility such as support groups; professional counseling may be indicated for some couples

**B. Priority nursing diagnoses:** Compromised family coping; Deficient knowledge; Anxiety; Situational low self-esteem

**C. Implementation and collaborative care**

1. Educational needs of the infertile couple will be extensive; the couple will need education on how to:

a. Perform various procedures (e.g., semen collection for analysis or post-coital exam)

b. The meaning of the results of tests and assessments

c. Self-monitoring during medication administration, and how assisted reproductive technologies (ART) are performed

2. Hormonal therapy is used for induction of ovulation in preparation for in vitro fertilization; the client and/or her partner must be taught how to give subcutaneous and/or intramuscular injections

3. Medications are used to achieve induction of ovulation in cases of **anovulatory menstrual cycles** (menstrual cycles without ovulation) or to achieve multiple ova prior to in vitro fertilization

a. Clomiphene citrate (Clomid, Serophene) is often used to increase FSH and LH secretion, thereby stimulating ovulation; if this is not successful,

**Practice to Pass**

The semen analysis of the male client indicates that he is ejaculating no sperm. What options exist for this couple to achieve pregnancy?

**NCLEX!**

**Practice to Pass**

The infertile couple client reports marital difficulty caused by the stress of the infertility treatments they are undergoing. How should the nurse respond to this information?

| Table 2-1 | Factor | Value |
|---|---|---|
| **Normal Semen Analysis Results** | Volume | > 2.0 mL |
| | pH | 7.0 to 8.0 |
| | Total sperm count | > 20 million per mL |
| | Motility | 50% or greater |
| | Normal forms | 50% or greater |

Pergonol, Humegon, Repronex, or Fertinex may be used; these medications are given via daily injections

b. In some cases, one intramuscular dose of human chorionic gonadotropin (hCG) is administered to stimulate release of the ova from the follicles

c. Risks of ovulation induction include multiple births and ovarian hyperstimulation, which can result in enlarged ovaries, abdominal distention, pain, and occasionally ovarian cysts

4. Sperm washing for intrauterine insemination (IUI): the client's ejaculate is centrifuged to concentrate the spermatozoa, which are then rinsed in saline to remove the seminal fluid; the spermatozoa are again centrifuged, and then used for either in vitro or intrauterine artificial insemination

**NCLEX!**

5. Intrauterine insemination is a form of **artificial insemination,** whereby:

a. Sperm that have been collected within 3 hours of coitus are inserted via a catheter into the uterus

b. Donor sperm may be used if the male partner's sperm count or motility is low or for single women who desire to become pregnant

c. The identity of the sperm donor is kept confidential

**NCLEX!**

6. **In vitro fertilization (IVF):** multiple ova are harvested via a large-bore needle and syringe transvaginally under ultrasound guidance; the ova are then mixed with spermatozoa, and up to 4 of the resultant embryos are returned to the uterus 2 to 3 days later; extra embryos can be frozen for implantation at a later date; side effects include cysts on the ovaries, multiple births related to multiple embryos, and ovarian hyperstimulation

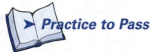

**▶ Practice to Pass**

The client is undergoing ovulation induction in preparation for IVF. She has business commitments and wants to know when to schedule her meetings around the IVF procedure. What should the nurse tell her?

a. Preprocedure care includes instructing the client to give synthetic FSH injections subcutaneously in the abdomen, thigh, or upper arm to stimulate the ovary to produce multiple ova for 5 to 6 days prior to the procedure, giving sedation for the ova retrieval procedure, observing the client for about 2 hours after egg retrieval, and instructing the woman to limit activity for the next 24 hours

b. Postprocedure care following embryo placement in the uterus includes instructing the client to have minimal activity for 24 hours and progesterone supplementation is commonly prescribed

7. **Gamete intrafallopian transfer (GIFT):** harvested ova and sperm are mixed and placed via large bore needle and syringe under ultrasound guidance into the ovarian end of the fallopian tube

8. **Tubal embryo transfer (TET):** in vitro fertilized embryos are placed into the fallopian tube via large-bore needle and syringe under ultrasound guidance; performed 42 to 72 hours after egg retrieval

9. **Zygote intrafallopian transfer (ZIFT):** ova fertilized in vitro are placed into the fallopian tube via large-bore needle and syringe under ultrasound guidance; performed 18 to 24 hours after egg retrieval

10. Micro-epididymal sperm aspiration (MESA) is a micro-surgical technique to obtain a specimen of sperm from the epididymis; it is done as an outclient procedure under sedation and/or local anesthesia

10. Percutaneous epididymal sperm aspiration (PESA) utilizes a small needle under local anesthesia to aspirate sperm from the epididymis

**D. Evaluation:** the couple's knowledge of diagnostic studies, their infertility problem(s), and infertility treatment options is increased; the clients experience decreased anxiety regarding infertility; the clients share their feelings openly; the clients make an informed decision about pursuing or not pursuing treatment for infertility

---

**Case Study**

The client is a 38-year-old woman with primary infertility. The client and her husband are in today for a first appointment at the infertility clinic where you work.

❶ What medical and surgical history questions will you ask of the woman?

❷ What medical and surgical history questions will you ask of the client's husband?

❸ When the client asks you what to expect in the initial assessment of her infertility, how will you answer?

❹ What information about the couple's sexual activity do you need to obtain?

❺ How will the woman's age affect the couple's probable infertility treatment?

*For suggested responses, see pages 336–337.*

---

# Posttest

**1** The nursing plan of care for the infertile client and partner should include:

(1) Assistance in resolving feelings of guilt.
(2) Past year medical and surgical history of both partners.
(3) Brief answers to questions asked and issues raised.
(4) Referral to another clinic for a second opinion.

**2** The client is scheduled for a hysterosalpingogram. Which of the following should be included in the preoperative assessment?

(1) History of sexually transmitted infections
(2) Allergy to shellfish
(3) Presence of metal implants
(4) Difficulty swallowing

**3** The client is considering in vitro fertilization (IVF) and gamete intrafallopian transfer (GIFT). Which of the following statements indicates the need for additional information?

(1) "I will give myself injections of medications to cause my ovaries to ripen more than one egg."
(2) "My husband will need to produce a sample of his sperm the day my eggs are retrieved."
(3) "I will be in the hospital overnight for this procedure."
(4) "I can expect to have some discomfort after the procedure."

**4** The client is seeking to become pregnant through artificial insemination using donor sperm. In teaching the client about this procedure, which information should the nurse plan to include?

(1) The client will be able to find out who the father of her baby is from the sperm bank prior to conception.
(2) The client's child will be able to find out who its father is from the sperm bank when the child turns 18.
(3) The identity of the sperm donor who becomes the father of this child is confidential and will not be released to the client or her child.
(4) The identity of the sperm donor who becomes the father of this child is unknown, as sperm banks do not keep this kind of medical record.

**5** Which of the following statements made by the client indicates that she and her husband are having difficulty coping with their infertility regimen?

(1) "I am never going to consider pregnancy a spontaneous event again."
(2) "I don't like giving myself shots, but I'll do it to get pregnant."
(3) "We had to take out a home equity loan to pay for these treatments."
(4) "My husband just hates having to plan when we make love."

**6** The client, who has a complete bicornate uterus with two vaginas, will:

(1) Be unable to achieve pregnancy.
(2) Be at increased risk for preterm labor.
(3) Need to be artificially inseminated to conceive.
(4) Need to be delivered via cesarean section.

**7** Which client needs to be seen first in the infertility clinic?

(1) 27-year-old woman being seen for an initial infertility exam
(2) 34-year-old man in for semen analysis results
(3) 32-year-old woman on Pergonal and hCG complaining of severe abdominal pain
(4) 30-year-old woman in for pregnancy test following implantation of in vitro fertilization and GIFT

**8** The nurse has explained to the client that the results of the hysterosalpingogram revealed bilateral tubal blockage. The nurse determines further education is needed when the client asks:

(1) "Will the surgery to unblock my tubes be done in the hospital or the surgery center?"
(2) "Will the acupuncture treatments I am getting interfere with the surgical procedure?"
(3) "Will this plug in my fallopian tubes go away forever after I become pregnant?"
(4) "Will long-distance running and a low percentage of body fat affect the success of the surgery?"

**9** The client is a long-distance runner, with 9.0 percent body fat. Which of the following would you expect to see?

(1) Regular menses and a BBT that indicates ovulation
(2) Irregular menses and a BBT that indicates ovulation
(3) Regular menses and a BBT that indicates lack of ovulation
(4) Irregular menses and a BBT that indicates lack of ovulation

**10** The client is a 43-year-old nullipara who is in for her first intrauterine insemination of her partner's washed semen. The nurse determines teaching has been effective when the client states:

(1) "If I get pregnant, I'll see an increase in my BBT."
(2) "If I do not become pregnant, I'll see an increase in my BBT."
(3) "If I get pregnant, I'll see a decrease in my BBT."
(4) "If I do not get pregnant, I'll see a dip and then an increase in my BBT."

*See pages 47–48 for Answers and Rationales.*

# Answers and Rationales

## Pretest

**1** **Answer: 1** *Rationale:* A flat BBT graph indicates lack of ovulation, as the BBT will raise 0.5 to 1.0°F 24 to 48 hours after ovulation.
*Cognitive Level:* Analysis
*Nursing Process:* Assessment; *Test Plan:* HPM

**2** **Answer: 2** *Rationale:* Chlamydial PID causes scarring of the fallopian tubes, thus increasing the incidence of ectopic pregnancy. All other options are incorrect.
*Cognitive Level:* Application
*Nursing Process:* Assessment; *Test Plan:* PHYS

**3** **Answer: 2** *Rationale:* A vas deferens blockage will prevent the sperm from being ejaculated. All other options are incorrect.
*Cognitive Level:* Analysis
*Nursing Process:* Implementation; *Test Plan:* HPM

**4** **Answer: 4** *Rationale:* Options 1, 2, and 3 all increase the likelihood of conception by timing intercourse around the expected time of ovulation. Option 4 does not and indicates a need for further teaching.
*Cognitive Level:* Analysis
*Nursing Process:* Evaluation; *Test Plan:* HPM

**5** **Answer: 1** *Rationale:* Inadequate number or motility of sperm and tubal anomaly or blockage are the most common causes of infertility. Semen analysis will provide information on number and motility of sperm, and hystersalpingogram will detect uterine or tubal anomalies or blockage. The other options are either partially incorrect (option 2) or completely incorrect (options 3 and 4).
*Cognitive Level:* Application
*Nursing Process:* Planning; *Test Plan:* HPM

**6** **Answer: 1** *Rationale:* Infertile couples must deal with guilt, shame, and other psychosocial issues. The nurse's role is to be supportive, facilitate sharing of feelings between the couple, and provide guidance through the infertility assessment and treatment process. History-taking and vital signs are a small part of the infertility clinic nurse role. The client should decide whether adoption or infertility treatment is the best choice, not the nurse.
*Cognitive Level:* Application
*Nursing Process:* Implementation; *Test Plan:* HPM

**7** **Answer: 2** *Ratlonale:* Tubal blockage will prohibit sperm from traveling through the fallopian tubes to reach an ovum and fertilize it. In vitro fertilization involves harvesting ova and placing them with sperm in a petri dish. The resultant embryos are then returned to the uterus.
*Cognitive Level:* Analysis
*Nursing Process:* Analysis; *Test Plan:* HPM

**8** **Answer: 3** *Rationale:* Hysterosalpingograms are performed in the follicular phase of the cycle to avoid interrupting an early pregnancy. The other options do not address this point.
*Cognitive Level:* Application
*Nursing Process:* Planning; *Test Plan:* HPM

**9** **Answer: 4** *Rationale:* Three to four embryos are implanted in the uterus or fallopian tube following in vitro fertilization to maximize the chance of achieving pregnancy while minimizing the risk of multifetal pregnancy.
*Cognitive Level:* Application
*Nursing Process:* Evaluation; *Test Plan:* HPM

**10** **Answer: 3** *Rationale:* Anti-sperm antibodies can develop in the vaginal and cervical secretions. Inserting the sperm directly into the uterus via intrauterine insemination bypasses the secretions so that the sperm are not destroyed. The other options are incorrect.
*Cognitive Level:* Analysis
*Nursing Process:* Assessment; *Test Plan:* HPM

## Posttest

**1** **Answer: 1** *Rationale:* Either partner may experience feelings of guilt when faced with infertility. If the problem is with one partner, that partner's feelings of guilt are often more intense.
*Cognitive Level:* Application
*Nursing Process:* Planning; *Test Plan:* PSYC

**2** **Answer: 2** *Rationale:* Iodine-based dye is instilled into the uterus and watched on X-ray to detect uterine anomalies or lack of tubal patency. An allergy to shellfish, high in iodine content, should alert the nurse to a potential allergic response to the iodine-based dye used for the procedure.
*Cognitive Level:* Application
*Nursing Process:* Assessment; *Test Plan:* HPM

**3** **Answer: 3** *Rationale:* Ova retrieval and GIFT are outclient procedures. The client will not be hospitalized overnight. The other options are true.
*Cognitive Level:* Application
*Nursing Process:* Evaluation; *Test Plan:* HPM

**4** **Answer: 3** *Rationale:* The identity of sperm donors is confidential information. Donors are assigned

random numbers to identify their sperm, and the listing of donors and numbers is kept locked.
*Cognitive Level:* Application
*Nursing Process:* Planning; *Test Plan:* HPM

5  **Answer: 4** *Rationale:* To maximize the chances of conception through achieving the greatest number of motile sperm, couples must abstain for 2 to 3 days prior to expected ovulation and then have intercourse on the day of ovulation or the date of artificial insemination or in vitro fertilization. Because of this, the client's husband must be a willing participant in the infertility regime.
*Cognitive Level:* Application
*Nursing Process:* Assessment; *Test Plan:* HPM

6  **Answer: 2** *Rationale:* A complete bicornate uterus is two complete and separate unicornate uteri. Because of the shape of the uteri being long and narrow (instead of pear-shaped), the maximum uterine volume is often less than a normally shaped uterus. Risks of bicornate uterus include multiple pregnancy losses, preterm labor, and breech presentation. Becoming pregnant is not an issue; carrying the pregnancy to term is the problem.
*Cognitive Level:* Application
*Nursing Process:* Analysis; *Test Plan:* HPM

7  **Answer: 3** *Rationale:* Severe abdominal pain during a cycle of induced ovulation may indicate hyperstimulation of the ovaries. The ovaries could potentially rupture, leading to death.
*Cognitive Level:* Application
*Nursing Process:* Analysis; *Test Plan:* HPM

8  **Answer: 3** *Rationale:* Bilateral tubal blockage requires surgical intervention. The client will not become pregnant until the tubes are cleared. The client does not understand her situation and requires further education.
*Cognitive Level:* Analysis
*Nursing Process:* Evaluation; *Test Plan:* HPM

9  **Answer: 4** *Rationale:* 14 percent body fat is considered adequate to have regular menses and regular ovulation. A client with less than 10 percent body fat will ovulate and menstruate very irregularly or not at all.
*Cognitive Level:* Analysis
*Nursing Process:* Assessment; *Test Plan:* HPM

10  **Answer: 1** *Rationale:* Pregnancy is characterized by a 0.5 to 1.0°F persistent increase in BBT.
*Cognitive Level:* Application
*Nursing Process:* Evaluation; *Test Plan:* HPM

## References

Bergman, R., Afifi, A., Miyauchi, R. Unicornate Uterus. *Virtual Hospital: Illustrated Encyclopedia of Human Anatomic Variation.* Retrieved January 15, 2001 from the World Wide Web: http://vh.org/Providers/Textbooks/AnatomicVariants/AnatomyHP.html.

Dickason, E., Silverman, B., & Kaplan, J. (1998). *Maternal-infant nursing care* (3rd ed.). St. Louis: Mosby, Inc., pp. 45–131.

Kozier, B., Erb, K., Wilkinson, J., & Van Leuven, K. (1998). *Fundamentals of nursing* (Updated 5th ed.). Menlo Park, CA.: Addison Wesley Longman, Inc.

Lowdermilk, D., Perry, S., & Boback, I. (2000) *Maternity and women's health care* (7th ed.). St. Louis: Mosby, Inc., pp. 206–224.

McKinney, E., Ashwill, J., Murray, S., James, S., Gorrie, T., & Droske, S. (2000). *Maternal-child nursing.* Philadelphia: W. B. Saunders Company, p. 209.

Olds, S., London, M., & Ladewig, P. (2000) *Maternal newborn nursing: A family and community-based approach* (6th ed.). Upper Saddle River, NJ: Prentice Hall Health, pp. 69, 140–142, 147–148, 178–194.

Pilliteri, A. (1999). *Maternal and child health nursing* (3rd ed.). Philadelphia: Lippincott, p. 124.

Planned Parenthood. (1996). *The Planned Parenthood women's health encyclopedia.* New York: Crown Trade Paperbacks, pp. 234–237.

Sherwen, L., Scoloveno, M., & Weingarten, C. (1999). *Maternity nursing: Care of the childbearing family* (3rd ed.). Stamford: Appleton & Lange, pp. 103–132.

## CHAPTER 3

# Family Planning and Contraception

Rita S. Glazebrook, PhD, RN, CNP
Patricia Posey-Goodwin, MN, RN
Angela F. Wood, PhD, RN, C

## CHAPTER OUTLINE

## OBJECTIVES

▪ Identify the goals of family planning.

▪ Compare the advantages, disadvantages, and effectiveness of various contraceptives.

▪ Describe nursing responsibilities related to client education regarding contraception.

**[ Media Link ]**

*Use the CD-ROM enclosed with this text, or log onto the address given to access the free, interactive Companion Website created for this series. The CD-ROM and Companion Website accompanying this book offer additional practice opportunities and information—NCLEX Review, Case Studies, Glossary, In Depth with NCLEX, and more.*

**www.prenhall.com/hogan**

## REVIEW AT A GLANCE

**abstinence** *refraining voluntarily from sexual intercourse*

**calendar method** *method of contraception in which a woman abstains from intercourse during the fertile period, also known as rhythm method*

**cervical cap** *a small cap made of soft rubber that is placed over the cervix to block the entry of sperm into the cervix*

**coitus interruptus** *withdrawal of the penis and ejaculation away from the vagina*

**contraceptive sponge** *a small, round polyurethane sponge containing a spermicide*

**Depo-Provera** *long-acting progestin administered by injection every 3 months for contraception*

**diaphragm** *flexible, dome-shaped rubber device to cover the cervix and prevent conception*

**female condom** *disposable, polyurethane sheath with a flexible ring at each end; the closed end is placed into the vagina to prevent sperm from entering the vagina*

**intrauterine device (IUD)** *a plastic or metal device placed into the uterus for long periods of time to prevent implantation of a fertilized egg or cause changes in the lining of the endometrium*

**male condom** *sheath made of latex, plastic, or natural membranes and placed on an erect penis prior to inserting into the vagina to collect the contents of ejaculation*

**mittelschmerz** *mid-cycle pain experienced at the time of ovulation; may last from 1 to 2 days and may be accompanied by pressure, aching felt into the rectum, or distention*

**oral contraceptives** *birth control pills that contain estrogen and progestin, or progestin alone to prevent ovulation and promote thinning of the endometrium*

**postcoital contraception** *emergency contraception initiated within 72 hours of unprotected intercourse or contraceptive failure to prevent pregnancy*

**spermicide** *chemical agent contained in a variety of forms and used to kill sperm*

*or neutralize vaginal secretions to immobilize sperm; commonly nonoxynol-9 and oxynol-9*

**subdermal implants** *Norplant, trade name for six flexible capsules filled with synthetic progestin, that are surgically inserted on the inner side of a woman's upper arm to prevent pregnancy by thickening cervical mucus, changing the endometrium, and reducing transportation of sperm*

**symptothermal method** *a fertility awareness method of contraception which assesses and records daily the primary and secondary signs of ovulation and a coital history on a menstrual cycle calendar and includes the abstinence from intercourse during the period of fertility*

**tubal ligation** *surgical intervention to cut, tie, cauterize, or band the fallopian tubes to block the passage of eggs from the ovary to the uterus*

**vasectomy** *resection of the vas deferens to prevent sperm from being ejaculated outside the body*

## *Pretest*

**1** The client is making her first visit to the contraceptive clinic to discuss family planning. When teaching the client about family planning, the nurse should instruct the client that the goals of family planning include:

(1) Giving the client control over preventing pregnancy.
(2) Increasing fertility in some clients.
(3) Providing oral contraceptives for sexually active women.
(4) Screening for possible birth defects.

**2** The client has come to the family planning clinic to discuss the use of contraceptives. The nurse should do which of the following to facilitate a productive discussion?

(1) Only discuss contraceptive options with the married client if her partner is present.
(2) Instruct the client in which contraceptive option she should use.
(3) Inform the client about use, side effects, and effectiveness of different contraceptive options so that the client can select one that meets her needs.
(4) Avoid discussion of side effects as this might frighten the client and result in her not using a contraceptive.

**3** The client, who has been married for 3 years and sexually active but not yet ready to begin having children, has expressed a desire to use a natural method of family planning. Based on this information, which of the following would be the best choice for this client?

(1) Total abstinence
(2) Basal body temperature method
(3) Male condoms
(4) Female condoms with a spermicide

**4** Which of the following statements by a male client would indicate that he understands the instructions for use of a condom?

(1) "I should lubricate the condom with an oil-based product to avoid friction that could rupture the condom."
(2) "I should unroll the condom and check it for holes before applying it."
(3) "I should hold the rim of the condom while withdrawing my penis from the vagina to avoid leakage."
(4) "I should begin sexual intercourse without the condom and don the condom just before ejaculation."

**5** After counseling your client concerning several contraception options, the client tells you that she has decided to use female condoms. You will know the client understood the information if she says:

(1) "I understand that I shouldn't apply the condom more than 1 hour before having sex."
(2) "I understand that if I develop a latex allergy I will need to find a different type of birth control."
(3) "I understand that this will provide protection against sexually transmitted diseases for me and my partner."
(4) "I understand that my doctor will measure me for the condoms, and then I will purchase them at the drug store."

**6** In counseling a client about the use of a diaphragm, which of the following would be important assessment data to collect?

(1) Willingness of the client to touch her genitals
(2) Frequency of sexual contact
(3) Regularity of menses
(4) Current lactation status

**7** When reviewing the assessment data of the client, which of the following would lead the nurse to recommend a method of contraception other than oral contraceptives?

(1) Family history of ovarian cancer
(2) Insulin-dependent diabetic
(3) History of iron-deficiency anemia
(4) Fibrocystic breast disease

**8** The client is interested in having a subdermal implant (Norplant) inserted. Which of the following side effects should the client be informed of?

(1) Irregular bleeding
(2) Increased risk of pelvic inflammatory disease
(3) Increased production of thin cervical and vaginal mucus
(4) Incomplete emptying of the bladder

**9** A male client has come to the clinic to discuss having a vasectomy. Which of the following indicates the client understands teaching about the procedure?

(1) "I will be able to return to my job as a construction worker immediately following the procedure."
(2) "The procedure should be performed in a hospital, preferably under general anesthesia."
(3) "It will be safe for me to have unprotected sex 1 week following the procedure."
(4) "The procedure will not affect my sexual function."

**10** A pregnant client, who is considering a tubal ligation following her delivery, asks the nurse about the effectiveness of the method. The nurse's best response would be:

(1) "Like all methods of contraception, the effectiveness depends on client compliance."
(2) "Effectiveness depends on whether the tubes are clipped, banded, or plugged."
(3) "The method is very effective. Only 1 to 4 women per 1,000 get pregnant after a tubal ligation."
(4) "If you have a tubal ligation, you won't ever have to worry about getting pregnant again because the procedure is 100 percent effective."

*See page 74 for Answers and Rationales.*

## I. Overview of Family Planning and Contraception

**A. Goal of family planning:** to assist clients with reproductive decision making, enabling the client to have control in preventing pregnancy, limiting the number of children, spacing the time between children, and voluntarily interrupting pregnancy as desired

**B. Decision to use a contraceptive:** may be made individually by a man or woman, or jointly by a couple

**C. Legal issues related to family planning and contraception**

1. Laws pertaining to the provision of contraceptives to minors without parental consent vary from state to state

2. Some states may require consent from the client's spouse regarding sterilization and voluntary interruption of pregnancy

**NCLEX!**

3. Because of the potentially serious complications associated with many of the contraceptive methods, informed consent is obtained

    a. The nurse is responsible for documenting information provided and the understanding of the information by the client

    b. The mnemonic BRAIDED shown in Box 3-1 may be useful to the nurse when counseling a client about family planning and contraceptive methods

4. Decisions about family planning and contraception should be made voluntarily with knowledge of advantages, disadvantages, effectiveness, side effects, risks, contraindications, and long-term effects of a method

## II. Nursing Process in Family Planning and Contraception

**A. Assessment**

1. A history is obtained to identify the client's past and current health status and potential risk factors

2. Additional information is obtained through a sexual history regarding the client's reproductive health and future plans for childbearing

3. Psychosocial data provides information regarding the client's lifestyle, motivation, religious beliefs, cultural influences, and financial factors that may affect selection, access, and use of a particular method; the nurse should not assume the client is heterosexual

4. Knowledge of and concerns about contraceptive methods need to be determined and are necessary for the nurse to identify potential deficits and the need for accurate or additional information

---

**Box 3-1**

**Acronym for Informed Consent with Contraception: BRAIDED**

**B** = Benefits: information about advantages
**R** = Risks: information about disadvantages
**A** = Alternatives: information about other methods available
**I** = Inquiries: opportunity for the client to ask questions
**D** = Decisions: opportunity for the client to decide or change mind
**E** = Explanations: information about the selected method and how to use it
**D** = Documentation: information given and client's understanding of the information

**B. Priority nursing diagnoses:** Health-seeking behaviors; Deficient knowledge; Potential for self-concept, disturbance in body image; Anxiety; Risk for ineffective sexuality patterns

**C. Planning and implementation**

1. Identify actual or potential problems from the client assessment

2. Provide privacy to facilitate discussion; include the partner, if desired

3. Establish mutual goals that facilitate client understanding, compliance, and method effectiveness

4. Provide information about risks, benefits, use, side effects, and cost to facilitate decision making

5. Utilize educational materials designed at the client's level of comprehension; provide information that progresses from simple to complex

6. Assist the client to select a contraceptive method that meets both physiological and psychosocial needs

**D. Evaluation**

1. The client expresses satisfaction and willingness to comply with the selected method of contraception

2. Desired changes in client knowledge or behavior are demonstrated

3. Pregnancy is prevented

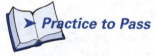
**Practice to Pass**

How might a nurse modify a teaching plan for a client with low literacy skills?

## III. Natural Methods of Family Planning and Contraception

**A. Natural methods:** safe, situational methods requiring increased self-awareness and self-control to be effective

**B. Types of natural family planning methods**

1. **Abstinence** is the practice of avoiding sexual intercourse

   **a.** Advantages

   1) The method is safe, free, and available to all clients

   2) 100 percent effective in preventing pregnancy and sexually transmitted infections when consistently practiced

   3) Can be initiated at any time

   4) Encourages communication between partners

   **b.** A disadvantage is that both participants must practice self-control

   **c.** Client education

   1) Teach alternative methods of obtaining sexual pleasure

   2) Provide positive feedback to clients who desire and maintain abstinence

2. **Coitus interruptus** (withdrawal)

   **a.** Coitus interruptus requires the male to withdraw the penis from the female's vagina when the urge to ejaculate occurs and ejaculate away from the external female genitalia

NCLEX!

**b.** Clients who choose this method must utilize self-control, as the most pleasurable moment during sexual intercourse may coincide with the time to withdraw the penis

**c.** Advantages

1) Coitus interruptus can be practiced at any time during the menstrual cycle

2) The method is free

**d.** Disadvantages

1) One of the oldest but least reliable contraceptive method; 80 percent effective with typical use

2) Some pre-ejaculatory fluid, which may contain sperm, may escape from the penis during the excitement phase prior to ejaculation

3) At the peak of sexual excitement, exercising self-control may be difficult

**e.** Client education

1) Before engaging in sexual intercourse, the male should urinate and wipe off the tip of the penis to decrease the potential of introducing sperm into the vagina

2) Conception may occur if pre-ejaculatory fluid containing sperm enters the introitus

3) A spermicide or post-coital contraceptive may be needed if the female partner is exposed to sperm

## IV. Fertility Awareness Methods of Family Planning and Contraception

**A. These methods are based on an understanding of the woman's ovulation cycle and the timing of sexual intercourse**

**B. All methods attempt to identify the period of female fertility and to avoid unprotected intercourse during that time period**

**C. Advantages**

1. Free, safe, and acceptable to couple's whose religious beliefs prohibit other methods, such as Roman Catholics

2. Increases awareness of the woman's body

3. Encourages couple communication

4. Can be used to prevent or plan a pregnancy

**D. Disadvantages**

1. Requires extensive initial counseling and education

2. May interfere with sexual spontaneity

3. May be difficult or impossible for women with irregular menstrual cycles

4. Used alone, offers no protection against sexually transmitted infections

5. Theoretically reliable, but less effective in actual use

**E.** *Calendar method*

    **1.** Also known as the rhythm method and is based on the assumption that ovulation occurs 14 days (plus or minus 2 days) prior to the next menses, sperm are viable for 5 days, and the ovum is capable of being fertilized for 24 hours

    **2.** The calendar method is the least reliable of the fertility awareness methods, 91 percent effective with perfect use, 75 percent effective with typical use

    **3.** Client education

        **a.** Teach the woman to maintain a menstrual calendar for 6 to 8 months to identify the shortest and longest cycles

        **b.** With the first day of menstruation as the first day of the cycle, calculate the fertile period by subtracting 18 days from the length of the shortest cycle through the length of the longest cycle minus 11 days

        **c.** Counsel the woman to avoid intercourse during the fertile period

**F. Basal body temperature (BBT) method**

    **1.** Based on the thermal shift in the menstrual cycle, the temperature drops just prior to ovulation, rises and fluctuates at a higher level until 2 to 4 days prior to the next menses, then falls if no conception; 97 percent effective with perfect use, 75 percent effective with typical use

    **2.** Client education

        **a.** Instruct the woman to take her temperature with a basal body thermometer, which shows tenths of a degree, and record the findings on a temperature chart

        **b.** Teach the client to take her temperature each morning prior to getting out of bed or beginning activity

        **c.** Counsel the client to avoid intercourse on the day the temperature drops and for 3 days thereafter

        **d.** Inform the client that reliability of the method can be affected by:

            1) A decrease in the BBT that is too small to detect

            2) Factors that may raise or lower the BBT such as illness, stress, fatigue, consumption of alcohol the prior evening, or sleeping in a heated waterbed

            3) Intercourse just prior to the drop in the temperature may result in pregnancy

**G. Cervical mucus method**

    **1.** Also known as the ovulation or Billings method, this method is based on the cervical mucus changes that occur during the menstrual cycle; effectiveness is the same as the BBT method

    **2.** Cervical mucus changes in response to levels of estrogen and progesterone are shown in Table 3-1

    **3.** Client education

        **a.** Teach the woman to assess her cervical mucus daily for amount, color, consistency, and viscosity

| Table 3-1 | | Menstrual cycle phase | |
|---|---|---|---|
| **Cervical Mucus Assessment** | **Factors to assess** | *Luteal phase (infertile period)* | *Follicular phase/ ovulation (fertile period)* |
| | Dominant hormone | Progesterone | Estrogen |
| | Vaginal characteristics | Dryness | Wetness |
| | Cervical mucus characteristics | | |
| | Amount | Scant | Profuse |
| | Color | Cloudy, white to yellow | Clear |
| | Consistency | Thick, sticky | Thin, watery, slippery |
| | Viscosity | None | Stretchable, spinnbarkheit Present at ovulation |
| | Microscopic appearance | No ferning | Ferning |

**NCLEX!**

    **b.** Counsel the woman to avoid intercourse when she first notices the cervical mucus becoming more clear, elastic, and slippery and for about 4 days

    **c.** Convey sensitivity as women who are uncomfortable touching their genitals may find this method unacceptable

    **d.** Instruct the client that cervical mucus can be affected by:

        1) Douches and vaginal deodorants

        2) Semen

        3) Blood and discharge from vaginal infections

        4) Contraceptive gels, foams, film, or suppositories

        5) Antihistamine drugs

**H. *Symptothermal method***

    **1.** The **symptothermal method** incorporates the assessment of multiple indicators of ovulation, and recording findings and coital history on a menstrual calendar, then abstaining from intercourse during the fertile period; effectiveness with perfect use is 98 percent, typical use effectiveness is 75 percent

    **2.** Client education

        **a.** Instruct the client to assess and record the primary indicators of ovulation

            1) Basal body temperature

            2) Cervical mucus

        **b.** Teach the client to become self-aware of and record secondary indicators of ovulation

            1) Increased libido

            2) Abdominal bloating

            3) **Mittelschmerz:** mid-cycle abdominal pain

            4) Breast or pelvic tenderness

            5) Pelvic or vulvar fullness

6) Slight dilatation of the cervical os

7) Softer cervix located higher in the vagina

c. Counsel the client to avoid unprotected sexual intercourse during the fertile period

d. Teach the client that this method provides no protection against sexually transmitted infections

## V. Mechanical Methods of Family Planning and Contraception

**A. Mechanical methods:** provide a physical or chemical barrier to block sperm from entering the cervix; some barrier devices are made from latex and should be avoided by those with latex allergies

**B. *Male condom***

1. The **male condom** is a sheath made of latex, plastic, or natural membranes, which is placed over an erect penis to collect semen; effectiveness is 97 percent with perfect use, 86 percent with typical use

2. Client education

a. Instruct the client to check the expiration date on package, and if it is past the date, obtain another condom

b. Teach the client to avoid using oil-based lubricants but contraceptive foam or water-based lubricants may be used

c. Instruct the client to put on a condom by placing the unrolled condom on the tip of the erect penis, leaving enough room at the tip to collect the sperm, then unrolling the condom from the tip to the base of the erect penis

d. Counsel the client that after intercourse, the erect penis should be withdrawn from the vagina while holding the rim of the condom to prevent leakage

e. Advise the client to inspect the used condom for tears or holes as a break in the integrity of the sheath will decrease effectiveness

f. Teach the client to discard the used condom in a disposable waste container; do not flush in the toilet

3. Advantages

a. Males are able to participate in contraception

b. Sexual intercourse may be prolonged

c. Condoms are available in a variety of sizes and styles at low cost

d. Partners can participate in placing the condom to enhance enjoyment

e. All condoms except those made of natural skins offer protection against pregnancy and sexually transmitted infections; natural skin condoms have pores which can allow the passage of viruses

4. Disadvantages

a. The penis must be erect before placing the condom

b. To prevent spillage of semen, the male must withdraw after ejaculating, while the penis is still erect

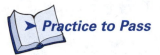
**Practice to Pass**

Discuss the changes that occur during ovulation to be included in a teaching plan for a client who wants to use a fertility awareness method.

    **c.** Condoms can rupture or leak, increasing the potential for semen to escape into the vagina

    **d.** Oil-based lubricants can decrease the effectiveness of the condom

    **e.** Condoms are for single use only

    **f.** Misplacement, perineal or vaginal irritation, or dulled penile sensation are possible

**C. Female condom**

  **1.** The **female condom** is a thin, polyurethane sheath with flexible rings at each end, which covers the cervix, lines the vagina, and partially shields the perineum; effectiveness is 95 percent with perfect use, 79 percent with typical use

  **2.** Client education

    **a.** Instruct the client to insert the closed end of the condom into the vagina so the ring fits loosely against the cervix

    **b.** Counsel the client to have her partner insert his penis into the open end leaving approximately 1 inch of the sheath from the flexible ring outside of the introitus

    **c.** Advise the client that after intercourse, she should remove the condom before standing up by squeezing and twisting the outer ring to close the sheath while gently pulling it out of the vagina

  **3.** Advantages

    **a.** The condom may be inserted up to 8 hours before intercourse

    **b.** Clients who are sensitive to latex can use the female condom

    **c.** Both partners are protected against sexually transmitted infections during intercourse

    **d.** Female condoms are available without a prescription

    **e.** The use of lubricants will not decrease effectiveness

    **f.** Breast-feeding women can safely use condoms

  **4.** Disadvantages

    **a.** These condoms may twist or slip during intercourse

    **b.** If the penis is placed outside of the condom, effectiveness is jeopardized

    **c.** Improper removal results in the risk of ejaculate leaking out of the condom

    **d.** The outer ring may irritate external genitalia

    **e.** The high cost, noise produced with intercourse, or altered sensation are unacceptable for some couples

    **f.** Initially, insertion may be difficult or awkward

**D. Spermicides**

  **1. Spermicides** form a chemical barrier preventing pregnancy by killing sperm or neutralizing vaginal secretions and are available in a variety of forms including creams, gels, melting suppositories, foaming tablets, aerosol foams, and vaginal contraceptive film

2. When used alone, effectiveness with perfect use is 94 percent and with typical use effectiveness is 74 percent; when spermicides and other methods are combined, the contraceptive and anti-microbial benefits are increased

3. The most common spermicidal agents are nonoxynol-9 and octoxynol-9; allergic response is possible

4. Client education

   a. Instruct the client to apply spermicide inside the vagina and close to the cervix before the penis is placed near the introitus

   b. Advise that spermicides must be applied with each act of sexual intercourse

   c. Teach the client that the onset of spermicidal action varies; when used alone effectiveness lasts no longer than 1 hour

   d. Counsel the client that contraceptive foams, creams, and gels are effective immediately

   e. Counsel the client that vaginal contraceptive film and suppositories become effective 15 minutes after insertion into the vagina

5. Advantages

   a. No prescription is required to purchase spermicides

   b. Spermicides may be used alone, with a diaphragm, or with a condom

   c. Foams, gels, and suppositories may add additional lubrication and moisture

   d. The penis can remain in the vagina following ejaculation

   e. The method is safe for breast-feeding women

   f. A variety of forms offers clients additional choices in selecting a spermicide

6. Disadvantages

   a. The spermicide may be irritating to one or both clients

   b. Some forms may be perceived as messy

   c. This method may interfere with spontaneity, as it is inserted before each act of intercourse and may require an interval of time before the onset of action

E. **Diaphragm**

1. The **diaphragm** is a dome-shaped appliance made of rubber with a flexible rim that fits over the cervix, is used with spermicidal cream or jelly, and prevents sperm from entering the cervix; effectiveness with perfect use is 94 percent; effectiveness with typical use is 80 percent

2. Client education

   a. Utilize models and visual aides when demonstrating insertion and removal of the diaphragm

   b. Teach the client to insert and remove the diaphragm (Figure 3-1)

      1) Apply about a teaspoon of spermicidal cream or jelly around the rim and inside the cup

**Figure 3-1**

Inserting the diaphragm.
A. Apply jelly to rim and center, B. Insert diaphragm, C. Push diaphragm rim under symphysis pubis, D. Check placement; cervix should be felt through diaphragm.

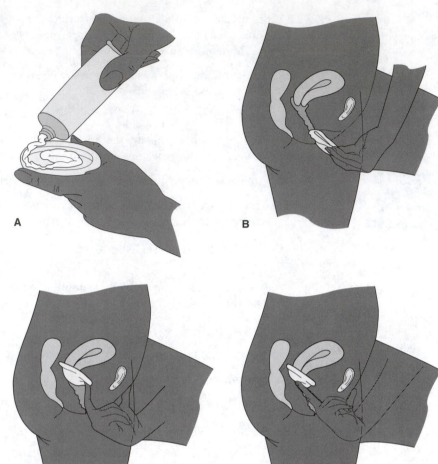

A

B

C

D

2) Squeeze the sides of the diaphragm together, insert through the vagina, place the side of the device containing spermicide over the cervix, and push the upper edge under the symphysis pubis

3) Remove the diaphragm by grasping the rim to dislodge from the cervix and pull down to remove through the vagina

c. Encourage the client to practice insertion and removal when the healthcare provider is present to check for proper placement in the vagina

d. Teach the client the diaphragm remains effective if inserted up to 4 hours before sexual intercourse and should be left in place at least 6 hours after coitus

e. Counsel the client that if the diaphragm is placed more than 4 hours prior to intercourse or coitus is desired again within 6 hours, a condom should be used or additional spermicide should be inserted into the vagina without disturbing the diaphragm

f. Instruct the client that the device should be removed at least once during a 24-hour period to decrease the risk of toxic shock syndrome

**g.** Advise the client to clean the diaphragm with mild soap and water and inspect for tears, punctures, and thinning, avoid the use of oil-based lubricants which weaken the rubber, and replace the diaphragm if any damage is observed

**h.** Teach the client to dry the device thoroughly, dust with cornstarch, and store in the carrying case away from light and heat

**i.** Advise the client that use during the menstrual period or when abnormal vaginal discharge is present should be avoided to decrease the risk of toxic shock syndrome

**j.** Instruct the client to contact the healthcare provider if experiencing any warning signs as shown in Table 3-2

NCLEX!

| Table 3-2 | Method | Warning Signs and Symptoms |
|---|---|---|
| **Warning Signs and Symptoms Associated with Various Methods of Contraception** | Cervical cap, diaphragm, and contraceptive sponge | Toxic Shock Syndrome<br>• Elevation of temperature >101.4°F<br>• Diarrhea and vomiting<br>• Weakness and faintness<br>• Muscle aches<br>• Sore throat<br>• Sunburn-type rash<br>Difficult or painful urination<br>Abdominal or pelvic fullness<br>Foul-smelling vaginal discharge |
| | IUD | Acronym **PAINS**<br>**P** = Period late (pregnancy), abnormal spotting or bleeding<br>**A** = Abdominal pain, pain with intercourse<br>**I** = Infection exposure (STI), abnormal vaginal discharge<br>**N** = Not feeling well, fever >100.4°F, chills<br>**S** = String missing, shorter or longer than usually felt |
| | Oral contraceptives | Acronym **ACHES**<br>**A** = Abdominal pain<br>**C** = Chest pain, cough, and/or shortness of breath<br>**H** = Headaches, dizziness, weakness or numbness<br>**E** = Eye problems (blurring or change in vision) and speech problems<br>**S** = Severe leg, calf, and/or thigh pain |
| | Vasectomy | Fever > 100.4°F<br>Excessive pain<br>Difficulty urinating<br>Redness, swelling, bruising, drainage, or skin edges of the incision that are not closed<br>Bleeding at the site |
| | Tubal ligation | Fever > 100.4°F<br>Excessive pain<br>Difficulty with defecation or urination<br>Nausea or vomiting<br>Redness, swelling, bruising, drainage, or skin edges of the incision that are not closed |

**3.** Advantages

   **a.** Using a diaphragm gives the woman control

   **b.** The barrier provides some protection against sexually transmitted infections

   **c.** A partner may insert the diaphragm if the client has trouble with placement or as part of foreplay

   **d.** The diaphragm contains no hormones and is safe for the breast-feeding client

   **e.** The penis can remain inside the vagina after ejaculation

**4.** Disadvantages

   **a.** The diaphragm must be fitted by a qualified healthcare provider and re-placed annually

   **b.** Refitting or replacement may be needed following pregnancy or a 15-pound weight gain or loss

   **c.** Some clients may have difficulty learning to correctly place the diaphragm

**5.** Contraindications

   **a.** A history of urinary tract infections; pressure from the diaphragm on the urethra may interfere with complete emptying of the bladder and increase the risk of infection related to stasis of urine

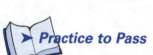

**Practice to Pass**

What patient education is indicated to reduce the potential of toxic shock syndrome for a client using a diaphragm?

   **b.** A history of toxic shock syndrome; if the diaphragm is left in place for a long period of time this may increase the risk of infection

**F. Cervical cap**

**1.** The **cervical cap** is a small thimble-shaped device made of soft rubber that fits over the cervix, is held in place by suction, and acts as a barrier between sperm and the cervix (see Figure 3-2)

**2.** Effectiveness is influenced by the childbearing history of the woman; effectiveness with perfect use for nulliparous women is 91 percent, with typical use effectiveness is 80 percent; in parous women perfect use effectiveness is 74 percent and typical use effectiveness is 60 percent

**Figure 3-2**

**A cervical cap.**

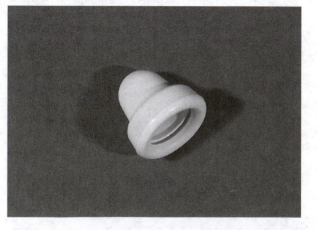

3. Client education

   a. Teach the client to apply spermicide inside the cap

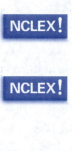

   b. Instruct the client to insert the cap at least 20 minutes but not longer than 4 hours prior to intercourse

   c. Advise the client that the cervical cap may be left in place up to 48 hours

   d. Counsel the client that reapplication of spermicide with repeated intercourse is not needed

   e. Teach the client not to use the cap during menstruation or if any abnormal vaginal discharge is present

   f. Instruct the client to contact the healthcare provider if warning signs develop as listed in Table 3-2

4. Advantages of the cervical cap are similar to those of the diaphragm

5. Disadvantages

   a. The cervical cap may be more difficult to fit because of limited sizes

   b. The cervical cap must be fit by a qualified healthcare provider and should be replaced annually

   c. Clients will need to be rechecked for fit following pregnancy or a 15-pound weight gain or loss; effectiveness is reduced for parous women

   d. If the device dislodges, or slips during sexual intercourse, the risk for contraceptive failure or acquiring a sexually transmitted infection is increased

   e. Some clients may have difficulty inserting and removing the cervical cap

   f. Instruct the client not to use the cervical cap during menstruation or if any signs or symptoms of infection or inflammation are present

G. **Contraceptive sponge**

   1. The **contraceptive sponge** is a small, round polyurethane sponge containing nonoxynol-9 spermicide

   2. Effectiveness in nulliparous women is 91 percent with perfect use and 80 percent with typical use; in parous women, perfect use effectiveness is 80 percent, and with typical use the effectiveness is 60 percent

   3. Client education

      a. Moisten the sponge with water prior to insertion into the vagina to activate the spermicide

      b. Place the concave side of the sponge next to the cervix for a better fit

      c. Leave the sponge in place for at least 6 hours after intercourse

      d. Remove by pulling the polyester loop on the non-concave side of the sponge downward and out of the vagina

      e. Advise that the sponge provides protection up to 24 hours and for repeated acts of intercourse

      f. Leaving the sponge in place for >24 to 30 hours should be avoided because of the increased risk of toxic shock syndrome

      g. Contact the healthcare provider if warning signs develop as listed in Table 3-2

**4.** Advantages

    **a.** Same as for the diaphragm

    **b.** Low cost

**5.** Disadvantages

    **a.** Some clients perceive the sponge as bulky or awkward when in place

    **b.** Some clients perceive the presence of the sponge as uncomfortable during intercourse

    **c.** Effectiveness is reduced for parous women

**H. Intrauterine device (IUD)**

**1.** The specific action of the IUD is unknown; contraception is achieved by immobilizing sperm and impeding their travel from the cervix to the fallopian tubes

**2.** Types of IUDs available in the United States (see Figure 3-3)

    **a.** The Progesterone T (Progestasert) is recommended for women who are allergic to copper and must be changed annually

    **b.** The Copper T380A (ParaGard) is recommended for women who have at least one child; it can be left in place for 10 years; to be avoided for women with an allergy to copper

    **c.** Effectiveness with perfect use is 98.5 to 99.4 percent; typical use effectiveness ranges from 98 to 99.2 percent

    **d.** Preferred candidates for use include parous women in a stable monogamous relationship [low risk for sexually transmitted infection (STI)] with no history of pelvic inflammatory disease (PID) and normal uterine anatomy; nulliparous women at low risk for STI or women with a history of PID who are in a stable monogamous relationship and have had a pregnancy since the PID episode may also be considered on an individual basis

**3.** Client education

    **a.** Teach that cramping or intermittent bleeding may occur for 2 to 6 weeks after insertion

    **b.** Advise that the first few menses after placement may be irregular

    **c.** Instruct that follow-up examination is suggested in 4 to 8 weeks

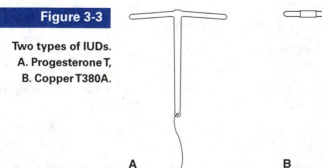

**Figure 3-3**

Two types of IUDs.
A. Progesterone T,
B. Copper T380A.

A        B

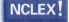

d. Instruct the woman to check for the presence of the string protruding through the cervix by inserting a finger into the vagina once a week for the first month and then after each menstrual period.

e. Counsel the woman to contact the healthcare provider if she is exposed to a sexually transmitted infection or if warning signs known as PAINS develop as shown in Table 3-2

4. Advantages

   a. IUDS are highly effective and provide continuous contraceptive protection

   b. They do not interact with medications

   c. Provide a good contraceptive option for women who cannot use hormone contraceptives, are breast-feeding, or are smokers >35 years of age

5. Disadvantages

   a. The IUD must be inserted by a qualified healthcare professional

   b. Some women experience discomfort, bleeding, and cramping, both during and between menses

   c. The client is at increased risk of pelvic infection for the first 3 weeks following insertion

   d. The uterus may perforate during insertion

   e. The IUD may be expelled spontaneously

   f. IUDs do not protect clients from acquiring sexually transmitted infections

   g. Adolescents rarely meet the criteria for IUD candidates

## VI.  Hormonal Methods of Family Planning and Contraception

A. *Oral contraceptives* **(birth control pills):** act by inhibiting the release of an ovum, blocking the cyclical release of gonadotropin-releasing hormone, and changing cervical mucus

1. Types of oral contraceptives

   a. Combined oral contraceptives contain both estrogen and progestin and are available in 21-day and 28-day packages; effectiveness with perfect use is 99.1 percent; typical use effectiveness is 95 percent

   b. The progestin-only pill, also known as the mini-pill, does not contain estrogen, contains less progestin than combination pills, and may be used by lactating women, women with mild hypertension, and those who experienced side effects from oral contraceptives containing estrogen; effectiveness with perfect use is 95.5 percent; typical use effectiveness is 95 percent

2. Client education

   a. When starting oral contraceptives, instruct the client to begin pills on the first Sunday after the onset of the menstrual period and take one pill at the same time each day

   b. If a 28-day pack is prescribed or the client is taking progestin-only pills, advise the client not to skip days between packages

    **c.** Clients using a 21-day pack should wait 7 days before starting the next cycle of pills

    **d.** Instruct the client what to do if progestin-only oral contraceptives are missed

       1) If the client misses one pill at any time during the cycle, the missed pill should be taken immediately and the next pill taken at the regular time

       2) Any time a pill is missed, the client should use an additional method of contraception through the end of that cycle

    **e.** Instruct the client what to do if combination oral contraceptives are missed

       1) If one pill is missed at any time during the cycle, the client should take the missed pill immediately, the next pill at the regular time, and no back-up method is needed

       2) If two pills are missed during the first 2 weeks, the client is advised to take two pills for the next 2 days and resume taking pills on the regular schedule

       3) If two pills are missed during the third week, the client is advised to take one pill daily until Sunday, then begin a new pack on Sunday without missing any days

       4) If three or more pills are missed at any time, the client is advised to take one pill daily until Sunday, then begin a new pack on Sunday without missing any days

       5) If two or more pills are missed at any time, a back-up method should be used for 1 week or emergency contraception considered, if unprotected intercourse occurs

    **f.** Observe for side effects of oral contraceptives, which can be estrogen-related (such as thromboembolic disease, headache, fluid retention and nausea) or progestin-related (including acne, increased HDL cholesterol level, depression, and hirsutism)

    **g.** Contact the healthcare provider immediately if warning signs develop, which are known as ACHES and are shown in Table 3-2

**3.** Advantages

    **a.** Use of the method is not directly related to the act of sexual intercourse

    **b.** Menstrual periods are usually more regular and predictable

    **c.** The amount of menstrual flow and pre-menstrual symptoms are decreased

    **d.** The incidence or degree of iron-deficiency anemia may be reduced

    **e.** Oral contraceptives are safe throughout the reproductive years for women who do not smoke

    **f.** Non-contraceptive benefits include a decreased risk of ectopic pregnancy, fibrocystic breast disease and ovarian and endometrial cancers; improvement of acne; and some protection against the development of functional ovarian cysts

4. Disadvantages

   a. The risk of ectopic pregnancy is increased if the client conceives while taking the progestin-only pill

   b. Progestin-only pills are more likely to cause irregular bleeding or amenorrhea

   c. Offer no protection against sexually transmitted infections

   d. Clients need to remember to take a pill at the same time each day

   e. Clients with preexisting medical problems may not be candidates for this method

   f. Oral contraceptives may decrease the effectiveness of insulin and oral anticoagulants such as warfarin (Coumadin)

   g. The effectiveness of oral contraceptives may be decreased when taken with other drugs such as phenytoin (Dilantin), carbamazepine (Tegretol), primidone (Mysoline), topirimate (Topamax), griseofulvin (Grisactin), rifampin (Rifadin), ampicillin (Omnipen), and tetracycline (Achromycin)

5. Contraindications

   a. Combined oral contraceptives should not be taken by women with a history of thromboembolic or cardiovascular disorders, breast cancer, or estrogen-dependent neoplasms

   b. Combined oral contraceptives should not be used if the woman is currently pregnant, lactating of <6 weeks duration, smokes >20 cigarettes per day and is >35 years old, has headaches with focal neurological symptoms, experiencing prolonged immobility or surgery on the legs, or has hypertension of >160/100 or diabetes mellitus of 20 or > years duration with vascular disease

**B. Subdermal implants (Norplant)**

1. Consist of six silastic capsules containing levonorgestrel, a progestin, implanted subdermally into the woman's upper inner arm during the first 7 days of the menstrual cycle

2. Act by preventing ovulation and stimulating production of thick cervical mucus, which prevents penetration of sperm

3. Client education

   a. Inform client of possible side effects such as spotting, irregular bleeding, amenorrhea, weight gain, headache, fluid retention, mood changes, and depression

   b. Provide client with information regarding signs and symptoms of infection indicating the need for post-procedure followup

4. Advantages

   a. Not user-dependent for effectiveness; perfect and typical use effectiveness is 99.95 percent in the first year, 98.9 percent cumulative over 5 years

   b. Provides continuous contraception not related to sexual intercourse

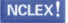

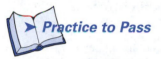

**Practice to Pass**

A client calls the clinic reporting that she "forgot to take her birth control pills for the last two days." How would the nurse advise this client?

      **c.** Does not contain estrogen

      **d.** Effective immediately within 24 hours and for up to 5 years

    **4.** Disadvantages

      **a.** Requires minor surgery to insert and remove the implants

      **b.** May be visible under the skin

      **c.** Irregular or prolonged menses may be unacceptable to the client

      **d.** Cost may be prohibitive

      **e.** Offers no protection against sexually transmitted infections

      **f.** Slightly higher failure rates have been reported in women >154 pounds in the fifth year of use

**C. Long-acting progestin injections**

    **1.** The injectable contraceptive hormone contains medroxyprogesterone acetate (**Depo-Provera**) 150 mg, a long-acting progestin that blocks the luteinizing hormone surge, prevents pregnancy by suppressing ovulation, and thickens the cervical mucus to prevent penetration of sperm with a perfect and typical use effectiveness of 97.7 percent

    **2.** Client education

      **a.** Inform the client of potential side effects such as menstrual irregularities, headache, weight gain, breast tenderness, and depression

      **b.** Teach the importance of following the 3-month injection regimen to maintain contraceptive effects; subsequent dose must be given 80 to 90 days after the previous dose for continuous contraceptive protection

      **c.** Instruct the client to contact the healthcare provider if she experiences any of the warning signs of ACHES as identified in Table 3-2

    **3.** Advantages

      **a.** Contraception is not related to sexual intercourse

      **b.** Safe for lactating women

      **c.** Does not contain estrogen

      **d.** Requires administration only every 3 months

    **4.** Disadvantages

      **a.** The injection must be repeated within 80 to 90 days to maintain effectiveness

      **b.** Clients with cardiovascular disorders or breast cancer are not candidates for the contraceptive hormone injection

      **c.** Return of fertility may be delayed up to 1 year after stopping the method

**D. Postcoital contraception**

    **1.** Measures that may be utilized when the woman is concerned about becoming pregnant because of unprotected intercourse or when a contraceptive method fails

2. Postcoital contraception should be considered an emergency method and not be used by the client on a frequent or regular basis

3. Methods of postcoital contraception should be initiated as soon as possible after unprotected intercourse or contraceptive failure; average reduction in pregnancy rates of 75 to 85 percent, with higher effectiveness if emergency contraception is initiated within 12 hours of unprotected intercourse

   a. Oral contraceptives (MAP, morning after pills): initiate within 72 hours of unprotected intercourse or contraceptive failure

      1) Procedure used with combined oral contraceptive pills includes one dose containing at least 100 mcg ethinyl estradiol and either 100 mg of norgestrel or 50 mg levonorgestrel and repeating the same dose 12 hours later

      2) Procedure for use with progestin-only oral contraceptive pills includes one dose containing 0.75 mg levonorgestrel or 1.5 mg norgestrel and repeating the same dose in 12 hours

      3) An antiemetic, such as metoclopramide (Reglan), can be given 1 hour prior to the administration of the oral contraceptives to control nausea; contraindicated in clients with epilepsy and adverse effects may include depression with suicidal thoughts

   b. Insertion of an IUD

      1) A device containing copper (ParaGard) can be inserted within 5 days of unprotected intercourse or contraceptive failure

      2) This method of emergency contraception is only recommended for women wanting long-term protection and meeting the criteria for an IUD

   c. Mifepristone (RU 486)

      1) A progesterone antagonist that prevents implantation of a fertilized ovum

      2) A 600-mg dose within 72 hours of unprotected intercourse or contraceptive failure is usually effective in preventing pregnancy

4. Client education

   a. Administration of oral contraceptives or insertion of an IUD may not be effective if the client is pregnant

   b. The next menses can be expected about 5 days after the last dose of oral contraceptives; if no bleeding occurs within 21 days, the client should be evaluated for pregnancy

   c. Nausea and vomiting are common side effects of oral contraceptives unless an antiemetic has been given

   d. If postcoital contraception is sought repeatedly, the reason for unprotected intercourse or contraceptive failure should be explored

   e. Counsel the client regarding safer and more reliable methods of contraception for regular use

   5. Advantages

      a. Offers an opportunity to prevent an unwanted pregnancy after forced sexual intercourse, mistake, or method failure

      b. Reduces anxiety about pregnancy prior to the next menses

      c. Provides an opportunity to teach and counsel about reliable contraceptive methods for long-term pregnancy protection

   6. Disadvantages

      a. Timing of next menses can be affected

      b. Amount of next menstrual flow increases in many women

      c. Provides no protection against sexually transmitted infections

## VII. Surgical Methods of Contraception

   A. **Surgical contraceptive methods:** result in voluntary sterilization of the male or female

   B. **Surgical consent:** obtained after the risks and benefits of the specific method are explained

   C. **Vasectomy**

      1. During a **vasectomy,** the vas deferens is resected through small incisions made in each side of the scrotum resulting in blockage of the passage of sperm

      2. Client education

         a. The procedure takes about 15 to 20 minutes and can be performed in a clinic setting under local anesthesia

         b. The client should refrain from driving immediately after the procedure and be discharged to someone who can drive and remain with the client for 24 hours after the procedure

         c. Rest with minimal activity should be encouraged for 48 hours

         d. Tub baths should be avoided for 48 hours

         e. A scrotal support should be worn to increase comfort

         f. Ice packs should be used intermittently to minimize discomfort and swelling

         g. Sitz baths can be used after 48 hours

         h. Strenuous activity should be avoided for 1 week

         i. The healthcare provider should be contacted if warning signs develop as listed in Table 3-2

         j. Sterility is not achieved until the semen is free of sperm, about 4 to 6 weeks or 6 to 36 ejaculations; until then, another contraceptive method should be used during this time

         k. Two or three semen samples should be analyzed to verify sterility prior to resuming unprotected intercourse

         l. Semen should be rechecked at 6 and 12 months to verify stertility has been maintained

4. Advantages

   **a.** The procedure is 99.85 percent effective

   **b.** Recovery time is short

   **c.** Simpler, safer, and more effective than female sterilization

   **d.** Complications are rare

   **e.** Sexual function is not affected

   **f.** Cost-effective and convenient

5. Disadvantages

   **a.** Although reversal of a vasectomy is possible in some cases, this method is considered permanent

   **b.** Potential complications include adverse reaction to anesthesia, infection, bleeding, sperm granuloma or spontaneous re-anastomosis of the vas deferens

   **c.** Fertility, in rare instances, may occur spontaneously due to recanalization of the vas deferens

**D. Tubal ligation**

1. During a **tubal ligation,** the fallopian tubes are accessed through two small incisions into the abdomen and visualized using a laparoscope, then cut, tied, cauterized, or banded to block the passage of sperm and prevent the ovum from becoming fertilized

2. Effectiveness ranges from 99.2 to 96.3 percent depending on the method used; younger women have been reported to experience higher failure rates

3. Client education

   **a.** The procedure takes approximately 30 minutes and is performed under general or local anesthesia

   **b.** The client may be asked to restrict food and fluid intake for several hours prior to the procedure, especially if general anesthesia is planned

   **c.** Pain may be experienced for several days after the procedure

   **d.** Tub baths should be avoided for 48 hours

   **e.** Avoid driving, lifting, and strenuous activity for 1 week

   **f.** The healthcare provider should be contacted if warning signs develop as listed in Table 3-2

4. Advantages

   **a.** Permanent and effective in preventing pregnancy

   **b.** May be performed at any time; immediately after childbirth is optimal because the uterus is enlarged and the fallopian tubes are easy to identify

   **c.** Sexual function and spontaneity are not affected

5. Disadvantages

   **a.** Procedure requires outpatient surgery

   **b.** Potential complications include adverse reaction to anesthesia, infection, and bleeding

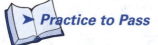
**Practice to Pass**

A client tells the nurse "I am so tired of using contraception. I think I'm ready for something permanent." What additional information should the nurse obtain before responding to the question?

c. If pregnancy occurs after tubal ligation, the risk of ectopic pregnancy increases

d. Reversal of the procedure may not be possible

e. Possible changes in menstrual pattern: "post-tubal ligation syndrome"

**Case Study**

A client comes to the reproductive health clinic seeking contraception. She says she is interested in birth control pills but has never used them and needs more information before making a decision regarding their use.

❶ What factors in the client's history would be contraindications to the use of oral contraceptives?

❷ What advantages of birth control pills should be shared with the client?

❸ What are the disadvantages of birth control pills that should be considered prior to use?

❹ How should the nurse teach the client to use birth control pills?

❺ What warning signs should the nurse teach the client to report immediately to the healthcare provider?

*For suggested responses, see page 337.*

## Posttest

**1** Which intervention would be most effective in teaching a client with low literacy skills how to insert a diaphragm?

(1) Assess the client's understanding of how a diaphragm works.
(2) Give the client a printed handout explaining use of the diaphragm.
(3) Provide the client with an opportunity to practice inserting and removing the diaphragm.
(4) Use an audio tape to explain use of the diaphragm.

**2** Which statement best demonstrates a male client understands how to correctly apply a condom?

(1) "I need to put it on before the penis is erect."
(2) "I should unroll the condom, then place it on the penis."
(3) "After putting on the condom, I need to leave some space at the tip to collect the sperm."
(4) "I can use oil-based lubricants if needed."

**3** A client with a history of toxic shock syndrome comes to the reproductive clinic seeking contraception. Based on this information, which method should the nurse avoid recommending for this client?

(1) Cervical cap
(2) Female condom
(3) Spermicide
(4) Norplant

**4** The rationale for the nurse to ensure that a client gives informed consent for contraception prior to use is based on knowledge that contraceptive methods:

(1) Are invasive procedures.
(2) Require a surgical procedure.
(3) May not be reliable.
(4) Have potentially dangerous side effects.

**5** The nurse should instruct the client who has had an IUD inserted to:

(1) Have the IUD replaced every 3 years.
(2) Check for the string periodically.
(3) Use another method of contraception for 2 weeks after insertion.
(4) Use a vinegar douche weekly for 4 weeks to decrease the risk of infection.

**6** Following a teaching session on how to use the diaphragm as a contraceptive method, the nurse evaluates the client's understanding. Which statement made by the client demonstrates the need for additional teaching?

(1) "If I chose a diaphragm, I won't need to use any spermicide."
(2) "I will need to inspect the diaphragm after I take it out and clean it."
(3) "When I want to get pregnant, I can just stop using my diaphragm."
(4) "I need to leave the diaphragm in for at least 6 hours after having intercourse."

**7** A client taking oral contraceptive pills calls the clinic and reports the presence of chest pain and shortness of breath. The nurse should instruct the client to:

(1) Go to the nearest emergency room to be evaluated.
(2) Wait for the physician to return a telephone call to the client.
(3) Stop taking the pills and use a non-hormonal contraceptive method.
(4) Eat smaller meals more frequently to prevent gastric distention.

**8** A client has decided to use a cervical cap for contraception. In providing instruction to the client on the correct use of this method, the nurse should tell the client to:

(1) Apply a spermicide to the outside of the cap.
(2) Insert the cap at least 20 minutes but not longer than 4 hours prior to intercourse.
(3) Remove the cap within 6 hours of sexual activity.
(4) Reapply spermicide with repeated acts of intercourse.

**9** The nurse is teaching a client how to correctly use progestin-only oral contraceptives. The nurse should include which information in the teaching plan?

(1) Take one pill at the same time each day.
(2) Take the pills with calcium-rich foods to promote absorption.
(3) Skip 5 days between the end of one pill cycle and the beginning of the next.
(4) An additional method of contraception is not needed through the end of the cycle if a pill is missed.

**10** A client comes to the family planning clinic for contraceptive advice. She states she has never used contraception before and does not know what options are available to her. The nurse determines the priority nursing diagnosis for this client to be:

(1) Anxiety related to fear of pregnancy.
(2) Ineffective coping related to unprotected intercourse.
(3) Deficient knowledge related to lack of information about contraceptives.
(4) Fear related to potential complications of contraception.

*See pages 74–75 for Answers and Rationales.*

# Answers and Rationales

## Pretest

**1 Answer: 1** *Rationale:* Family planning can help the client make decisions about avoidance of pregnancy, determining the number of children to conceive and the spacing of those children, and voluntary termination of pregnancy.
*Cognitive Level:* Application
*Nursing Process:* Implementation; *Test Plan:* HPM

**2 Answer: 3** *Rationale:* Contraceptive counseling is best done in private, assessing the client's needs, desires, and risk factors. This will result in a contraceptive method that best suits the needs and health of the client.
*Cognitive Level:* Application
*Nursing Process:* Planning; *Test Plan:* HPM

**3 Answer: 2** *Rationale:* Condoms, used with or without a spermicide, are mechanical methods of contraception. While abstinence is a natural method, since the woman is sexually active it will increase compliance if she only needs to be abstinent during fertile periods.
*Cognitive Level:* Analysis
*Nursing Process:* Planning; *Test Plan:* HPM

**4 Answer: 3** *Rationale:* Oil-based lubricants can break down latex condoms. The condom should be unrolled onto the penis, starting at the tip of the penis. Holding the rim keeps the condom from slipping off and leaking semen into the vagina. Small amounts of semen are released before ejaculation and can result in pregnancy.
*Cognitive Level:* Analysis
*Nursing Process:* Evaluation; *Test Plan:* HPM

**5 Answer: 3** *Rationale:* Female condoms can be applied up to 8 hours before intercourse, are not made of latex, and do not require that the client be measured for proper fit.
*Cognitive Level:* Analysis
*Nursing Process:* Evaluation; *Test Plan:* HPM

**6 Answer: 1** *Rationale:* The client will need to touch her genitals to insert the diaphragm. Frequency of sexual contact and regularity of menses are unrelated to diaphragm use. Diaphragms can be safely used by lactating or nonlactating women.
*Cognitive Level:* Application
*Nursing Process:* Assessment; *Test Plan:* HPM

**7 Answer: 2** *Rationale:* Oral contraceptives place the client at decreased risk for iron-deficiency anemia, ovarian cancer, and fibrocystic breast disease. Oral contraceptives can decrease the effectiveness of insulin.
*Cognitive Level:* Analysis
*Nursing Process:* Planning; *Test Plan:* PHYS

**8 Answer: 1** *Rationale:* Because of alteration of hormone levels, irregular bleeding and thickened cervical mucus can result. Norplant does not cause incomplete emptying of the bladder or increase the risk for pelvic inflammatory disease.
*Cognitive Level:* Application
*Nursing Process:* Implementation; *Test Plan:* HPM

**9 Answer: 4** *Rationale:* The procedure, usually performed in a clinic under local anesthesia, is not effective for 4 to 6 weeks. The client should rest with minimal activity for 48 hours following the procedure.
*Cognitive Level:* Application
*Nursing Process:* Evaluation; *Test Plan:* PHYS

**10 Answer: 3** *Rationale:* The pregnancy rate following tubal ligation is 1 to 4 per 1,000 women. Reversal of the procedure, not effectiveness, is affected by the method used for the procedure. The effectiveness of the method is not related to client behavior.
*Cognitive Level:* Application
*Nursing Process:* Implementation; *Test Plan:* HPM

## Posttest

**1 Answer: 3** *Rationale:* Option 1 is part of assessing the client's knowledge and should be performed before the teaching session. Printed materials may not be appropriate to the client's reading ability. Visual cues are provided by demonstration of the procedure. Practice sessions provide the nurse with an opportunity to give positive and corrective feedback integrating visual, auditory, and tactile senses.
*Cognitive Level:* Application
*Nursing Process:* Implementation; *Test Plan:* HPM

**2 Answer: 3** *Rationale:* Leaving space at the end of the condom to collect the semen can prevent breakage or spillage after ejaculation. The male condom is placed when the penis is erect, then rolled down. Water-based lubricants can be used to provide additional comfort, if needed.
*Cognitive Level:* Analysis
*Nursing Process:* Evaluation; *Test Plan:* HPM

**3** **Answer: 1** *Rationale:* The cervical cap increases the risk of toxic shock syndrome because it may be left in place for up to 48 hours. The other methods identified pose no additional risk to this client based on her history and could be considered for contraception.
*Cognitive Level:* Analysis
*Nursing Process:* Assessment; *Test Plan:* HPM

**4** **Answer: 4** *Rationale:* Ethical and legal considerations dictate that clients are knowledgeable of the benefits and risks of the contraceptive method. This empowers the client in making an informed decision. Not all contraceptive methods are invasive or require a surgical procedure. Informed consent is not related to the effectiveness of a method.
*Cognitive Level:* Application
*Nursing Process:* Implementation; *Test Plan:* SECE

**5** **Answer: 2** *Rationale:* Specific information about the type of IUD inserted is not provided; Progestasert needs to be replaced annually, the Copper T380A can be left in place for 10 years. The string should be checked once a week for the first month, then after the menses thereafter. Contraceptive effectiveness begins when the IUD is inserted. Although douching is sometimes used to treat vaginal infections, it is not a recommended practice to prevent infection.
*Cognitive Level:* Application
*Nursing Process:* Implementation; *Test Plan:* HPM

**6** **Answer: 1** *Rationale:* A spermicidal cream or jelly is applied to the rim and dome of the diaphragm before inserting the device to increase the contraceptive effectiveness of the device. Options 2, 3, and 4 are statements reflecting correct client behavior for effective diaphragm use.
*Cognitive Level:* Analysis
*Nursing Process:* Evaluation; *Test Plan:* HPM

**7** **Answer: 1** *Rationale:* Shortness of breath and chest pain can indicate a serious complication associated with the use of oral contraceptives and require immediate evaluation. Waiting for a return telephone call could delay evaluation and treatment jeopardizing the client's health. Changing the contraceptive method or food intake pattern does not reduce the immediate health risk to the client.
*Cognitive Level:* Analysis
*Nursing Process:* Implementation; *Test Plan:* PHYS

**8** **Answer: 2** *Rationale:* Spermicide should be applied to the inside of the cervical cap. The device may be left in place up to 48 hours after sexual activity. Reapplication of spermicide with repeated acts of intercourse is not needed.
*Cognitive Level:* Application
*Nursing Process:* Implementation; *Test Plan:* HPM

**9** **Answer: 1** *Rationale:* Every pill contains a low dose of hormone and should be taken daily; consistency in taking the pills ensures a constant serum level of the hormone to maximize effectiveness. The pills are absorbed with or without the presence of calcium. If a pill is missed, it should be taken immediately and an additional method of contraception utilized through the remainder of that cycle.
*Cognitive Level:* Application
*Nursing Process:* Planning; *Test Plan:* HPM

**10** **Answer: 3** *Rationale:* This client has a need for information about the various contraceptive methods available to her, their risks and benefits. No information is provided to determine if the client fears pregnancy or is engaging in unprotected sexual intercourse. If the client does not know what contraceptive methods are available, it is unlikely she knows or fears potential complications from using a method of contraception.
*Cognitive Level:* Analysis
*Nursing Process:* Analysis; *Test Plan:* HPM

# References

American Academy of Pediatrics. (1999). Contraception and adolescents. *Policy statements 104*(5): 1161–1166.

Dickason, E., Silverman, B., & Kaplan, J. (1998). *Maternal infant nursing care.* St. Louis: Mosby, Inc.

Hatcher, R. A. (1998). *Contraceptive technology* (17th ed.). New York: Irvington Publications, Inc.

Hatcher, R.A., Zieman, M., Watt, A. et al. (1999) *A pocket guide to managing contraception* (2nd ed.). Tiger, GA: Bridging the Gap Foundation, p. 85.

Lowdermilk, D. L., Perry, S. E., & Bobak, I. M. (2000). *Maternity and women's health care* (7th ed.). St. Louis: Mosby, Inc.

Nichols, F. H. and Zwelling, E. (1997). *Maternal-newborn nursing: Theory and practice.* Philadelphia: W.B. Saunders Co.

Olds, S. B., London, M. L., & Ladewig, P. A. (2000). *Maternal-newborn nursing: A family and community based approach* (6th ed.). Upper Saddle River, NJ: Prentice-Hall, Inc., pp. 32, 43–51, 53, 212.

Pillitteri, A. (1999). *Maternal and child health nursing: Care of the childbearing and childrearing family* (3rd ed.). Philadelphia: Lippincott.

Reeder, S. J., Martin, L. L., & Koniak-Griffin, D. (1997). *Maternity nursing: Family, newborn and women's health care* (18th ed.). Philadelphia: Lippincott.

Sherwen, L. N., Scoloveno, M. A., & Weingarten, C. T. (1999). *Maternity Nursing: Care of the childbearing family* (3rd ed.). Stamford, CT: Appleton & Lange, p. 201.

## CHAPTER 4

# Fetal Development

Pamela Pranke, MSN, RNC

## CHAPTER OUTLINE

## OBJECTIVES

- Describe the process of conception.
- Differentiate among the pre-embryonic, embryonic, and fetal stages of development.
- Identify the function of extra-embryonic structures—the amniotic fluid, umbilical cord, and placenta.
- Describe fetal circulation.
- Summarize fetal development from conception to birth.

[ *Media Link* ]

*Use the CD-ROM enclosed with this text, or log onto the address given to access the free, interactive Companion Website created for this series. The CD-ROM and Companion Website accompanying this book offer additional practice opportunities and information—NCLEX Review, Case Studies, Glossary, In Depth with NCLEX, and more.*

**www.prenhall.com/hogan**

## REVIEW AT A GLANCE

**amnion**  *the inner fetal membranes*

**blastocyst**  *inner mass of cells within the morula that implants in the uterus*

**chorion**  *outer membrane of the fetal membranes*

**decidua basalis**  *that part of the decidua that unites with the chorion to form the placenta*

**decidua capsularis**  *that part of the decidua that surrounds the chorionic sac*

**decidua vera**  *decidua lining the uterus other than the placenta*

**ductus arteriosus**  *a fetal cardiac connection between the pulmonary artery and the aorta to allow blood to bypass the pulmonary circulation*

**ductus venosus**  *a fetal circulatory adaptation to allow blood to bypass the liver*

**ectoderm**  *progenerators for neural and integument tissue*

**embryo**  *an early stage in prenatal development between the 2nd and 8th week of gestation*

**endoderm**  *progenerators for digestive and respiratory system*

**fertilization**  *union of the ovum and sperm*

**fetus**  *the period from 8 weeks until the end of intrauterine life*

**foramen ovale**  *an opening in the fetal heart between the right and left atriums allowing blood to bypass the pulmonary circulation*

**gamete**  *a haploid germ cell (i.e., sperm or ovum)*

**mesoderm**  *the intermediate layer of germ cells in the embryo that gives rise to connective tissue, bone marrow, muscles, blood, lymphoid tissue, and epithelial tissue*

**morula**  *an embryo in a 16-cell stage that resembles a mulberry*

**trophoblast**  *the outermost-layer of the developing blastocyst that comes into intimate relationship with the uterine endometrium becoming the placenta*

**Wharton's jelly**  *the gelatinous connective tissue of the umbilical cord*

**zygote**  *the fertilized ovum*

## Pretest

**1**  A couple visits the genetic counseling clinic regarding a family history of cystic fibrosis, an autosomal recessive disorder. They ask the nurse, "What are the chances that we will have a child with cystic fibrosis if we are both carriers?" The nurse explains that:

(1) They should not have children because they will all have cystic fibrosis.
(2) The disorder occurs at random, and there is no way to calculate the risk.
(3) There is a 50 percent chance that they will have a child with cystic fibrosis.
(4) There is a 25 percent chance that they will have a child with cystic fibrosis.

**2**  A nurse is counseling a couple about fertility awareness. The nurse determines they understand the ideal time for conception when the clients state:

(1) "Ovulation usually occurs 14 days after the beginning of the menstrual cycle."
(2) "The ovum survives for 24 hours after ovulation."
(3) "It is best to have intercourse 24 to 48 hours after ovulation."
(4) "The ovum must be in contact with sperm for 48 hours in order for fertilization to occur."

**3**  After completing a health history in a prenatal clinic, the nurse recognizes which client as having the greatest risk for potential birth anomalies?

(1) A 23-year-old pregnant woman at 7 months gestation with a urinary tract infection.
(2) A 15-year-old primigravida with a sister who has Down syndrome.
(3) A 35-year-old multigravida at 16 weeks gestation with a yeast infection.
(4) A 42-year-old multigravida at 5 months gestation with a cold.

**4**  A 30-year-old woman is pregnant with twins. She tells the nurse that twins run in her family. She has a twin brother, her mother is a twin, and many relatives have twins. The nurse explains that this type of twinning is most likely:

(1) Identical.
(2) Monozygotic.
(3) Dizygotic.
(4) Monoamniotic.

**5** A client appears in the clinic for her first prenatal clinic at 26 weeks of pregnancy. She states, "I didn't see any point in coming sooner since I felt fine." The nurse uses which of the following statements to explain why prenatal care in the first trimester is important?

(1) "We want to get to know our patients better. This gives us time to collect an accurate history and look for potential problems."
(2) "We need to monitor fetal lung maturity and fetal movement in case you go into labor early."
(3) "Important cellular growth happens in the first trimester. Early assessment and education promotes a healthy pregnancy during this time."
(4) "The most important thing is to see if you are even pregnant. Many women mistake a missed period for pregnancy."

**6** A woman at 7 months of pregnancy says that her 8-year-old daughter talks to the fetus and this calms the fetus when kicking her in the ribs. She asks the nurse if this is her imagination. The best response by the nurse is: .

(1) "No, this may very well be the case because the fetus begins to hear at 24 weeks."
(2) "We really don't know at what age the fetus begins to hear."
(3) "This is unlikely since the fetus doesn't hear until 8 months gestation."
(4) "You are both right and wrong. The fetus is able to hear, but it is silly to think your daughter's voice calms the fetus."

**7** A client at 8 months gestation is diagnosed with oligohydramnios. She asks the nurse if this can harm the fetus. The nurse's best response is:

(1) "Yes, oligohydramnios can lead to umbilical cord compression."
(2) "Yes, it means the fetus swallowed too much fluid."
(3) "No, this commonly occurs toward the end of pregnancy."
(4) "No, this is a sign that the lungs are maturing."

**8** After delivery the nurse examines the umbilical cord. She expects to find a cord with:

(1) One artery and two veins.
(2) Two arteries and one vein.
(3) Two arteries and two veins.
(4) One artery and one vein.

**9** During a prenatal class the nurse explains weight gain in pregnancy. She explains that the amniotic fluid in the third trimester weighs approximately:

(1) 1.5 kilograms.
(2) 150 grams.
(3) 75 grams.
(4) 1 kilogram.

**10** At a family planning clinic the nurse explains how a urine pregnancy test works and tells the client that the test detects an increase in the hormone:

(1) Estriol.
(2) Progesterone.
(3) Human chorionic gonadotropin (hCG).
(4) Human placental lactogen (hPL).

*See pages 98–99 for Answers and Rationales.*

## I. Conception

### A. Genetic principles

1. Hereditary material

   **a.** Each human somatic cell contains 46 chromosomes or 23 pairs; there are 22 pairs of autosomes plus one pair of sex chromosomes; chromosomes are made of DNA, tightly coiled strands of material containing all genetic material; they can be arranged in a particular order known as karyotype

   **b.** Sex chromosomes

      1) The maternal ovum carries an X chromosome

      2) The male sperm carries either an X or Y chromosome

      3) A female results when an X chromosome is contributed by the ovum and an X chromosome from the sperm

      4) A male results when an X chromosome is contributed by the ovum and a Y chromosome from the sperm

   **c.** Genes are made of DNA; alone or in combination, they are the smallest units of inheritance found on chromosomes; they perform a specific function in control of cellular activity

   **d.** Homozygous genes are a pair of genes carrying similar traits

   **e.** Heterozygous genes are a pair of genes carrying dissimilar traits

   **f.** The genome is the sum total of genes carried by all 46 chromosomes in the human

   **g.** Human Genome Project: Large coordinated effort to make a detailed map of human DNA and the genes that guide the development of a human being from a fertilized egg cell

2. Patterns of inheritance

   **a.** Mendelian inheritance (single gene inheritance)

      1) Autosomal dominant: a dominant gene is the one gene of a heterozygous pair that is expressed

         a) A heterozygous genotype parent who carries the trait will manifest the trait, express the phenotype

         b) If a heterozygous parent has an infant with a homozygous parent without the trait there are four possible ways to combine the four genes: dominant/recessive, dominant/recessive, recessive/recessive, and recessive/recessive; there is a 50 percent chance of the child expressing the trait and a 50 percent chance that the child will not

      2) Autosomal recessive genes are expressed only if homozygous

         a) When paired with a dominant gene it will not be expressed except in the genotype

         b) Autosomal recessive diseases include phenylketonuria (PKU), Tay-Sachs, and cystic fibrosis

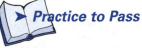

**Practice to Pass**

A client reveals that she has PKU. She asks what the chances are for passing on the disease if the father does not have PKU. Knowing that this is an autosomal recessive trait how would the nurse respond?

NCLEX!

      c) As an example, if a parent carries a gene for PKU, the parent will not have PKU; if both parents have a gene for PKU there are four possible ways to combine the genes: PKU/no PKU, PKU/no PKU, PKU/PKU, and no PKU/no PKU; there is a 25 percent chance of having a child with PKU, a 50 percent chance of the child being a carrier and a 25% chance that the child will not carry or have PKU

    3) X-linked recessive genes are carried only on the X chromosome; the female does not exhibit the disease if she has an X chromosome without the trait; the male will exhibit the trait because the recessive gene is unopposed by the Y chromosome; i.e., if a man has an X chromosome with a recessive trait for colorblindness, he will be colorblind because the Y chromosome has no comparable dominant gene to counteract the gene

    4) X-linked dominant: the gene is carried dominantly on the X chromosome; it manifests itself in both males and females with the trait; for example, vitamin D–resistant rickets is X-linked dominant—both males and females are affected

  **b.** Non-Mendelian inheritance is multifactorial; an interaction between the genetic material and the environment results in a trait, such as cleft palate

    1) Monosomy: one of an allele, an alternate form of a gene, is absent; an example is Turner's syndrome (XO); one of the sex chromosomes is missing so the individual has 45 chromosomes rather than 46

    2) Trisomy: An allele has an extra chromosome so the individual has 47 chromosomes rather than 46; examples include Klinefelter's syndrome (XXY) and Down syndrome (trisomy 21)

    3) Teratogens are nongenetic factors in the environment that can produce mutations, changes in DNA that alter genes, in the fetus; they include viruses and chemicals; the greatest risk is during weeks 2 to 8 of gestation

**B. Role of the nurse related to genetics**

  **1.** It is estimated that at least 50 percent of spontaneous abortions are caused by chromosomal abnormalities

  **2.** Genetic counseling and testing takes place in many contexts and settings, such as birthing unit, prenatal clinic, well-child clinic, and family planning clinic

  **3.** Genetic case finding and referral

  **4.** Client education and counseling

  **5.** Informed consent

  **6.** Confidentiality

  **7.** Communicating risks and dealing with uncertainty

  **8.** Recognizing social, religious and cultural differences

  **9.** Autonomous, client-based decision making

  **10.** Policy development

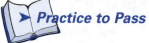

► *Practice to Pass*

Following an amniocentesis a client learns she is carrying a fetus with Down syndrome, trisomy 21. Explain this to the client.

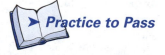

► *Practice to Pass*

A client learns that her fetus has anencephaly, a lethal congenital anomaly. What is the nurse's role in this situation?

**C. Sperm and ovum**

1.  A sexual reproductive cell, a **gamete,** is capable of uniting with a gamete of the opposite sex to form a new individual; gametes are also called germ cells

    a.  Female gamete is the ovum

    b.  Male gamete is the sperm

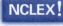

2.  Gametogenesis occurs through the cellular reproductive process of meiosis; through meiosis each gamete contains 23 chromosomes, the haploid state; this allows reshuffling of the maternal and paternal genomes creating new combinations of genes

3.  Oogenesis is the meiotic process by which female gametes are produced

    a.  Primordial germ cells develop in the ovary during fetal life; the neonate is born with a lifetime supply of oogonia, which soon after birth begin to grow in size

    b.  Oogonia that survive into the female's sexual maturation become primary oocytes

    c.  At sexual maturity, the oocytes advance into the first prophase of meiosis; when the hormonal changes of puberty occur initiating the menstrual cycle, one primary oocyte will continue through meiotic division in the graffian follicle producing one primary oocyte and one nonfunctioning polar body; each contains the haploid state of 23 chromosomes

    d.  Primary oocytes are released from the ovary during ovulation (Figure 4-1); the second meiotic division begins as the oocyte moves down the fallopian tube; the second division is completed with fertilization by a sperm resulting in a mature ovum and another polar body, each containing the haploid state

    e.  At the completion of meiotic division one oocyte results in three nonfunctioning polar bodies and one mature ovum

2.  Spermatogenesis is the meiotic process by which male gametes are produced

    a.  During puberty the germinal epithelium in the seminiferous tubules of the testes are stimulated to produce testosterone in the testes

    b.  As the diploid spermatogonium enters the first meiotic division, it is called the primary spermatocyte

    c.  Each primary spermatocyte results in four mature spermatozoon, or sperm; the primary spermatocytes replicate to form two secondary spermatocytes containing the haploid number of chromosomes; during the second meiotic division, they divide to form four spermatids, each with a haploid number of chromosomes

    d.  Spermatids continue to mature through the process of spermatogenesis to become the mature male gamete, spermatozoon or sperm

**D.** *Fertilization:* occurs when the sperm and ovum unite at conception (Figure 4-1)

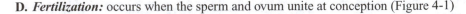

1.  Usually within 12 hours of ovulation if coitus (intercourse) occurs no more than 24 hours prior to ovulation

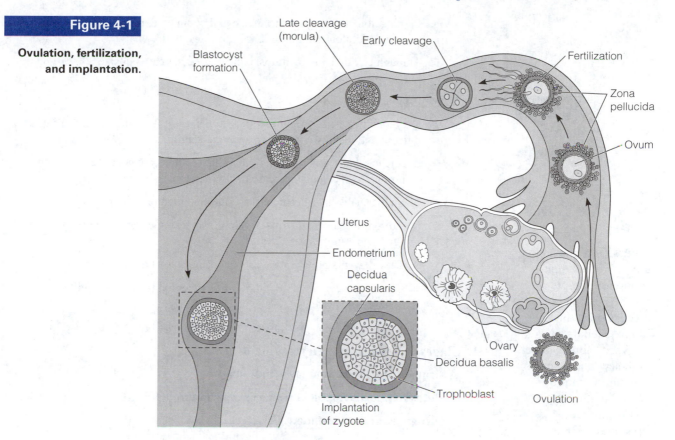

**Figure 4-1**

**Ovulation, fertilization, and implantation.**

2. During intercourse 200 to 400 million sperm are ejaculated into the vagina; they swim up into the fallopian tubes to meet the descending ovum, if present; only a few hundred sperm actually survive to the ampulla (outer third) of the fallopian tube where fertilization occurs

3. Sperm survive in the female reproductive tract for 24 to 48 hours but are most capable of fertilization for 24 hours

4. The ovum is enclosed in a glycoprotein matrix called the zona pellucida; the zona pellucida is surrounded by the corona radiata

   a. The zona pellucida binds the sperm and prevents additional sperm from penetrating the ovum

   b. The zona pellucida also initiates the acrosomal reaction after sperm binding has occurred mediating the entry of the sperm nucleus into the ovum; release of lytic enzymes causes a small perforation in the head of the sperm; enzymes escape to digest a path through the corona radiata and zona pellucida

   c. Capacitation occurs when the protective coating around the sperm is removed facilitated by enzymes in the fallopian tube

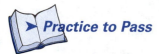

**Practice to Pass**

A client learning about fertility awareness asks, "When is the optimal time to have intercourse relative to ovulation?" How will the nurse explain this?

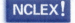

5. Fertilization occurs when the sperm and ovum fuse, resulting in a **zygote** containing the diploid number of chromosomes, or 46

6. Through cell division by mitosis, the zygote increases in size 200 billion times before birth

**E. Multiple pregnancies**

1. Dizygotic: fraternal or non-identical twins result from the release of two separate ova and fertilization by two separate sperm

   a. The incidence is 7 to 11 per 1,000 births and accounts for 2/3 of twin births; the incidence increases with maternal age

   b. They usually have separate placentas and membranes

2. Monozygotic: identical twins develop from a single fertilized ovum that splits into two separate zygotes

   a. They may share placentas and one or more fetal membranes

   b. If division occurs within 3 days of fertilization the zygotes will develop separate membranes

   c. Splitting of the zygote in later stages may result in conjoined twins

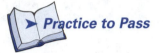

**▶ Practice to Pass**

A nurse is a guest speaker at a support group for parents of twins. The topic for discussion is the biological difference between monozygotic and dizygotic twins. What information should the nurse include in the presentation?

## II. Stages of Growth and Development

**A. Human development follows three stages**

**B. Intrauterine development from conception through birth is called gestation**

**C. Length of human gestation**

1. 40 weeks after the last menstrual period, or 280 days

2. 38 weeks after fertilization, or 266 days

## III. Pre-embryonic Development

**A. The first two weeks after fertilization:** a time of cellular multiplication and implantation

**B. Implantation:** the morula travels through the fallopian tube for approximately three days while it undergoes rapid mitotic division called cleavage

1. When the cells reach the uterus they are called a **morula** and float in the uterus for several days prior to implantation and are nourished by nutrients within the endometrial lining of the uterus

2. The solid inner mass of cells is called the **blastocyst**

3. The outer layer is the **trophoblast**

4. Adhesion occurs when the blastocyst aligns with and adheres to the uterine lining (endometrium)

5. Increased vascular permeability at the implantation site facilitates a union between the zygote and uterine tissues

6. The zygote implants in the upper posterior uterine wall approximately 7 to 9 days after fertilization; some women may experience spotting at this time and mistake it for menses

7. Trophoblasts grow into the endometrial lining and form finger-like projections called villi

C. **The endometrial lining:** rich in stored nutrients providing nourishment until the placenta is a functional unit of nutrient exchange

D. **Decidua:** layers of uterine tissue that grow around the blastocyst

1. **Decidua capsularis:** portion that covers the implanted blastocyst

2. **Decidua basalis:** portion directly under the blastocyst

3. **Decidua vera:** portion that lines the remainder of the uterine cavity

## IV. Embryonic Development

A. **2 to 8 weeks following fertilization:** characterized by rapid cell division and differentiation

B. **Major functions of the embryonic period**

1. Cell multiplication and growth

2. Cell differentiation into organs

   a. Organogenesis: critical periods of development occur as organ systems develop; this is a time when the embryo is particularly susceptible to teratogens and the development of birth anomalies

   b. Morphogenesis: development of shape

   c. By the end of the 8th week, every organ system and external structure is present

C. **Primary germ layers:** develop into all tissues, organs, and body systems

1. **Ectoderm:** forms the trophoblast that develops into the placenta, integument, neural tissue and glands

2. **Mesoderm:** forms muscles, bones, connective tissue, circulatory system, and genitourinary system

3. **Endoderm:** develops into the digestive, respiratory, and parts of the genitourinary systems

D. **Fetal membranes**

1. **Amnion:** innermost lining of the membrane that produces amniotic fluid

2. **Chorion:** outermost lining of the membrane that forms from trophoblasts; chorionic villi develop into the placenta

3. Membranes in multiple gestation

   a. Dizygotic twins: Both zygotes implant separately and usually have separate placenta and membranes; occasionally the zygotes implant so close together that the placenta and membranes fuse

   b. Monozygotic twins

      1) If the zygote separates at the two-cell stage, the two zygotes implant separately and have separate placentas and membranes

      2) Later splitting results in a common placenta; the chorion develops in the early blastocyste stage so the twins have a common placenta and chorion, but separate amnions

3) Twin transfusion syndrome occurs when twins have a common placenta and membranes resulting in unequal circulation; one twin receives little circulation and the other most of the circulation; the outcome is usually poor for both twins

4. Amniotic fluid is produced by the amnion and derived from maternal blood

   a. Functions

      1) Cushions the embryo and fetus

      2) Controls temperature

      3) Promotes symmetrical growth of the embryo and fetus

      4) Prevents fetal adherence to the amnion

      5) Allows freedom of movement within the amniotic cavity

   b. Amount

      1) 30 mL at 10 weeks

      2) 350 mL at 20 weeks

      3) 800 to 1,000 mL by 37 weeks

      4) Oligohydramnios is a condition of diminished amniotic fluid often related to renal system malfunction, intrauterine growth restriction, and postmaturity; it can contribute to skin and skeletal abnormalities, pulmonary hypoplasia, and cord compression

      5) Hydramnios is a condition of excess amniotic fluid often related to gastrointestinal malfunction

      6) Fetus swallows and urinates into the fluid after 23 to 25 weeks

   c. Contains fetal cells and many chemicals that can be used to diagnose fetal well-being

      1) Alkaline in pH

      2) DNA for genetic analysis

      3) Surfactant for lung maturity analysis

E. **Yolk sac:** develops in the blastocyst and forms early red blood cells during the embryonic stage; it is then integrated into the umbilical cord

F. **Body stalk:** connects the embryo to the yolk sac; as circulation develops in the stalk, it becomes the umbilical cord connecting the embryo to the placenta

G. **Placenta**

   1. Purpose is to connect the fetus to the uterine wall so nutritive, respiratory, and excretory exchange can occur between the mother and fetus

   2. Development begins in the 3rd week of gestation and begins early function by the 4th week

   3. Uterine circulation prior to implantation

      a. Uterine arteries encircle the uterus in a wreath called the arcuate arteries

      b. Radial arteries come off of these and divide into basal and spiral arteries

c. Spiral arteries are responsive to hormonal changes and grow during the luteal phase of the menstrual cycle

d. By the time of implantation, the spiral arteries are elongated and extend into the endometrium

e. The endometrium is rich in glycogen and protein to nourish the blastocyst

4. The ectoderm develops into the decidua basalis found directly below the implanted morula

5. Small arteries work their way through the entire decidua and open into the intervillous spaces of the developing placenta

6. Large venous sinuses develop

**NCLEX!**

**NCLEX!**

7. Uterine circulation after implantation (Figure 4-2)

a. Maternal and fetal circulation remains independent of one another separated by a thin membrane

b. Development of chorionic villi: the trophoblastic cells form intervillous spaces within the decidua for collection of maternal blood; as the villi grow into these spaces, fetal blood enters villi via arteries and returns to the fetus through fetal veins

c. Trophoblasts: by the end of 4 weeks, throphoblastic tissue has a radial appearance and contains a number of secondary and tertiary villi; the villi

**Figure 4-2** **Vascular arrangement of the placenta.**

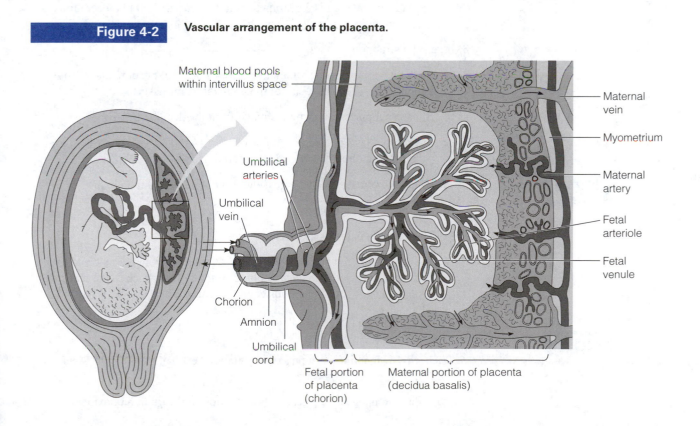

Maternal blood pools within intervillus space

Maternal vein

Myometrium

Maternal artery

Umbilical arteries

Umbilical vein

Fetal arteriole

Fetal venule

Chorion

Amnion

Umbilical cord

Fetal portion of placenta (chorion)

Maternal portion of placenta (decidua basalis)

are anchored in the mesoderm and attached peripherally to the maternal decidua

**d.** Prior to 12 weeks, there is little maternal blood in what will become the intervillous spaces

**e.** Capillaries develop, giving rise to a vascular system between the embryo and decidua that allows metabolic exchange but does not allow mixing of maternal and fetal blood

**f.** Maternal blood flows from uterine arteries into maternal sinuses surrounding the villi and then back into the uterine veins of the mother

**g.** Maternal blood enters the intervillous spaces through numerous spiral arteries

**h.** Blood enters deep into intervillous lakes and is drained away by the endometrial veins following metabolic exchange

**i.** Umbilical cord: two arteries and one vein

   1) Umbilical vessels are surrounded by **Wharton's jelly,** a gelatinous connective tissue that serves as a protective layer around the umbilical vessels

   2) Fetal circulation enters the placenta through arterial villi, then into capillary villi, finally returning to the fetus through the venous villi and umbilical vein following metabolic exchange.

   3) At birth the cord is 2 centimeters in diameter and 50 to 60 centimeters in length

**8.** Placental structure

**a.** By the beginning of the 4th month, a fetal placental portion, made from trophoblasts, becomes a unit of metabolic transfer tissue

**b.** A maternal placental portion is made from the decidua basalis

**c.** The trophoblasts and decidua intermingle in a junctional zone where trophoblasts are directly exposed to maternal blood flow

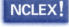

**d.** Metabolic transfer occurs across the trophoblastic cell membrane

**e.** Septums divide the placenta into sections called cotyledons

**f.** The placenta enlarges as the fetus grows

**g.** The umbilical cord has one vein that carries blood from the placenta to the fetus and two arteries that carry blood from the fetus back to the placenta, is surrounded by the gelatinous connective tissue of the cord, Wharton's jelly

**9.** Metabolic functions of the placenta

**a.** Begins to functions as a means of metabolic exchange by the 4th week and is fully functional by 8 weeks

**b.** Gases: exchange of oxygen, carbon dioxide, and carbon monoxide

c. Nutrients and electrolytes: amino acids, free fatty acids, carbohydrates, and vitamins

d. Excretory products transfer from the fetus to the mother

e. Production of hormones

1) Progesterone to maintain pregnancy

2) Estriol to stimulate uterine growth and mammary glands

3) Human chorionic gonadotropin (hCG) functions similar to luteinizing hormone

4) Human placental lactogen (hPL) functions similar to growth hormone; causes decreased insulin sensitivity resulting in a diabetogenic effect in the mother and stimulates maternal breast development

f. Immunologic

1) Transfer of maternal antibodies: immunoglobulin G (IgG)

2) Poorly understood immunologic suppression occurs through the actions of progesterone and hCG to protect the fetus from rejection

g. Mechanisms of metabolic transport of the placenta

1) Simple diffusion moves substances including oxygen, carbon dioxide, carbon monoxide, water, electrolytes, and some drugs, from an area of higher concentration to an area of lower concentration

2) Facilitated diffusion requires a carrier to move molecules from an area of greater concentration to lesser concentration, such as glucose

3) Active transport moves substances, including amino acids, calcium, iron, vitamins, and glucose against a gradient

4) Pinocytosis transfers large molecules, including albumin and IgG by engulfment

5) Hydrostatic and osmotic pressures regulate water balance

## V. Fetal Development

A. **Fetal period:** extends from the end of the 8th week until birth and is characterized by rapid growth and organ maturation

B. **Table 4-1:** summarizes organ system development from 2 to 40 weeks gestation

C. **Table 4-2:** lists important developmental highlights of interest to parents

D. **Growth and appearance**

1. Greatest increase in length occurs during the 3rd, 4th, and 5th months of pregnancy

   a. At 3 months the head is ½ of the length, at full gestation it is ¼ of the length

   b. Growth in length: 12 weeks—10 centimeters, 20 weeks—25 centimeters, 40 weeks—53 centimeters

| **Table 4-1** | **Summary of Organ System Development** |

*Age: 2-3 weeks*
**Length:** 2 mm C-R (Crown-to-Rump)
**Nervous system:** Groove forms along middle back as cells thicken; neural tube forms from closure of neural groove.
**Cardiovascular system:** Beginning of blood circulation; tubular heart begins to form during third week.
**Gastrointestinal system:** Liver begins to function.
**Genitourinary system:** Formation of kidneys beginning.
**Respiratory system:** Nasal pits forming.
**Endocrine system:** Thyroid tissue appears.
**Eyes:** Optic cup and lens pit have formed; pigment in eyes.
**Ear:** Auditory pit is now enclosed structure.

*Age: 4 weeks*
**Length:** 4-6 mm C-R
**Weight:** 0.4 g
**Nervous system:** Anterior portion of neural tube closes to form brain; closure of posterior end forms spinal cord.
**Musculoskeletal system:** Noticeable limb buds.
**Cardiovascular system:** Tubular heart beats at 28 days and primitive red blood cells circulate through fetus and chorionic villi.
**Gastrointestinal system:** Mouth: formation of oral cavity; primitive jaws present; esophagotracheal septum begins division of esophagus and trachea. Digestive tract: stomach forms; esophagus and intestine become tubular; ducts of pancreas and liver forming.

*Age: 5 weeks*
**Length:** 8 mm C-R
**Weight:** Only 0.5% of total body weight is fat (to 20 weeks).
**Nervous System:** Brain has differentiated and cranial nerves are present.
**Musculoskeletal system:** Developing muscles have innervation.
**Cardiovascular system:** Atrial division has occurred.

*Age: 6 weeks*
**Length:** 12 mm C-R
**Musculoskeletal system:** Bone rudiments present; primitive skeletal shape forming; muscle mass begins to develop; ossification of skull and jaws begins.
**Cardiovascular system:** Chambers present in heart; groups of blood cells can be identified.
**Gastrointestinal system:** Oral and nasal cavities and upper lip formed; liver begins to form red blood cells.
**Respiratory system:** Trachea, bronchi, and lung buds present.
**Ear:** Formation of external, middle, and inner ear continues.
**Sexual development:** Embryonic sex glands appear.

*Age: 7 weeks*
**Length:** 18 mm C-R
**Cardiovascular system:** Fetal heartbeats can be detected.
**Gastrointestinal system:** Mouth: tongue separates; palate folds. Digestive tract: stomach attains final form.
**Genitourinary system:** Separation of bladder and urethra from rectum.
**Respiratory system:** Diaphragm separates abdominal and thoracic cavities.

**Eyes:** Optic nerve formed; eyelids appear, thickening of lens.
**Sexual development:** Differentiation of sex glands into ovaries and testes begins.

*Age: 8 weeks*
**Length:** 2.5–3 cm C-R
**Weight:** 2 g
**Musculoskeletal system:** Digits formed; further differentiation of cells in primitive skeleton; cartilaginous bones show first signs of ossification; development of muscles in trunk, limbs, and head; some movement of fetus now possible.
**Cardiovascular system:** Development of heart essentially complete; fetal circulation follows two circuits—four extraembryonic and two intraembryonic.
**Gastrointestinal system:** Mouth: completion of lip fusion. Digestive tract: rotation in midgut; anal membrane has perforated.
**Ear:** External, middle, and inner ear assuming final forms.
**Sexual development:** Male and female external genitals appear similar until end of ninth week.

*Age: 10 weeks*
**Length:** 5–6 cm C-H (Crown-to-Heel)
**Weight:** 14 g
**Nervous system:** Neurons appear at caudal end of spinal cord; basic divisions of brain present.
**Musculoskeletal system:** Fingers and toes begin nail growth.
**Gastrointestinal system:** Mouth: separation of lips from jaw; fusion of palate folds. Digestive tract: developing intestines enclosed in abdomen.
**Genitourinary system:** Bladder sac formed.
**Endocrine system:** Islets of Langerhans differentiated.
**Eyes:** Eyelids fused closed; development of lacrimal duct.
**Sexual development:** Males: production of testosterone and physical characteristics between 8 and 12 weeks.

*Age: 12 weeks*
**Length:** 8 cm C-R; 11.5 cm C-H
**Weight:** 45 g
**Musculoskeletal system:** Clear outlining of miniature bones (12–20 weeks); process of ossification is established throughout fetal body; appearance of involuntary muscles in viscera.
**Gastrointestinal system:** Mouth: completion of palate. Digestive tract: appearance of muscles in gut; bile secretion begins; liver is major producer of red blood cells.
**Respiratory system:** Lungs acquire definitive shape.
**Skin:** Pink and delicate.
**Endocrine system:** Hormonal secretion from thyroid; insulin present in pancreas.
**Immunologic system:** Appearance of lymphoid tissue in fetal thymus gland.

*Age: 16 weeks*
**Length:** 13.5 cm C-R; 15 cm C-H
**Weight:** 200 g
**Musculoskeletal system:** Teeth beginning to form hard tissue that will become central incisors.

*(continued)*

| Table 4-1 | Summary of Organ System Development (*continued*) |
|---|---|

**Gastrointestinal system:** Mouth: differentiation of hard and soft palate. Digestive tract: development of gastric and intestinal glands; intestines begin to collect meconium.
**Genitourinary system:** Kidneys assume typical shape and organization.
**Skin:** Appearance of scalp hair; lanugo present on body; transparent skin with visible blood vessels; sweat glands developing.
**Eye, ear, and nose:** Formed.
**Sexual development:** Sex determination possible.

*Age: 18 weeks*
**Musculoskeletal system:** Teeth beginning to form hard tissue (enamel and dentine) that will become lateral incisors.
**Cardiovascular system:** Fetal heart tones audible with fetoscope at 16–20 weeks.

*Age: 20 weeks*
**Length:** 19 cm C-R; 25 cm C-H
**Weight:** 435 g (6% of total body weight is fat)
**Nervous system:** Myelination of spinal cord begins.
**Musculoskeletal system:** Teeth begining to form hard tissue that will become canine and first molar. Lower limbs are of final relative proportions.
**Gastrointestinal system:** Fetus actively sucks and swallows amniotic fluid; peristaltic movements begin.
**Skin:** Lanugo covers entire body; brown fat begins to form; vernix caseosa begins to form.
**Immunologic system:** Detectable levels of fetal antibodies (IgG type).
**Blood formation:** Iron is stored and bone marrow is increasingly important.

*Age: 24 weeks*
**Length:** 23 cm C-R; 28 cm C-H
**Weight:** 780 g
**Nervous system:** Brain looks like mature brain.
**Musculoskeletal system:** Teeth are beginning to form hard tissue that will become the second molar.
**Respiratory system:** Respiratory movements may occur (24–40 weeks). Nostrils reopen. Alveoli appear in lungs and begin production of surfactant; gas exchange possible.
**Skin:** Reddish and wrinkled, vernix caseosa present.

**Immunologic system:** IgG levels reach maternal levels.
**Eyes:** Structurally complete.

*Age: 28 weeks*
**Length:** 27 cm C-R; 35 cm C-H
**Weight:** 1200–1250 g
**Nervous system:** Begins regulation of some body functions.
**Skin:** Adipose tissue accumulates rapidly; nails appear; eyebrows and eyelashes present.
**Eyes:** Eyelids open (28–32 weeks).
**Sexual development:** Males: testes descend into inguinal canal and upper scrotum.

*Age: 32 weeks*
**Length:** 31 cm C-R; 38–43 cm C-H
**Weight:** 2000 g
**Nervous system:** More reflexes present.

*Age: 36 weeks*
**Length:** 35 cm C-R; 42–48 cm C-H
**Weight:** 2500–2750 g
**Musculoskeletal system:** Distal femoral ossification centers present.
**Skin:** Pale; body rounded, lanugo disappearing, hair fuzzy or woolly; few sole creases; sebaceous glands active and helping to produce vernix caseosa (36–40 weeks).
**Ears:** Ear lobes with little cartilage.
**Sexual development:** Males: scrotum small and few rugae present; descent of testes into upper scrotum to stay (36–40 weeks). Females: labia majora and minora equally prominent.

*Age: 40 weeks*
**Length:** 40 cm C-R; 48–52 cm C-H
**Weight:** 3200+ g (16% of total body weight is fat)
**Respiratory system:** At 38 weeks, lecithin-sphingomyelin (L/S) ratio approaches 2:1 (indicates decreased risk of respiratory distress from inadequate surfactant production if born now).
**Skin:** Smooth and pink; vernix present in skinfolds; moderate to profuse silky hair; lanugo hair on shoulders and upper back; nails extend over tips or digits; creases cover sole.
**Ears:** Ear lobes firmer due to increased cartilage.
**Sexual development:** Males: rugous scrotum. Females: labia majora well developed and minora small or completely covered.

*Note:* Age refers to gestational age of fetus/conceptus; fertilization age.
*Source:* Olds, S. B., London, M. L., & Ladewig, P. A. (2000). *Maternal-newborn nursing: A family and community-based approach* (6th ed.). Upper Saddle River, NJ: Prentice-Hall, Inc., p. 168–169.

2. Growth-weight: the greatest weight gain occurs in the 8th and 9th month of pregnancy

   **a.** < 23 week = < 1 pound

   **b.** 23 weeks = 1 pound

   **c.** 32 weeks = 3 pounds

   **d.** 36 weeks = 4.5 pounds

   **e.** 40 weeks = 7 pounds

| Table 4-2 | | |
|---|---|---|
| **Fetal Development: What Parents Want to Know** | 4 weeks | The fetal heart begins to beat. |
| | 8 weeks | All body organs are formed. |
| | 8–12 weeks | Fetal heart tones can be heard by Doppler device. |
| | 16 weeks | Baby's sex can be seen. Although thin, the fetus looks like a baby. |
| | 20 weeks | Heartbeat can be heard with a fetoscope. Mother feels movement (quickening). Baby develops a regular schedule of sleeping, sucking, and kicking. Hands can grasp. Baby assumes a favorite position in utero. Vernix (lanolinlike covering) protects the body, and lanugo (fine hair) keeps oil on skin. Head hair, eyebrows, and eyelashes present. |
| | 24 weeks | Weighs 1 lb 10 oz. Activity is increasing. Fetal respiratory movements begin. |
| | 28 weeks | Eyes begin to open and close. Baby can breathe at this time. Surfactant needed for breathing at birth is formed. Baby is two-thirds its final size. |
| | 32 weeks | Baby has fingernails and toenails. Subcutaneous fat is being laid down. Baby appears less red and wrinkled. |
| | 38–40 weeks | Baby fills total uterus. Baby gets antibodies from mother. |

*Source:* Olds, S. B., London, M. L., & Ladewig, P. A. (2000). *Maternal-newborn nursing: A family and community-based approach* (6th ed.). Upper Saddle River, NJ: Prentice-Hall, Inc., p. 174.

3. After 8 weeks, the fetus takes on a human appearance

   a. The eyes and ears are positioned on the face

   b. Limbs are relatively proportionate to the rest of the body although lower limbs are a bit short

**E. Integument**

1. Epidermis production begins at 3 weeks; by the 11th week, it has three layers, and four layers exist by the end of the 4th month; by 24 weeks the integument is fully present but immature

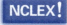

2. Lanugo forms at 13 weeks and begins to disappears at 36 weeks

3. Vernix caseosa appears at 5 months gestation when an earlier skin layer is shed and mixes with secretions from sebaceous glands; it protects the fetus from amniotic fluid skin maceration

4. At 24 weeks, the skin is red, wrinkled, and lacks underlying connective tissue

5. Brown fat is deposited after 28 weeks gestation in the neck, subscapula, axillae, mediastinum, and perineal tissues

6. Subcutaneous fat deposited during the last 2 months

7. Innervation develops in the 3rd month; it is greatest around the lips, sucking pad, and perioral zone

**F. Cardiac**

1. Heart begins beating 22 days after fertilization

2. Septation of the heart completed by the 5th week

3. Fetal heart rate at 20 weeks gestation averages 155 beats/minute; at term it averages 140 beats/minute

4. Primitive RBCs appear at 3 to 4 weeks gestation

5. Fetal hemoglobin compensates for low fetal oxygen content

   a. Fetal hemoglobin has 20 to 30 percent greater oxygen-carrying capacity than maternal hemoglobin

**b.** After 30 to 32 weeks gestation, fetal hemoglobin production slows and formation of adult hemoglobin begins

**6.** Anatomical structure of fetal circulation (Figure 4-3)

**a.** The lung and liver are nonfunctional so circulation bypasses these organs through special fetal circulatory structures

NCLEX!

**Figure 4-3**

**Fetal circulation.**

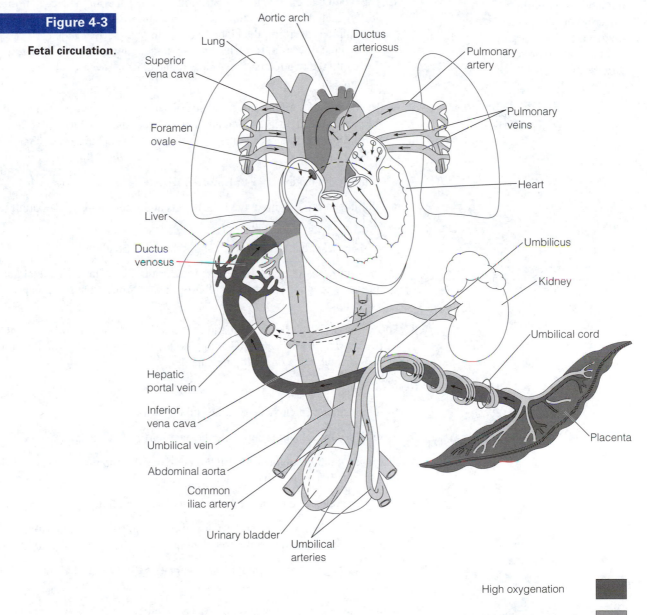

High oxygenation

Moderate oxygenation

Low oxygenation

Very low oxygenation

**Practice to Pass**

Some infants have a heart defect called patent ductus arteriosus. In this condition, the ductus arteriosus does not close after birth. Describe the consequences of maintaining this circulatory pattern after birth.

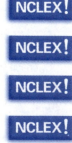

**b.** As blood returns from the placenta through the single umbilical vein, a majority of the blood supply bypasses the liver through the **ductus venosus** and goes directly to the inferior vena cava

**c.** As blood enters the right atrium from the inferior vena cava, most of it is directed across the right atrium into the left atrium through an opening called the **foramen ovale;** this enables oxygen-rich blood from the placenta to by-pass the lung and be circulated to the body

**d.** The blood that enters the right atrium from the superior vena cava is mostly deoxygenated and passes through the tricuspid valve into the right ventricle and pulmonary artery; the blood in the pulmonary artery mostly passes through the **ductus arteriosus** into the descending aorta; from there, it flows into the two fetal arteries back to the placenta where it becomes oxygenated

**e.** The umbilical cord has three vessels, two arteries that return fetal blood to the placenta and one vein that takes blood from the placenta and returns it to the fetus; infants born with only two vessels often have other fetal anomalies

**7.** Clotting ability begins at 11 to 12 weeks

   **a.** Fibrinogen production in the liver begins at 5 weeks and reaches adult levels by 30 weeks gestation

   **b.** By 13 weeks, platelet levels are about the same as adults

   **c.** Vitamin K levels are 50 percent of the adult because the sterile fetal gut is unable to produce the vitamin; after birth, gastrointestinal bacteria produce vitamin K

**8.** Formation of WBCs begins in the liver at 5 to 7 weeks gestation, spleen at 8 weeks, thymus at 10 weeks, and lymph nodes at 12 weeks; at birth, the number of WBCs is the same or greater than adults

**G. Respiratory**

**1.** Respiratory movements occur at the end of the 1st trimester

**2.** Respiratory movement is stimulated by tactile stimuli and asphyxia

**3.** Respiratory inhibition occurs during the 3rd and 4th month to prevent a collection of debris in the alveoli

**4.** Fluid is secreted into the lungs by the alveolar epithelium

**5.** At 22 weeks, the alveolar-capillary membrane comes into juxtaposition, allowing life outside the womb to be possible, although survival is unlikely

**6.** At 24 weeks gestation, terminal air sacs appear at the end of terminal bronchioles

**7.** Mean fetal $pO_2$ after oxygenation is only 30 mmHg; increased oxygen-carrying capacity of fetal hemoglobin prevents hypoxia

**8.** Surfactant secretion is detectable between 25 to 30 weeks gestation and is mature by 36 weeks

**9.** Lungs mature at 36 weeks

### H. Gastrointestinal

1. Anatomic development begins at 4 weeks

2. At 12 weeks, intestinal loops in the umbilical cord withdraw into the abdominal cavity

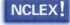

3. At the beginning of the 5th month the fetus swallows amniotic fluid.

4. During the last 2 to 3 months of pregnancy, gastrointestinal development approaches that of the term newborn

5. The liver is primarily hematopoetic; enzyme systems are immature at birth

6. Peristalsis is mature by the 3rd trimester

7. Meconium forms in the intestine beginning at 16 weeks composed of the unabsorbed residue of amniotic fluid and excretory products of gastrointestinal mucosa and glands

### I. Musculoskeletal

1. Primary ossification begins in long bones and the skull by 12 weeks

2. Minimal reflexive muscle movement noted by 12 weeks

3. Fetal movement clearly detected by the mother by 20 weeks

4. Bones are mostly unossified and cartilaginous until the last 4 weeks of gestation; rapid ossification occurs when half of the calcium and phosphate absorbed by the fetus occurs in the last month of pregnancy

### J. Neurologic

1. Neural folds appear 22 to 23 days after conception and fuse at 28 days to form the neural tube

    a. Closure of the tube begins at 22 days and progresses in a cephalocaudal direction

    b. Failure of closure results in neural tube defect

    c. The neural tube becomes the central nervous system, the brain, and spinal cord

2. Some reflex activity present by 12 weeks

3. Neuronal proliferation maximizes at 12 to 18 weeks gestation

4. Brain development

    a. Begins with lower levels such as basal ganglia, thalamus, midbrain, and brain stem

    b. Higher levels, cerebrum and cerebellum, form later

    c. Most neurons of the cerebrum are formed from 10 to 18 weeks

    d. At birth the brain is 27 percent the adult weight

5. Neural organization begins at about 6 months and continues into adulthood

6. Myelinization occurs in the 3rd trimester and continues into adulthood; it progresses from peripheral to central nervous system and motor to sensory

7. Some body regulation control occurs at 25 to 28 weeks

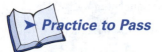

**► Practice to Pass**

While inquiring about the appearance of her fetus at 16 weeks gestation, a client wants to know the difference between an embryo and a fetus. How will the nurse respond to her inquiries?

### K. Urinary

1. Nephron development begins at 8 weeks and filtration at 10 weeks

2. The absolute number of nephrons reaches adult levels by 34 to 35 weeks but are functionally immature

**NCLEX!**

3. By the 5th month the fetus urinates into the amniotic fluid although the urine contains little waste; in the second half of pregnancy, urine makes up a major portion of amniotic fluid

**NCLEX!**

4. The ability to concentrate urine is 20 to 30 percent that of adults.

### L. Sexual

1. Testosterone production begins by the male fetal genital ridge at 7 weeks gestation; later, fetal testes produce it; it is responsible for male organ development

2. Without testosterone, the fetus appears female

**NCLEX!**

3. By 16 weeks, external genitalia are developed enough for identification by ultrasound

---

**Case Study**

A nurse working in a women's health clinic conducts prenatal classes. At each class, the nurse addresses a different topic related to prenatal development. The nurse includes information to support safe progression through pregnancy and assist parents to picture stages of fetal development.

❶ The nurse explains the stage of pre-embryonic development. Describe the significant events of this time period.

❷ The nurse explains organogenesis and critical periods of development in relationship to teratogens. Explain the connection between these concepts.

❸ A class participant asks about genetic transmission of birth defects. What is the nurse's response?

❹ The nurse includes information about the age of viability. When is this achieved and what developmental landmarks must be present for life outside of the womb?

❺ The nurse describes the appearance of the fetus at the end of each trimester. How does the fetus appear at each stage?

*For suggested responses, see pages 337–338.*

## *Posttest*

**1** The clients have one child with Tay-Sachs disease, an autosomal recessive trait. Neither of the clients have the disease. They are in the clinic for genetic counseling prior to conceiving another child. The nurse understands that the clients are undergoing:

(1) Decisional conflict related to knowledge deficit.
(2) Post-trauma syndrome related to care of a disabled child.
(3) Powerlessness related to transmission of genetic disease.
(4) Ineffective health maintenance related to ineffective family coping.

**2** Following an ultrasound at 6 weeks gestation the client comments, "The embryo doesn't look human." She asks, "When will it begin to look like a baby?" The nurse's best response is:

(1) "In one more week the embryo will take on a human appearance."
(2) "The embryo looks like a baby already. Let me show you again."
(3) "The embryo becomes a fetus and looks human after 8 weeks gestation."
(4) "You are right, the embryo doesn't look human. Is this important to you?"

**3** A woman decides to use natural family planning as a means of contraception and states, "The ovum is fertile for 48 hours after ovulation, the same as sperm." The nurse's best response is:

(1) "Correct, avoid intercourse during this time."
(2) "Sperm are fertile for 48 hours, while the ovum is fertile for 24 hours."
(3) "Actually, the ovum is fertile for 36 hours and sperm for 24 hours."
(4) "Let me explain again, the ovum may be fertile up to 72 hours."

**4** A nurse discusses teratogens with a client during pre-conceptual counseling. The client demonstrates understanding by stating:

(1) "I should stop taking all my medications while I am pregnant."
(2) "The fetus is at greatest risk for developing anomalies during the first 16 weeks of pregnancy."
(3) "After 12 weeks the placenta protects the fetus from teratogens."
(4) "Exposure to teratogens poses the greatest risk during the first 8 weeks."

**5** Following an amniocentesis the parents discover that their fetus has Down syndrome. The nurse should:

(1) Provide information about Down syndrome.
(2) Discuss the possibility of intrauterine surgery.
(3) Refer the parents for karyotyping.
(4) Refer the parents to their local public health agency.

**6** A pregnant client asks about the function of the placenta. Which of the following should the nurse include in the teaching plan?

(1) The placenta filters fetal urine.
(2) Fetal and maternal blood mix in the placenta to exchange nutrients.
(3) The placenta filters alcohol from the mother's blood.
(4) Substances are exchanged by the placenta without mixing maternal and fetal blood.

**7** At 36 weeks gestation, a primigravida enters the birthing unit in labor and is concerned about delivering early. The nurse reassures her by stating:

(1) "No need to worry, you are at term."
(2) "Everything is going to be fine. Your baby has a strong heart rate."
(3) "Many babies born at this age have lungs that are just about mature."
(4) "This is nothing. We deliver babies at this age all of the time."

**8**  A nurse evaluates understanding of fetal development in a prenatal class. The nurse knows more
teaching is required when one of the group members responds:

(1) "Smoking will help me have an easy labor because
the baby will be small."
(2) "I should not smoke at all during pregnancy."
(3) "Infants born to mothers who smoke may suffer lung
problems."
(4) "Chemicals from smoking pass through the placenta
to the fetus."

**9**  A client is pregnant with twins, a boy and a girl,
and she asks if they will be identical. The nurse's
best response is:

(1) "They are not identical because the ultrasound
showed one was bigger than the other."
(2) "I'll discuss this with the doctor and give you a call
later."
(3) "We won't know until the babies are delivered."
(4) "The twins are not identical. Identical twins are always the same sex."

**10**  The nurse assesses a woman at 20 weeks gestation,
and expects the woman to report:

(1) Nausea related to hCG production.
(2) Symptoms of diabetes as human placental lactogen is
released.
(3) Feeling fetal kicks.
(4) Spotting related to placental implantation.

*See pages 99–100 for Answers and Rationales.*

# Answers and Rationales

## Pretest

**1  Answer: 4  *Rationale:*** A carrier for cystic fibrosis is
an individual who does not have the illness but is heterozygous for the abnormal gene. It is not until two
carriers mate and produce children that the abnormal
gene will be manifested in the offspring. The affected
offspring must carry two of the abnormal genes to be
affected. There is a 25 percent chance of this occurring, a 50 percent chance that the offspring will be a
carrier without the disease, and a 25 percent chance
of not having the gene at all. With this knowledge the
clients will be able to make a more informed decision
regarding childbearing.
***Cognitive Level:*** Analysis
***Nursing Process:*** Analysis; ***Test Plan:*** HPM

**2  Answer: 2  *Rationale:*** Ovulation usually occurs 14
days prior to the first day of the menstrual period.
The ovum survives 24 hours after ovulation. If sperm
are introduced 24 hours after ovulation, the ovum
cannot be fertilized. Sperm are most capable of fertilization 24 hours after introduction into the female's
reproductive tract.
***Cognitive Level:*** Application
***Nursing Process:*** Evaluation; ***Test Plan:*** PHYS

**3  Answer: 4  *Rationale:*** The risk of Down syndrome
increases markedly after the age of 40. The 42-year-
old woman is at great risk, while the 15-year-old is at
lesser risk. Infection is more likely to result in a birth
anomaly if it occurs in the first trimester.
***Cognitive Level:*** Analysis
***Nursing Process:*** Analysis; ***Test Plan:*** HPM

**4  Answer: 3  *Rationale:*** Dizygotic twins, also known
as fraternal or non-identical, do run in families. The
pregnancy results from the fertilization of two different ova by two different sperm. The zygotes develop
separately and carry their own distinct genetic code
and develop their own placentas and amniotic sacs.
Monozygotic, also known as identical, result from a
single fertilized ovum. They share the same genetic
code and often share placentas and amniotic sacs.
This type of twinning occurs at random.
***Cognitive Level:*** Application
***Nursing Process:*** Implementation; ***Test Plan:*** HPM

**5  Answer: 3  *Rationale:*** It is important to establish a
relationship with clients, obtain a history, verify pregnancy, and monitor fetal well-being. However, the
reason for early prenatal care relates to the critical periods of development that occur in the first trimester

and to promote safety during this particularly vulnerable time of pregnancy.
*Cognitive Level:* Application
*Nursing Process:* Implementation; *Test Plan:* PHYS

**6** **Answer: 1** *Rationale:* The ears ossify at 20 weeks gestation and the fetus hears at 24 weeks.
*Cognitive Level:* Application
*Nursing Process:* Implementation; *Test Plan:* PHYS

**7** **Answer: 1** *Rationale:* Oligohydramnios is an abnormal condition occurring when amniotic fluid volume is less than expected for a given stage of pregnancy. While the exact cause is unknown, oligohydramnios is associated with postmaturity, intrauterine growth retardation, and fetal malformations of the urinary tract. An insufficient amount of amniotic fluid impairs the normal functions of the fluid, resulting in potential complications such as fetal skin and skeletal abnormalities, pulmonary hypoplasia, and cord compression.
*Cognitive Level:* Application
*Nursing Process:* Implementation; *Test Plan:* PHYS

**8** **Answer: 2** *Rationale:* There are two umbilical arteries that carry blood from the fetal common iliac artery to the placenta. These two arteries are twisted around a large umbilical vein that carries blood from the placenta to the fetal heart. About 1 percent of umbilical cords contain only two vessels. This condition is more likely to be associated with congenital malformations.
*Cognitive Level:* Analysis
*Nursing Process:* Assessment; *Test Plan:* PHYS

**9** **Answer: 4** *Rationale:* At term the amniotic fluid volume ranges from 700 to 1,000 milliliters (mL). Each mL weighs about 1 gram (g), so the amniotic fluid contributes about 700 to 1,000 g to the weight of pregnancy. This is the same as .7 to 1 kilogram (kg) since 1,000 g equals a kilogram.
*Cognitive Level:* Application
*Nursing Process:* Assessment; *Test Plan:* PHYS

**10** **Answer: 3** *Rationale:* Once the fertilized egg implants in the uterus, it secretes the hormone hCG. The function of hCG is to support corpus luteum secretion of progesterone. As the placenta develops and matures, it takes over the task of producing progesterone. Most pregnancy tests detect the presence of hCG in the urine.
*Cognitive Level:* Application
*Nursing Process:* Implementation; *Test Plan:* PHYS

## Posttest

**1** **Answer: 1** *Rationale:* Families with genetic disease are faced with difficult decisions regarding pregnancy. One of the purposes of genetic counseling is to provide the best information available so families can make knowledgeable decisions. The fact that the family is seeking professional help is evidence that they feel some power regarding the situation. There is no evidence one way or another regarding their coping abilities with a disabled child.
*Cognitive Level:* Analysis
*Nursing Process:* Analysis; *Test Plan:* HPM

**2** **Answer: 3** *Rationale:* The embryonic phase of development is a time of organogenesis. By the end of 8 weeks gestation, all of the tissue and organ foundations have developed. Once this occurs, the embryo appears human and enters the fetal phase. The fetal phase is one of organ maturation.
*Cognitive Level:* Analysis
*Nursing Process:* Implementation; *Test Plan:* HPM

**3** **Answer: 2** *Rationale:* Ova are capable of being fertilized for 24 hours after ovulation. Sperm live for 48 to 72 hours after coitus but are most capable of fertilization in the first 24 hours.
*Cognitive Level:* Analysis
*Nursing Process:* Evaluation; *Test Plan:* HPM

**4** **Answer: 4** *Rationale:* Organogenesis and cell differentiation occurs during the first 8 weeks of pregnancy. This makes the embryo particularly sensitive to teratogens during this time. Although medications may have teratogenic effects, each medication's risk versus benefit needs to be evaluated by the physician.
*Cognitive Level:* Analysis
*Nursing Process:* Evaluation; *Test Plan:* HPM

**5** **Answer: 1** *Rationale:* The nurse is in an ideal position to provide information, educate families, and review what has been discussed in genetic counseling sessions. The nurse provides information about Down syndrome. Karyotyping is not indicated because they have a diagnosis. Intrauterine surgery cannot cure a chromosomal anomaly. Referral to public health may be indicated after the parents makes a decision regarding the pregnancy.
*Cognitive Level:* Application
*Nursing Process:* Implementation; *Test Plan:* HPM

**6** **Answer: 4** *Rationale:* Fetal gas exchange occurs in the intervillous spaces of the placenta through simple diffusion of oxygen, carbon dioxide and carbon

monoxide. Substance exchange between the maternal and fetal blood occurs without mixing of the blood. Fetal waste products are excreted via the placenta, but urine is excreted by the fetus into the amniotic fluid. While the placenta is capable of filtering some substances, most substances consumed by the mother are exchanged with the fetus, including alcohol.
*Cognitive Level:* Analysis
*Nursing Process:* Planning; *Test Plan:* HPM

7   **Answer: 3** *Rationale:* Surfactant with a lecithin to sphingomyelin ratio of 2:1 is required for mature lung function. This occurs at about 36 weeks gestation. An infant born prior to 38 weeks gestation is considered preterm. A reassuring fetal heart rate is not indicative of lung maturity.
*Cognitive Level:* Application
*Nursing Process:* Implementation; *Test Plan:* PHYS

8   **Answer: 1** *Rationale:* Smoking causes vasoconstriction that can interfere with placental circulation. The infant may suffer negative effects including growth restriction. Any chemical the mother is exposed to during pregnancy has the potential to pass through the placenta to the fetus.
*Cognitive Level:* Application
*Nursing Process:* Evaluation; *Test Plan:* HPM

9   **Answer: 4** *Rationale:* Twins of opposite sex are always fraternal because it indicates two sperm were involved in fertilization, one carrying a Y chromosome and one carrying an X chromosome. Identical twins develop from one ovum and one sperm. Therefore, the genotype is the same, including sex. Identical twins may be different sizes because one twin may receive a greater amount of placental circulation than the other.
*Cognitive Level:* Application
*Nursing Process:* Implementation; *Test Plan:* HPM

10   **Answer: 3** *Rationale:* Fetal movement begins early in pregnancy but is not felt by the mother until 16 to 20 weeks.
*Cognitive Level:* Application
*Nursing Process:* Assessment; *Test Plan:* HPM

## References

Andrews, L. B., Fullarton, J. E., Holtzman, N. A., & Motulsky, A. G. (Eds.) (1994). *Assessing genetic risks: Implications for health and social policy.* Washington D.C.: National Academy Press.

Blackburn, S. T. & Loper D. L. (1992). *Maternal, fetal, and neonatal physiology: A clinical perspective.* Philadelphia: W.B. Saunders Company.

Blank, R. & Merrick, J. (1995). *Human reproduction, emerging technologies, and conflicting rights.* Washington D.C.: A Division of Congressional Quarterly, Inc.

Caruthers, B. (1999). Fetal lung development. *The Surgical Technologist 31*(3): 22–25.

Caruthers, B. (1999). Kidney development and functions in the fetus. *The Surgical Technologist 31*(1): 16–20.

Cefalo, R. C. & Moos, M-K. (1995). *Preconceptual health care: A practical guide* (2nd ed.). St. Louis: Mosby.

Cooper, N. G. (Ed.) (1994). *The human genome project: Deciphering the blueprint of heredity.* Mill Valley, CA: University Science Books.

Coticchio, G. & Fishel, S. (1998). Conception to implantation. In G. Chamberlain, F. Broughton Pipkin (Eds.) *Clinical physiology in obstetrics* (3rd ed.). Osney Mead, Oxford: Blackwell Science, Ltd.

Cruz, Y. P. (1997). Mammals. In S. F. Gilbert & A. M. Raunio (Eds.), *Embryology: Constructing the organism.* Sunderland, MA: Sinauer Associates, pp. 459–492.

Guyton, A. C. & Hall, J. E. (2000). *Textbook of medical physiology* (10th ed.). Philadelphia: W.B. Saunders Company.

Harrison, J. M. (2000). The events of early pregnancy. *British Journal of Midwifery 8*(3): 137–142.

Jones, O. W. & Cahill, T. C. (1994). Basic genetics and patterns of inheritance. In R. K. Creasy & J. Resnick (Eds.), *Maternal-fetal medicine: Principles and practice* (3rd ed.). Philadelphia: W.B. Saunders Company, pp. 3–60.

Kalthoff, K. (1996). *Analysis of biological development.* New York: McGraw-Hill, Inc.

Larsen, W. J. (1998). *Essentials of human embryology.* New York: Churchill Livingston.

Levitt, P., Reinoso, B., & Jones, L. (1998). The critical impact of early cellular environment on neuronal development. *Preventive Medicine, 27*(2): 180–183.

Lowdermilk, D. L., Perry, S. E., & Bobak, I. M. (2000). *Maternity and women's health care* (7th ed.). St. Louis: Mosby, pp. 329–330.

Moore, K. L. & Persand, T. V. N. (1998). *Before we are born: Essentials of embryology and birth defects* (5th ed.). Philadelphia: W. B. Saunders Company.

Moore, K. L. & Persand, T. V. N. (1998). *The developing human: Clinically oriented embryology* (6th ed.). Philadelphia: W. B. Saunders Company.

Olds, S. B., London, M. L., & Ladewig, P.A. (2000). *Maternal-newborn nursing: A family and community-based approach* (6th ed.). Upper Saddle River, NJ: Prentice Hall-Inc., pp. 141–208, 237, 463, 646–647.

Polin, R. A. & Fox, W. W. (1992). *Fetal and neonatal physiology (Vol 1)*. Philadelphia: W.B. Saunders Company.

Sadler, T. W. (1995). *Langman's medical embryology* (7th ed.). Baltimore: Williams & Wilkins.

Scalon, C. & Fibison, W. (1995). *Managing genetic information: Implications for nursing practice*. Washington, D.C.: American Nurses Association.

Thomas, C. L. (Ed.), (1997). *Taber's cyclopedic medical dictionary* (18th ed.). Philadelphia: F. A. Davis Company.

Williams, J. K. (1996). *Genetic issues for perinatal nurses*. White Plains, NY: Education & Health Promotion Department March of Dimes Birth Defects Foundation.

Wolpert, L., Beddington, R., Brockes, J., Jessell, T., Lawrence, P., & Meyerowitz, P. (1998). *Principles of development*. London: Current Biology LTD.

Wong, D. L. & Perry, S. E. (1998). *Maternal child nursing*. St. Louis: Mosby, pp. 61, 71.

## CHAPTER 5

# The Normal Prenatal Experience

Angela F. Wood, PhD, RN, C

## CHAPTER OUTLINE

*Nursing Care of the Prenatal Client*
*Essential Concepts of Pregnancy*

*Signs and Symptoms of Pregnancy*
*Physiologic Changes of Pregnancy*

*Nutritional Needs*
*Psychosocial Changes of Pregnancy*

## OBJECTIVES

▉ Describe the nursing care provided to the maternity client during the first prenatal visit.

▉ Identify assessment needs of maternity clients during subsequent prenatal visits.

▉ Differentiate between presumptive, probable, and positive signs of pregnancy.

▉ Describe the physical changes that occur in each body system of the pregnant woman.

▉ Identify discomforts commonly experienced in pregnancy and related nursing interventions.

▉ Describe the content areas that nurses should include in an educational program for a pregnant client.

[ **Media Link** ]

*Use the CD-ROM enclosed with this text, or log onto the address given to access the free, interactive Companion Website created for this series. The CD-ROM and Companion Website accompanying this book offer additional practice opportunities and information—NCLEX Review, Case Studies, Glossary, In Depth with NCLEX, and more.*

**www.prenhall.com/hogan**

## REVIEW AT A GLANCE

**Chadwick's sign** *a bluish color of the vaginal mucous membrane resulting from increased vascularity; it can be seen beginning at about the fourth month of pregnancy*

**chloasma** *increased pigmentation, commonly seen over the nose and cheeks during pregnancy; sometimes called the "mask of pregnancy"*

**colostrum** *a thin, bluish-white breast secretion that appears before the onset of lactation; comprised mainly of serum and white blood corpuscles, the fluid is high in protein and contains immune properties*

**estimated date of birth (EDB)** *sometimes called the "due date" or "estimated date of confinement," this is the date in the pregnancy when birth is expected*

**fetal heart tones** *sounds produced by the fetal heart; can be counted to determine the fetal heart rate*

**fundal height** *the distance, in centimeters, from the symphysis pubis to the top edge of the fundus; this measurement can be used to calculate gestational age*

**Goodell's sign** *a softening of the cervix that begins in the second month of pregnancy*

**gravida** *term used to indicate a pregnant woman; sometimes used to indicate the number of times a woman has been pregnant*

**linea nigra** *a dark line of pigment extending from the umbilicus to the pubis, sometimes seen in the later part of pregnancy*

**McDonald's method** *procedure used to determine gestational age by measuring the fundal height; it is most accurate between 22 and 34 weeks; it can also be used serially to monitor fetal growth; can be inaccurate in the presence of maternal obesity, uterine fibroids, and polyhydramnios*

**Nägele's Rule** *a commonly used method for determining the estimated date of birth; it is calculated by determining the first day of the last menstrual period, subtracting 3 months from that date, and then adding 7 days*

**para** *a woman who has delivered an infant who had reached the age of viability*

**positive signs of pregnancy** *findings that confirm pregnancy such as auscultation of fetal heart tones, fetal movement, and visualization of the fetus*

**presumptive signs of pregnancy** *findings reported by the mother that suggest the presence of a pregnancy such as cessation of menses, morning sickness, and quickening*

**probable signs of pregnancy** *findings noted by the healthcare provider that suggest a pregnancy is present including Goodell's sign, McDonald's sign, enlargement of the abdomen, and palpation of the fetal outline*

**quickening** *the first fetal movement felt by the pregnant woman, usually between 16 to 18 weeks gestation*

**striae gravidarum** *shiny red lines on the skin of breasts, abdomen, thighs, and buttocks as a result of stretching of the skin*

## Pretest

**1** During the client's initial prenatal visit, which of the following would indicate a need for further assessment?

(1) History of diabetes for 6 years
(2) Exercises three times a week
(3) Occasional use of over-the-counter pain relievers
(4) Maternal age 30 years

**2** The low-risk client, who is 16 weeks pregnant, should be told to return to the prenatal clinic in:

(1) 1 week.
(2) 2 weeks.
(3) 3 weeks.
(4) 4 weeks.

**3** The client has completed an at-home pregnancy test with positive results. Which of the following indicates that the client understands the meaning of the test results?

(1) "I understand that this means I have ovulated in the past 24 hours."
(2) "I understand that this means I am not pregnant."
(3) "I understand that this means I might be pregnant."
(4) "I understand that this means I am pregnant."

**4** The client is pregnant and reports that her last menstrual period began July 10. Her expected date of birth is:

(1) April 3.
(2) April 17.
(3) October 3.
(4) October 17.

5 The pregnant client reports that she has a 3-year-old child at home who was born at term, had a miscarriage at 10 weeks gestation, and delivered a set of twins at 28 weeks gestation that died within 24 hours. In the prenatal record, the nurse should record:

(1) Gravida 2, para 1.
(2) Gravida 3, para 3.
(3) Gravida 4, para 2.
(4) Gravida 5, para 4.

6 The client, who is 36 weeks gestation, calls her prenatal care provider because she is concerned about a thin, bluish-white fluid leaking from her breasts. The nurse's best response is:

(1) "This probably indicates an infection in your breasts. You will need to come into the office."
(2) "This usually happens when you are going into premature labor. You should go to the hospital."
(3) "This normally occurs as your breasts prepare for breast-feeding. You should continue to wear a good-fitting bra."
(4) "This is an indication that you may have some problems with breast-feeding. I will have the lactation consultant call you."

7 The client's prenatal education includes danger signs to report. Which of the following, if reported, would indicate that the client understood the teaching?

(1) Dizziness and blurred vision
(2) Occasional nausea and vomiting
(3) No bowel movement for 3 days
(4) Ankle edema

8 The client, a pregnant 20-year-old single woman, tells the nurse that she wants to keep her baby, but she isn't sure she can manage by herself. The best response by the nurse is:

(1) "It is hard to raise a child by yourself. I will need to contact Child Protective Services."
(2) "Oh, don't worry, lots of women manage by themselves."
(3) "I can see you are concerned, let's talk about possible support systems."
(4) "If you are having some concerns, maybe you should talk to an adoption agency."

9 The nurse is planning a childbirth education class for women in their first trimester of pregnancy. Which of the following topics will be most appropriate?

(1) Breathing techniques for pain relief in labor
(2) Choosing a prenatal care provider
(3) Postpartum self-care
(4) Care of the newborn infant

10 The client, who was an appropriate weight for height at the time she became pregnant, is 20 weeks pregnant and has gained a total of 12 pounds. She is concerned about weight gain. The best response by the nurse is:

(1) "I will tell the doctor that you are worried. He will tell you what to do."
(2) "Your weight gain is about average for this point in your pregnancy. What concerns you about it?"
(3) "You really have gained at lot. I will consult the nutritionist for you."
(4) "A lot of your weight gain is probably fluid. Why don't you decrease your salt intake and see if that will help."

*See pages 118–119 for Answers and Rationales.*

## I. Nursing Care of the Prenatal Patient

**A. First prenatal visit:** should begin by finding out why the woman is seeking care and should include a complete health history and physical examination

1. History should be collected on pre-pregnant health including weight; nutrition; exercise pattern; over-the-counter, prescription, and illicit drug use; allergies;

potential teratogens; history of surgery or present disease states, especially those with known implications for pregnancy, such as viral infections, diabetes, hypertension, cardiovascular disease, renal problems, and thyroid or bleeding disorders; gynecologic history including date of last Pap smear; previous infections; age at menarche and menstrual, contraceptive, and obstetric histories are obtained

2. Physical assessment

**NCLEX!**

    **a. Fetal heart tones** (FHT), the fetal heart rate per minute, can be assessed by fetoscope (beginning at about 16 weeks) or by ultrasonic Doppler device (beginning at about 8 weeks); FHT's are useful in determining gestational age and fetal well-being; fetal heart rate normally ranges from 120 to 160 beats per minute

**NCLEX!**

    **b. Fundal height,** the measurement from the symphysis pubis to the top of the uterine fundus (in centimeters) can be used to assess gestational age and fetal growth (see Figure 5-1)

**NCLEX!**

    **c.** Complete maternal physical examination should be done including vital signs; height and weight; thyroid; heart and breath sounds; and reproductive organs including pelvic musculature, size of uterus, and adequacy of pelvis for delivery

    **d.** Laboratory assessment should include hematocrit and hemoglobin; blood type, Rh and irregular antibody; rubella titer; tuberculin skin test, renal function tests, urinalysis and culture; screening for sexually transmitted diseases; Pap test and offer of HIV test

**Figure 5-1**

**Fundal height during pregnancy.**

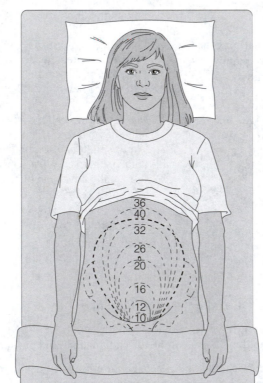

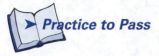

**Practice to Pass**

The client has just had her pregnancy confirmed by ultrasound. When she begins to cry, how should the nurse respond?

    **e.** Priority nursing diagnosis: Health-seeking behaviors

    **f.** Planning and implementation

        1) Prepare for the exam by telling the woman what to expect

        2) Provide information about the prenatal care program, setting, and personnel

        3) Provide information about physiologic changes to be expected in pregnancy as well as danger signs to report

    **g.** Evaluation: client verbalizes knowledge of procedures for the physical exam, future prenatal care, and expected changes related to normal and abnormal aspects of pregnancy

  **3.** Psychosocial assessment

    **a.** Assess client for emotions such as excitement, anxiety, and/or ambivalence about the pregnancy

    **b.** Explore available support systems

    **c.** Assess stability and functional level of client's immediate and extended family

    **d.** Assess economic support adequate for housing, daily needs, and medical expenses

    **e.** Discuss cultural preferences including practices to be used or avoided during pregnancy, preference of caregiver gender, and preferred support person(s)

**B. Follow-up prenatal visits**

  **1.** Frequency

    **a.** Every 4 weeks during the first 28 weeks gestation

    **b.** Every 2 weeks until 36 weeks

    **c.** Every week until delivery

  **2.** Priority nursing diagnoses: Potential ineffective health maintenance; Progressive normal fetal growth and development

  **3.** Planning and implementation

    **a.** Visits should include teaching as well as assessment of maternal and fetal well-being

    **b.** Instruct the mother concerning physical changes associated with pregnancy, such as **quickening** (the first fetal movements felt) and colostrum production, as well as the danger signs of pregnancy presented in Table 5-1

    **c.** The mother should be assessed for acceptance of the pregnancy and adjustment to the maternal role, changes from baseline measurement of vital signs, weight gain, nutritional status, and presence of glucose and/or protein in the urine

    **d.** Blood levels of alpha-fetoprotein (AFP) to screen for fetal neural tube defects should be assessed at 16 to 18 weeks; maternal blood glucose level should be assessed at 24 to 28 weeks to screen for gestational diabetes

    **e.** The fetus should be assessed at each visit for growth as measured by fundal height, movement, and heart rate

| Table 5-1 | Danger Sign | Possible Cause |
|---|---|---|
| **Danger Signs in Pregnancy** | Gush of fluid from vagina | Rupture of membranes |
| | Vaginal bleeding | Abruptio placentae, placenta previa, bloody show |
| | Abdominal pain | Premature labor, abruptio placentae |
| | Temperature > 101°F | Infection |
| | Persistent vomiting | Hyperemesis gravidarum |
| | Visual disturbances | Hypertension, preeclampsia |
| | Edema of hands and face | Hypertension, preeclampsia |
| | Severe headache | Hypertension, preeclampsia |
| | Epigastric pain | Preeclampsia |
| | Dysuria | Urinary tract infection |
| | Decreased fetal movement | Compromised fetal well-being |

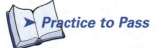

**Practice to Pass**

The client has come to the clinic for her first prenatal visit at 18 weeks gestation. After the nurse explains the prenatal visit schedule, the client states, "I don't really see any need to come back until I go into labor." How should the nurse respond?

4. Evaluation: the client reports whether or not she is engaged in positive health behaviors; maternal health indicators and uterine growth are comparable to normal parameters

**C. Childbirth education**

1. Childbirth classes provide information on pregnancy and childbirth to facilitate families in optimal decision making; topics should be timed to the progress of pregnancy as illustrated in Table 5-2

2. In addition, classes can be planned for special groups such as grandparents, siblings, adolescents, and clients who will deliver by cesarean section

3. Exercise is an important topic for childbirth education; women should be encouraged to participate in regular (three times per week) exercise during pregnancy

   a. Benefits of exercise include maintaining muscle tone and bowel function, as well as fewer complications during labor and delivery

   b. Exercises especially helpful for childbirth include pelvic tilt, partial sit-ups, Kegel exercises, and exercises to stretch the inner-thigh muscles

4. Classes on preparation for the birth process provide information on selection of birthing method and relaxation techniques

| Table 5-2 | Trimester | Educational Topic |
|---|---|---|
| **Childbirth Education Topics by Trimester** | First | Physical and psychosocial changes of pregnancy |
| | | Self-care in pregnancy |
| | | Protecting and nurturing the fetus |
| | | Choosing a care provider and birth setting |
| | | Prenatal exercise |
| | | Relief of common early pregnancy discomforts |
| | Second | Planning for breast-feeding |
| | | Sexuality in pregnancy |
| | | Relief of common later-pregnancy discomforts |
| | Third | Preparation for childbirth |
| | | Development of a birth plan |
| | | Relaxation techniques |
| | | Postpartum self-care |
| | | Infant stimulation |
| | | Infant care and safety |

| | Method | Characteristics | Breathing techniques |
|---|---|---|---|
| **Table 5-3**<br><br>**Comparison of Common Birthing Methods** | Lamaze | Uses education about fetal growth and changes associated with pregnancy along with training in exercises that strengthen muscles used during labor and delivery to decrease fear and help the mother cope with the pain of labor | Patterned, paced |
| | Bradley | Relies on partner or husband to coach the laboring woman; promotes relaxation through abdominal breathing and exercises | Primarily abdominal |
| | Kitzinger | Prepares the woman for birth through the use of sensory memory and the Stanislavsky acting method to teach relaxation | Chest breathing with abdominal relaxation |

**► *Practice to Pass***

The client, who is a gravida 3, para 2, tells the nurse that she didn't go to childbirth classes with her previous pregnancies and that she and the babies did fine. The client asks why she should go to classes with this pregnancy. How should the nurse respond?

**NCLEX!**

a. Commonly taught birthing methods include the Lamaze, Kitzinger, and Bradley methods of prepared childbirth; see Table 5-3 for a comparison of these methods

b. Relaxation techniques commonly taught to be used in labor include touch, disassociation, and progressive relaxation

5. Classes geared toward knowledge that will be needed after delivery include sessions on postpartum self-care, newborn care, infant stimulation, and infant safety needs

D. **Management of common discomforts of pregnancy (see Tables 5-4 and 5-5)**

1. Discomforts occur as a result of the physiologic or anatomic changes of pregnancy; they differ from trimester to trimester

2. While not dangerous, they constitute a significant problem for the client and present an opportunity for nursing intervention

## II. Essential Concepts of Pregnancy

A. *Estimated date of birth* (EDB) or "due date": can be determined by several methods

1. **Nägele's Rule** is used to determine the EDB by taking the first day of the last menstrual period, subtracting 3 months and adding 7 days; this date is most accurate when the woman remembers her last menstrual period, has menses every 28 days, and was not taking oral contraceptives

| | Discomfort | Management |
|---|---|---|
| **Table 5-4**<br><br>**Management of Discomforts in Early Pregnancy** | Nausea and vomiting | Avoid strong odors<br>Drink carbonated beverages<br>Avoid drinking while eating<br>Eat crackers or toast before getting out of bed<br>Eat small, frequent meals<br>Avoid spicy or greasy foods |
| | Breast tenderness | Wear a well-fitting, supportive bra |
| | Urinary frequency | Increase daytime fluid intake<br>Decrease evening fluid intake<br>Empty bladder as soon as urge is felt |
| | Fatigue | Plan a rest period or nap during the day<br>Go to bed as early as possible |
| | Ptyalism | Use gum, mints, hard candy, or mouthwash |
| | Nasal stuffiness/bleeding | Use cool air vaporizer |

| Table 5-5 | Discomfort | Management |
|---|---|---|
| **Management of Discomforts in Late Pregnancy** | Heartburn | Eat small, frequent meals |
| | | Avoid spicy or greasy foods |
| | | Refrain from laying down immediately after eating |
| | | Use low-sodium antacids |
| | Constipation | Increase fluid and fiber intake |
| | | Exercise |
| | | Develop regular bowel habits |
| | | Use stool softeners as needed |
| | Hemorrhoids | Avoid constipation |
| | | Apply topical anesthetics, ointments, or ice packs |
| | | Use sitz baths or warm soaks |
| | | Reinsert into rectum, if necessary |
| | Backache | Practice good body mechanics |
| | | Practice pelvic tilt exercise |
| | | Avoid high heels, heavy lifting, overfatigue, and excessive bending or reaching |
| | Leg cramps | Dorsiflex feet |
| | | Apply heat to affected muscle |
| | | Evaluate calcium to phosphorus ratio in diet |
| | Varicose veins | Elevate legs |
| | | Wear support hose |
| | | Avoid crossing legs at the knee, restrictive clothing, and standing for long periods of time |
| | Ankle edema | Practice frequent dorsiflexion of feet |
| | | Avoid standing for long periods of time |
| | | Elevate legs when sitting or resting |
| | Faintness | Arise slowly |
| | | Avoid prolonged standing |
| | | Maintain hematocrit and hemoglobin |
| | Flatulence | Avoid gas-forming foods |
| | | Chew food thoroughly |
| | | Establish regular bowel habits |

2. **McDonald's method** uses uterine size to indicate gestational age by measuring, in centimeters, the distance from the symphysis pubis to the top of the uterine fundus

   a. This distance, **fundal height,** correlates well with the number of weeks gestation between 22 and 34 weeks

   b. The formula for calculation of gestational age based on fundal height is

   $$\frac{\text{distance in centimeters} \times 8}{7} = \text{total weeks of gestation}$$

   c. Prediction of EDB using this method can be affected by maternal height, irregular fetal growth, multiple gestation, and abnormal amounts of amniotic fluid

3. Quickening, feeling of fetal movement by the mother, usually occurs between 16 and 18 weeks; because of the wide range of times this is experienced, this method gives a less accurate EDB

4. Auscultation of fetal heart rate can occur as early as 8 weeks gestation using a ultrasonic Doppler device but is more commonly heard between 10 and 12 weeks; this variation can result in a less accurate date

5. Ultrasound examination may be used for estimation of the EDB when the date of the last menstrual period is unknown or the uterine size is inconsistent with the EDB calculated with Nägele's Rule or McDonald's method

**B. Gravida and para**

1. Gravida and para are terms to describe a woman's childbearing history

2. **Gravida** is the number of times the woman has been pregnant

3. **Para** is the number of infants delivered after 20 weeks gestation, born dead or alive; multiple births count as one delivery regardless of the number of infants delivered

4. TPAL is a more detailed description of para

   a. T is the number of infants born after 37 weeks

   b. P is the number of infants born between 20 and 37 weeks

   c. A is the number of pregnancies that end in spontaneous or therapeutic abortion prior to 20 weeks

   d. L is the number of children currently alive

**III. Signs and Symptoms of Pregnancy (see Box 5-1)**

A. *Presumptive* (subjective) *signs of pregnancy:* signs and symptoms that the woman reports, which may or may not be associated with pregnancy

---

**Box 5-1**

**Signs and Symptoms of Pregnancy**

**Presumptive Signs**
   amenorrhea
   nausea and vomiting
   fatigue
   urinary frequency
   breast changes
   quickening

**Probable Signs**
   Hegar's sign
   McDonald's sign
   enlargement of abdomen
   pigmentation changes
   abdominal striae
   ballottement
   positive pregnancy test
   palpation of fetal outline

**Positive Signs**
   fetal heartbeat
   fetal movement palpable by the examiner
   visualization of the fetus by ultrasound

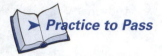

**Practice to Pass**

The client, who states that she and her partner use condoms "most of the time," presents with amenorrhea for 1 month, fatigue, and breast tenderness. The client suspects that she is pregnant. How can this be confirmed?

**B.** *Probable* (objective) *signs of pregnancy:* noted by the examiner, which may or may not be associated with pregnancy

**C.** *Positive* (diagnostic) *signs of pregnancy:* noted by the examiner and can only be caused by pregnancy

## IV. Physiologic Changes of Pregnancy

### A. Reproductive

1. Uterus: during pregnancy, the uterus, which takes on an ovoid shape, increases in capacity from 10 mL to 5 L; this increase is primarily caused by an increase in size of the cells (hypertrophy) in response to estrogen, as well as distention caused by the growing fetus; by the end of the pregnancy, the uterus and its contents require up to one-sixth of the total maternal blood flow

2. Cervix: under the influence of estrogen, the cervix secretes mucus that forms a plug at the opening of the endocervical canal to limit bacteria entering the uterus; increased blood flow to the cervix results in **Goodell's sign** (softening of the cervix) and **Chadwick's sign** (bluish color of the cervix during pregnancy)

3. Vagina: under the influence of estrogen, vaginal mucosa thickens and connective tissue relaxes; vaginal secretions thicken and increase in amount during pregnancy; the pH is acidic, 3.6 to 6.0

4. Breasts: estrogen and progesterone cause the breasts to increase in size and to increase in the number of glands; **colostrum** (a thin bluish-white secretion high in protein and immune properties) is produced and may be expressed during the last trimester

### B. Cardiovascular

1. Cardiac output increases 30 to 40 percent over non-pregnant output with an increase in pulse of 10 to 15 beats

2. Pulmonary and peripheral vascular resistance decreases 40 to 50 percent, resulting in a decrease in blood pressure throughout the first and second trimesters of pregnancy; in the third trimester, it begins to increase to prepregnant levels; postural hypertension may result as the pregnant uterus presses on pelvic and femoral vessels limiting blood return to the heart

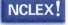

3. Vena cava syndrome results as the gravid uterus compresses the vena cava resulting in decreased blood flow to the right atrium and a decrease in blood pressure

   a. Symptoms include pallor, dizziness, and clammy skin

   b. Problem can be prevented or treated by positioning the woman on her left side with a pillow under her right hip

4. Blood volume increases 45 percent over pre-pregnant levels

   a. Red blood cells (RBC) increase 18 to 30 percent depending on the degree of iron supplementation

   b. Plasma volume increases 50 percent

   c. The greater increase in plasma over RBCs results in physiologic anemia and is seen in a 7 percent decrease in hematocrit

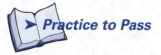

**Practice to Pass**

The client, who is 28 weeks gestation, complains of fatigue. She reports difficulty sleeping. She says that she slept on her back before becoming pregnant, but now she feels like she is going to faint in that position. How should the nurse respond?

**C. Respiratory**

1. Volume of air breathed increases 30 to 40 percent because of decreased airway resistance that occurs in response to progesterone

2. Intrathoracic volume remains unchanged, even though the enlarged uterus presses up on the diaphragm, because the rib cage flares and chest circumference increases

**D. Neurologic:** no known changes

**E. Musculoskeletal**

1. Relaxation of the pelvic joints results in the classic "waddling" gait often seen in pregnancy

2. Physiologic lordosis (Figure 5-2) develops as the curvature of the lumbar spine increases to compensate for the weight of the gravid uterus; this can result in low back pain

3. Diastasis recti, separation of the rectus abdominis muscle, can result as the uterus enlarges

**F. Gastrointestinal**

1. During the first trimester, human chorionic gonadotropin (hCG) increases and can cause nausea and vomiting

2. Increased progesterone levels relax smooth muscles, resulting in decreased peristalsis as evidenced by bloating, reflux of gastric secretions, and constipation; gastrointestinal problems are worsened as the gravid uterus presses on the intestines

3. Constipation and increased pressure on blood vessels in the rectum can result in hemorrhoids

**Figure 5-2** **Postural changes during pregnancy.**

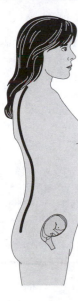 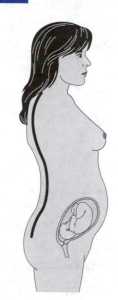 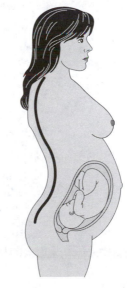 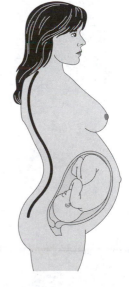

12 weeks     20 weeks     28 weeks     36 weeks     40 weeks

#### G. Renal

1. In the first trimester, the gravid uterus presses on the bladder causing urinary frequency; relieved in the second trimester by the uterus moving into the abdominal area, this problem returns in the third trimester as the presenting part presses on the bladder

2. Glomerular filtration increases 50 percent during the second trimester and remains elevated until delivery; the kidneys may not be able to reabsorb all of the glucose filtered resulting in glycosuria

#### H. Integumentary

1. In response to increased levels of estrogen, some areas of the skin have an increase in pigmentation; this is seen primarily in areas with increased pigmentation such as the areola, nipples, and vulva

   a. **Chloasma,** mask of pregnancy, is an increase in pigmentation on the forehead and around the eyes; it is seen most often in women of color and is aggravated by sun exposure

   b. **Linea nigra** is a darkly pigmented line that extends from the umbilicus to the public area

   c. **Striae gravidarum,** or stretch marks, appear as reddish streaks on trunk and thighs; they result from stretching of connective tissue caused by increased adrenal steroid levels; while these generally change to a shiny gray-white color after delivery, they do not disappear

2. Sweat and sebaceous gland activity increases during pregnancy

#### I. Endocrine

1. Metabolism

   a. Average weight gain is 3 to 5 pounds in the first trimester and 12 to 15 pounds in each of the following trimesters

   b. Water retention occurs during pregnancy caused by increased sex hormones and decreased serum protein

2. Hormones in pregnancy

   a. Secreted by the trophoblast early in pregnancy, human chorionic gonadotropin (hCG) stimulates progesterone and estrogen production; it is thought to support the pregnancy and to cause nausea and vomiting in the first trimester

   b. Human placental lactogen, also known as chorionic somatomammotropin or hPL, is an insulin antagonist; it promotes lipolysis, resulting in increased amounts of circulating free fatty acids available for maternal metabolic use

   c. Estrogen and progesterone are produced by the corpus luteum for the first 7 weeks of pregnancy and then by the placenta

      1) Estrogen stimulates uterine development to support fetal growth and stimulates the ductal system of the breast for lactation

2) Progesterone maintains the endometrium, decreases uterine contractility, stimulates development of the breast acini and lobules, and causes relaxation of smooth muscle

d. Relaxin, primarily made by the corpus luteum, decreases uterine contractility, contributes to the softening of the cervix, and has long-term effects on collagen

e. Prostaglandins, lipids that are found throughout the female reproductive system, contribute to the decrease seen in the placental vascular system, and probably contribute to the onset of labor

## V. Nutritional Needs

### A. Requirements are affected by a variety of factors

1. Pre-pregnancy nutritional status: women who are underweight or overweight may need more or less calories for adequate fetal weight gain, respectively

2. Maternal age: teenage mothers may need increased caloric intake to allow for maternal and fetal growth

3. Maternal parity: number of pregnancies and the interval between them can affect nutritional needs

### B. Maternal nutrition

1. The normal pregnant woman requires an additional 300 calories per day

2. Other nutritional requirements are increased during pregnancy, as illustrated in Table 5-6

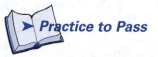

**Practice to Pass**

The client, who is 24 weeks gestation, is concerned about her weight. She has gained a total of 26 pounds over her pre-pregnant weight. She tells the nurse that she usually eats lunch at a fast food restaurant and frequently snacks in the afternoon. How should the nurse respond?

**NCLEX!**

| **Table 5-6** | | |
|---|---|---|
| **Nutritional Requirements during Pregnancy** | | |

| Nutritional Element | Requirements | |
| | *Pregnant* | *Non-pregnant\** |
|---|---|---|
| Protein | 60 g | 46 g |
| Vitamin A | 800 mcgR | 800 mcgR |
| Vitamin D | 10 mcg | 10 mcg |
| Vitamin E | 10 mcg | 8 mcg |
| Vitamin K | 65 mcg | 60 mcg |
| Vitamin C | 70 mg | 60 mg |
| Thiamine | 1.5 mg | 1.1 mg |
| Riboflavin | 1.6 mg | 1.3 mg |
| Niacin | 17 mg NE | 15 mg NE |
| Vitamin B$_6$ | 2.2 mg | 1.6 mg |
| Folate | 400 mcg | 180 mcg |
| Vitamin B$_{12}$ | 2.2 mcg | 2.0 mcg |
| Calcium | 1200 mg | 1200 mg |
| Phosphorus | 1200 mg | 1200 mg |
| Magnesium | 320 mg | 280 mg |
| Iron | 30 mg | 15 mg |
| Zinc | 15 mg | 12 mg |
| Iodine | 175 mcg | 150 mcg |
| Selenium | 65 mcg | 55 mcg |

\*Requirement for females age 19–24.

| Maternal Structure | Increase in Weight Gain |
|---|---|
| Fetus, placenta, and amniotic fluid | 11 pounds |
| Uterus | 2 pounds |
| Increased blood volume | 4 pounds |
| Breast tissue | 3 pounds |
| Maternal stores | 5 to 10 pounds |

**Table 5-7**

**Maternal Weight Gain Distribution**

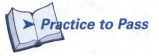

**Practice to Pass**

The client, who has a full-time job outside the home and is the mother of a 2-year-old and a 4-year-old, is 24 weeks gestation. The woman seems very tired and reports little help at home from her husband. The client states, "If things continue like this, I just don't know what I'm going to do!" How should the nurse respond?

3. Appropriate pregnancy weight gain averages 25 to 35 pounds for women with a normal pre-pregnant weight

   a. 10 to 13 pounds in the first 20 weeks

   b. About 1 pound per week after the 20th week

4. Maternal weight gain is distributed to a variety of structures (see Table 5-7)

**VI. Psychosocial Changes of Pregnancy**

A. **Role changes:** occur as decisions are made concerning whether or not the mother will continue or return to work and who will meet household responsibilities

B. **Anxieties:** related to the birthing process, well-being of the mother and baby, and finances

C. **Family strengths in coping with the psychosocial changes of pregnancy:** communication skills, ability to resolve conflict and reach compromise, and willingness to seek and utilize support systems

D. **Priority nursing diagnosis:** Potential interrupted family processes

E. **Planning and implementation**

   1. Discuss with client the psychosocial processes that occur during pregnancy such as role changes, anxieties related to well-being of mother and infant, and additional financial responsibilities

   2. Explore family coping mechanisms, communication skills, and support systems

**Case Study**

The client, who is a primigravida in her second trimester, has come in for a scheduled prenatal visit. When the nurse asks how things are going, the client replies, "Not very well. It seems like I'm just falling apart. I have heartburn after I eat, my ankles swell, I'm constipated all the time, and I think I may be getting hemorrhoids."

❶ What questions should the nurse ask the client regarding the problems described?

❷ What objective data should the nurse collect regarding the problems described?

❸ What nursing diagnoses are appropriate for this client?

❹ What teaching is needed in this situation?

❺ How should the nurse follow-up with this client?

*For suggested responses, see page 338.*

# Posttest

**1** The nurse has given the client information on maternal serum alpha-fetoprotein screening. Which of the following statements by the mother would indicate that she understood the information?

(1) "If this test is negative, it means that my baby doesn't have any birth defects."
(2) "It is best if this test is done before I reach 12 weeks gestation."
(3) "If the level of alpha-fetoprotein is elevated, it could indicate a problem with the baby's spinal cord."
(4) "If my alpha-fetoprotein level is below normal, I won't need any further testing."

**2** Which of the following would be the best indicator of normal fetal growth?

(1) Maternal weight gain 7 pounds at 22 weeks gestation.
(2) Fundal height 22 centimeters at 25 weeks gestation.
(3) Maternal waist circumference 41 inches at 36 weeks gestation.
(4) Maternal intake 1,500 calories per day.

**3** The nurse is planning an educational program for a client who is in her third trimester of pregnancy. Which of the following childbirth education topics would be most appropriate?

(1) Childbirth healthcare provider selection
(2) Morning sickness management
(3) Nutritional needs during pregnancy
(4) Pain relief during labor and delivery

**4** Following confirmation of pregnancy, the client has come into the clinic for her first prenatal visit. The client reports having a 5-year-old child who was born at 40 weeks gestation, a set of 3-year-old triplets who were born at 34 weeks gestation, and a first trimester abortion when she was in college. On the client's medical record, the nurse would make which of the following entries?

(1) gravida 4, para 1114
(2) gravida 3, para 1314
(3) gravida 4, para 4014
(4) gravida 3, para 3112

**5** The client has come to the clinic because she suspects that she is pregnant. Which of the following would be the most definitive way to confirm the diagnosis?

(1) Client's report of amenorrhea for 3 months
(2) Positive Hegar's sign
(3) Pigmentation changes of the breasts
(4) Palpation of fetal movement by the care provider

**6** The client, who is 34 weeks gestation, says to the nurse, "I had hoped to use the Lamaze method when my baby is born, but my husband doesn't want to . . . so I guess I'll just have an epidural." The best response by the nurse would be:

(1) "Oh, don't worry, your husband will probably change his mind when delivery time gets closer."
(2) "Well, that prepared childbirth stuff is really overrated if you ask me."
(3) "Have you and your husband discussed what he thinks his role would be in being your coach in childbirth?"
(4) "Why don't you just ask your mother or someone else to be your support person?"

**7** The client is concerned about facial chloasma that has developed since her last prenatal visit. The best response by the nurse is:

(1) "You should apply a facial skin bleach twice a day."
(2) "Avoiding sun exposure may keep the pigmentation from getting any darker."
(3) "This is a permanent condition caused by hormonal changes. You may be able to cover it with makeup."
(4) "This is a condition associated with the development of skin cancer. I will make an appointment for you with a dermatologist."

8   The client, who is 32 weeks gestation, complains of severe heartburn, especially at night. Following instruction by the nurse, which of the following statements by the client indicates that she understands the best course of management?

(1) "I should eat small, frequent meals."
(2) "I should try to lay down and rest after eating."
(3) "I should avoid using antacids because medication can hurt the baby."
(4) "Heartburn is a common discomfort in pregnancy; there is really nothing to do about it."

9   The client, who is 8 weeks gestation, is experiencing frequent nausea and vomiting. Following instruction by the nurse, which of the following statements by the client demonstrates that she understands the best course of management?

(1) "I should plan to arise early so that I will have time to eat a full breakfast."
(2) "I should avoid carbonated beverages as they can cause gas."
(3) "I should eat crackers or toast before arising."
(4) "I should avoid eating more frequently than every 4 hours."

10   Which of the following statements would indicate acceptance of pregnancy?

(1) "I just can't seem to shake this feeling of hopelessness I've had since I found out I was pregnant."
(2) "I still can't believe I let my husband talk me into having unprotected sex. This baby is really not what I need right now."
(3) "I've thrown up every day for the last week, but I guess it will be worth it when I have that tiny baby in my arms."
(4) "This pregnancy is causing so many changes in my life, I'm just not sure I'm going to be able to deal with it."

*See page 119 for Answers and Rationales.*

## Answers and Rationales

### Pretest

1   **Answer: 1** *Rationale:* Maternal diabetes places both the mother and infant at risk during pregnancy.
*Cognitive Level:* Analysis
*Nursing Process:* Analysis; *Test Plan:* PHYS

2   **Answer: 4** *Rationale:* The risk for the mother and fetus increases as the pregnancy progresses. Therefore, clients are seen more frequently as pregnancy nears term. Visits every 4 weeks for low-risk clients are appropriate until 28 weeks of gestation.
*Cognitive Level:* Application
*Nursing Process:* Planning; *Test Plan:* HPM

3   **Answer: 3** *Rationale:* A positive at-home pregnancy test indicates the presence of growing trophoblastic tissue and not necessarily a uterine pregnancy.
*Cognitive Level:* Analysis
*Nursing Process:* Analysis; *Test Plan:* PHYS

4   **Answer: 2** *Rationale:* Using Nägele's Rule, the estimated date of birth is calculated by subtracting 3 months from the first day of the last menstrual period and then adding 7 days to that date.
*Cognitive Level:* Application
*Nursing Process:* Analysis; *Test Plan:* HPM

5   **Answer: 3** *Rationale:* Counting the current pregnancy, the client has been pregnant a total of 4 times for gravida 4. Para is the number of pregnancies that have reached viability, in this case 2.
*Cognitive Level:* Analysis
*Nursing Process:* Analysis; *Test Plan:* HPM

6   **Answer: 3** *Rationale:* The fluid leaking from her breasts is colostrum. It normally leaks from the breasts during the last trimester.
*Cognitive Level:* Application
*Nursing Process:* Implementation; *Test Plan:* PHYS

7   **Answer: 1** *Rationale:* Dizziness and blurred vision can be symptoms of pregnancy-induced hypertension, a complication which requires further assessment and medical management.
*Cognitive Level:* Application
*Nursing Process:* Evaluation; *Test Plan:* PHYS

8   **Answer: 3** *Rationale:* The client has expressed a realistic concern. The nurse needs to help her explore what support systems are available for her and her child.
*Cognitive Level:* Application
*Nursing Process:* Planning; *Test Plan:* PSYC

**9** **Answer: 2** *Rationale:* Topics should be timed to present information that the woman needs at that specific stage of pregnancy. The items identified in the other options can be covered later in the pregnancy.
*Cognitive Level:* Application
*Nursing Process:* Planning; *Test Plan:* HPM

**10** **Answer: 2** *Rationale:* For women of normal prepregnant weight, the recommended pattern of weight gain during pregnancy is 3 to 5 pounds during the first trimester and 1 pound per week thereafter. Nutritional counseling is an appropriate action for the nurse or the nurse should make a referral for the client to meet with the nutritionist. Salt intake during normal pregnancy should be moderate but not restricted.
*Cognitive Level:* Application
*Nursing Process:* Implementation; *Test Plan:* HPM

## Posttest

**1** **Answer: 3** *Rationale:* If the maternal level of alpha-fetoprotein is elevated, it could indicate that fetal alpha-fetoprotein from a fetal neural tube defect has leaked into the maternal serum. The test is most sensitive between 16 to 18 weeks gestation. It is not definitive enough to make a diagnosis and is best used as a screening tool.
*Cognitive Level:* Application
*Nursing Process:* Implementation; *Test Plan:* HPM

**2** **Answer: 2** *Rationale:* In singleton births with fetal growth within normal limits, fundal height in centimeters multiplied by 8 and divided by 7 should correlate with gestational age in weeks.
*Cognitive Level:* Analysis
*Nursing Process:* Evaluation; *Test Plan:* HPM

**3** **Answer: 4** *Rationale:* Childbirth education should be geared to the time in pregnancy. In the third trimester, the pregnant woman begins to focus on labor, delivery, and newborn care.
*Cognitive Level:* Analysis
*Nursing Process:* Planning; *Test Plan:* HPM

**4** **Answer: 1** *Rationale:* The first number, gravida, represents the total number of pregnancies including the current one. In this case that equals 4. Para is represented by using the TPAL system. T represents the number of term births, 1; P represents the number of preterm births, 1; A represents the number of therapeutic or spontaneous abortions, 1; and L represents the number of living children, 4. Multiple births do not affect the parity in the T, P, or A categories; they are counted in the L category.

*Cognitive Level:* Analysis
*Nursing Process:* Implementation; *Test Plan:* HPM

**5** **Answer: 4** *Rationale:* Palpation of fetal movement is considered to be a completely objective sign of pregnancy that cannot have any other cause. The other signs listed here could have another etiology.
*Cognitive Level:* Analysis
*Nursing Process:* Assessment; *Test Plan:* PHYS

**6** **Answer: 3** *Rationale:* The husband can take on a variety of roles during labor and delivery including coach, teammate, and observer. Exploring both partner's expectations may help to clarify reasons for the husband's hesitancy in participating in the birth. This could result in improved communication and family coping.
*Cognitive Level:* Application
*Nursing Process:* Implementation; *Test Plan:* PSYC

**7** **Answer: 2** *Rationale:* Increased pigmentation during pregnancy is a response to increased estrogen levels. It can be worsened by the sun, is harmless, and generally fades after the pregnancy ends.
*Cognitive Level:* Application
*Nursing Process:* Implementation; *Test Plan:* PHYS

**8** **Answer: 1** *Rationale:* Heartburn is usually caused by gastric reflux. Remaining in an upright position, not overeating, and using low-sodium antacids all help relieve the problem.
*Cognitive Level:* Application
*Nursing Process:* Evaluation; *Test Plan:* PHYS

**9** **Answer: 3** *Rationale:* Nausea and vomiting, probably related to hormonal changes, usually disappear by the 12th week of pregnancy. Small frequent meals, carbonated beverages, and crackers or toast sometimes relieve the symptoms.
*Cognitive Level:* Application
*Nursing Process:* Evaluation; *Test Plan:* PHYS

**10** **Answer: 3** *Rationale:* While some ambivalence is common during pregnancy, the client should also have some feelings of happiness, tolerance of physical discomforts, and a feeling that she can deal with the changes and problems related to the pregnancy.
*Cognitive Level:* Analysis
*Nursing Process:* Assessment; *Test Plan:* PSYC

# References

Bailey, C. (1998). Assessing health during pregnancy. In E. Youngkin & M. Davis (Eds.), *Women's health: A primary care clinical guide* (2nd ed.). Stamford, CT: Appleton & Lange, pp. 441–477.

Barry, D. (1999). The expectant family at risk: Second and third trimesters. In L. Sherwin, M. A. Scoloveno, & C. Weingarten, (Eds.), *Maternal nursing care of the childbearing family* (3rd ed.). Stamford, CT: Appleton & Lange, pp. 585–644.

Bungum, T. & Jackson, A. (2000). Exercise during pregnancy and type of delivery in nulliparae. *Journal of Obstetric, Gynecologic, and Neonatal Nursing 29*(3): 258–264.

Cannella, B. (1999). Community-based nursing during pregnancy. In L. Sherwin, M. A. Scoloveno & C. Weingarten (Eds.), *Maternal nursing care of the childbearing family* (3rd ed.). Stamford, CT: Appleton & Lange, pp. 647–659.

Corder-Mabe, J. (1998). Complications of pregnancy. In E. Youngkin & M. Davis (Eds.), *Women's health: A primary care clinical guide* (2nd ed.). Stamford, CT: Appleton & Lange, pp. 533–600.

Costello, M. (1999). Nutrition during childbearing. In L. Sherwin, M. A. Scoloveno & C. Weingarten (Eds.), *Maternal nursing care of the childbearing family* (3rd ed.). Stamford, CT: Appleton & Lange, pp. 379–404.

Dickason, E., Silverman, B., & Kaplan, J. (1998). *Maternal-infant nursing care* (3rd ed.). St. Louis: Mosby, Inc., pp. 184–273.

Doenges, M. & Moorhouse, M. (1999). *Maternal/newborn plans of care guidelines for individualizing care* (3rd ed.). Philadelphia: F. A. Davis Co., pp. 38–89.

Fuqua, M. (1998). Assessing fetal well-being. In E. Youngkin & M. Davis (Eds.), *Women's health: A primary care clinical guide* (2nd ed.). Stamford, CT: Appleton & Lange, pp. 601–638.

Gill, E. (2000). Nutrition for the childbearing years. *Journal of Obstetric, Gynecologic, and Neonatal Nursing 29*(1): 43–55.

House, J. (1999). Stopping neural tube defects. *Lifelines 3*(3): 10.

Ladewig, P., London, M., & Olds, S. (1998). *Maternal-newborn nursing care: The nurse, the family, and the community* (4th ed.). Menlo Park, CA: Addison Wesley, pp. 153–336.

Lowdermilk, D. (1999). Anatomy and physiology of pregnancy. In D. Lowdermilk, S. Perry, & I. Bobak (Eds.), *Maternity nursing* (5th ed.). St. Louis: Mosby, Inc., pp. 185–202.

Lowdermilk, D., Perry, S., & Bobak, I. (2000). *Maternity & women's health care*. St. Louis: Mosby, Inc., pp. 333–443.

Moore, M., (1999). Maternal and fetal nutrition. In D. Lowdermilk, S. Perry, & I. Bobak (Eds.), *Maternity nursing* (5th ed.). St. Louis: Mosby, Inc., pp. 258–272.

Menendez, A. M. (1998). Adaptation to pregnancy. In E. Dickason, B. Silverman, & J. Kaplan (Eds.), *Maternal-infant nursing care* (3rd ed.). St. Louis: Mosby, Inc., pp. 160–180.

Olds, S., London, M., & Ladewig, P. (2000). *Maternal newborn nursing: A family and community-based approach* (6th ed.). Upper Saddle River, NJ: Prentice Hall Health, pp. 217–287, 332.

Phelan, S. (1998). Preconception and antepartum care. In J. Mattox (Ed.), *Core textbook of obstetrics & gynecology*. St. Louis: Mosby, Inc., pp. 47–62.

Remich, M. (1998). Promoting a healthy pregnancy. In E. Youngkin & M. Davis (Eds.), *Women's health: A primary care clinical guide* (2nd ed.). Stamford, CT: Appleton & Lange, pp. 477–532.

Riordan, J. (1998). Predicting breast-feeding problems. *Lifelines 2*(6): 31–33.

Saunders, R. (1999). Nursing care during pregnancy. In D. Lowdermilk, S. Perry, & I. Bobak (Eds.), *Maternity nursing* (5th ed.). St. Louis: Mosby, Inc., pp. 206–252.

Sherwin, L., Scoloveno, M. A., & Weingarten, C. (1999). *Maternal nursing care of the childbearing family* (3rd ed.). Stamford, CT: Appleton & Lange, pp. 239, 407–582.

## CHAPTER 6

# Common Laboratory and Diagnostic Tests

Angela F. Wood, PhD, RN, C

## CHAPTER OUTLINE

*Laboratory and Diagnostic Testing during the First Prenatal Visit*

*Laboratory and Diagnostic Testing during Follow-up Prenatal Visits*

*Other Diagnostic Tests and Nursing Care Implications*

## OBJECTIVES

▍ Describe laboratory tests used to evaluate the status of the pregnant client.

▍ Describe diagnostic tests used to assess fetal well-being.

[ **Media Link** ]

*Use the CD-ROM enclosed with this text, or log onto the address given to access the free, interactive Companion Website created for this series. The CD-ROM and Companion Website accompanying this book offer additional practice opportunities and information—NCLEX Review, Case Studies, Glossary, In Depth with NCLEX, and more.*

**www.prenhall.com/hogan**

## REVIEW AT A GLANCE

**alpha-fetoprotein (AFP)** *a fetal antigen leaked into amniotic fluid and absorbed into the maternal circulation; measurement at 16 to 18 weeks is used as a screening tool for body wall defects, especially of the neural tube*

**amniocentesis** *a procedure for collection of amniotic fluid via a needle inserted through the maternal abdominal wall; used to assess fetal well-being and maturity*

**biophysical profile** *an assessment of fetal well-being that uses ultrasound to determine fetal breathing movements, body movements, muscle tone, heart rate reactivity, and amniotic fluid volume; based on the assessment findings, scores range from 0 to 10*

**chorionic villus sampling (CVS)** *collection of a specimen from the fetal side of the placenta, obtained transcervically or transabdominally and used for fetal genetic testing*

**contraction stress test (CST)** *an assessment of the ability of the fetus to withstand the stress of uterine contractions, which occur spontaneously or are artificially induced by oxytocin or nipple stimulation*

**Doppler blood flow analysis** *an assessment of fetal blood flow across the placenta;*

*noninvasive and useful for detection of intrauterine growth restriction*

**glucose tolerance test (GTT)** *a screening test for gestational diabetes at 24 to 28 weeks gestation; 50-g oral glucose is administered followed by venous plasma glucose assessment in one hour; results >140 mg/dL are abnormal and indicate the need for further testing*

**karyotype** *schematic arrangement of chromosomes used to assess chromosome number and morphology*

**lecithin to sphyngomyelin (L/S) ratio** *used to denote the ratio of lecithin to sphingomyelin in amniotic fluid and assess fetal lung maturity; a ratio of 2:1 or > indicates probable lung maturity*

**nonstress test (NST)** *an assessment of fetal well-being that analyzes the response of the fetal heart rate to fetal movement*

**oral glucose tolerance test (OGTT)** *diagnostic test for gestational diabetes and indicated following an abnormal GTT; glucose levels are assessed at 1, 2, and 3 hours following a 3-day high-carbohydrate diet, 8-hour fast, fasting glucose assessment and administration of 100 g of oral glucose*

**phosphatidylglycerol (PG)** *a phospholipid found in pulmonary surfactant; evidence of it in amniotic fluid is an indicator of fetal lung maturity*

**sexually transmitted infections (STIs)** *a group of infections that are spread by sexual contact including human papillomavirus (HPV), human immunodeficiency virus (HIV), group B streptococcus (GBS), syphilis, gonorrhea, and chlamydia; also called sexually transmitted or venereal diseases*

**TORCH infections** *a group of infections caused by viruses or protozoa that cause serious fetal problems when contracted by the mother during pregnancy including toxoplasmosis (T), other infections such as hepatitis (O), rubella (R), cytomegalovirus (C), and herpes simplex virus (H)*

**triple-screen test** *a screening test for Down syndrome (trisomy 21), trisomy 18, and neural tube defects that measures maternal alpha-fetoprotein, human chorionic gonadotropin, and unconjugated estriol*

**ultrasound** *use of high-frequency sound waves for the identification of maternal and fetal tissues, bones, and fluids*

## *Pretest*

**1** The client, a 42-year-old pregnant woman, is 6 weeks pregnant and has requested genetic testing. During your counseling session, the client asks the nurse what the advantages of chorionic villus sampling (CVS) are over amniocentesis. The nurse's best response is:

(1) "CVS can be done earlier in your pregnancy, and the results are available more quickly."
(2) "CVS is a safer procedure for you and the baby."
(3) "CVS provides more information than amniocentesis."
(4) "You will need anesthesia for amniocentesis, but not for CVS."

**2** The client, who is 1 week past her due date, is to have a nonstress test. After explaning the test, which of the following statements by the client would indicate a need for further teaching?

(1) "I understand that you will start an IV containing medicine to cause me to have contractions."
(2) "During the test I will need to push a button when I feel the baby move."
(3) "I won't need to be admitted to the hospital for this test."
(4) "The test should take 20–30 minutes."

**3** The client, who is in her first trimester, is scheduled for an abdominal ultrasound. When explaining the reason for early pregnancy ultrasound, the nurse should tell the client which of the following?

(1) "The test will help to determine if your baby is in a good position for delivery."
(2) "The test will help to determine how many weeks you have been pregnant."
(3) "The test will help to determine if your baby has intrauterine growth restriction."
(4) "The test will help to determine if you have enough amniotic fluid."

**4** The gravid client is to be screened for gestational diabetes with a 50-g oral glucose load. At what point in the pregnancy should the nurse advise the client to schedule this test?

(1) 12 weeks gestation
(2) 16 weeks gestation
(3) 24 weeks gestation
(4) 36 weeks gestation

**5** The nurse is reviewing results from the client's initial prenatal visit and notes that the urine contained an increased number of white blood cells, nitrites, and greater than 10,000 bacteria/mL of urine. These findings lead the nurse to suspect which of the following?

(1) Renal failure
(2) Contamination of the urine with amniotic fluid
(3) Urinary tract infection
(4) Nothing unusual, this is a normal finding in pregnancy

**6** The client is considering having maternal alpha-fetoprotein (AFP) screening. She asks the nurse how a test on her blood can indicate a fetal birth defect. The best reply by the nurse is:

(1) "We aren't sure why this test works, but it does."
(2) "Neural tube defects are passed in genetic material so it is possible to know if it was passed to your baby by examining the amount of alpha-fetoprotein in your DNA."
(3) "When babies have a neural tube defect, some of their alpha-fetoprotein leaks out and is absorbed into your blood which causes your level to rise. This test detects that rise."
(4) "When a fetus has a neural tube defect, not enough alpha-fetoprotein is produced so some of your alpha-fetoprotein moves across the placenta into the baby's circulation. This makes your level decrease, and that is reflected in the level we measure in your blood."

**7** The client's test for syphilis has come back positive. In talking with the woman about how the infection is spread, the client should be taught that syphilis can be contracted through:

(1) Shaking hands, kissing, and oral-genital sexual contact.
(2) Kissing, oral-genital or genital-genital sexual contact, and biting.
(3) Exposure to contaminated toilet seats and oral-genital sexual contact.
(4) Only oral-genital sexual contact.

**8** In explaining to the client who has come in for her initial prenatal exam why it is important to test pregnant women for gonorrhea, the nurse should tell the client that gonorrhea can cause neonatal:

(1) Vaginal discharge.
(2) Eye infections.
(3) Liver damage.
(4) Congenital anomalies.

**9** Which of the following signs or symptoms would indicate a need for colposcopy and biopsy for human papillomavirus?

(1) Rash on the palms of the hands and soles of the feet
(2) Chancre sore noted on the vulva
(3) A crusted ulcer inside the vagina
(4) 2 to 3 mm soft, papillary swellings either singly or in clusters noted on the genitalia

**10** The client has come in for her initial prenatal visit. When the testing that will be done at this visit is explained, the client asks why it all has to be done today. The nurse's best response is:

(1) "We do it all on the first visit in case the patient does not come back."
(2) "Insurance won't pay for testing unless it is done in the first trimester."
(3) "It is best to find any current problems so that they can be treated as early as possible."
(4) "You don't need to worry about what we're doing, your doctor knows what is best for you and your baby."

*See page 139 for Answers and Rationales.*

**I. Laboratory and Diagnostic Testing during the First Prenatal Visit:** testing done at the initial visit can be analyzed for abnormal results; intervention can be implemented as soon as possible or at follow-up visits, as indicated

    **A. Complete blood count (CBC):** a series of tests done on peripheral blood that provide information on the hematologic system as well as other body systems; advantages of the CBC include that it is inexpensive, easy to perform, and the results are quickly available; for individual tests, their purpose, normal results, and changes in pregnancy see Table 6-1

        **1.** Test procedure: after explaining the procedure to the client, obtain 5 to 7 mL of blood in a lavender-top tube; mix well but avoid hemolysis

        **2.** Interfering factors

            **a.** Changes in fluid balance

            **b.** Living at a high altitude

            **c.** Drugs including antibiotics, methyldopa, hydantoins, antineoplastic drugs, aspirin, and quinidine

            **d.** Abnormalities in RBC size

            **e.** Strenuous exercise may affect platelet levels

**Table 6-1**    **Complete Blood Count**

| Test | Purpose | Normal Results | Changes in Pregnancy |
|---|---|---|---|
| RBC Count | A count of the number of circulating RBCs in 1 mm$^3$ of peripheral venous blood; can be used to evaluate the client for anemia | 4.2–5.4 million/mm$^3$ | 5–6.25 million/mm$^3$ |
| Hemoglobin | A measure of the total amount of hemoglobin in the peripheral blood and indicates the oxygen-carrying capacity of the blood | 12–16 g/dL | >11g/dL |
| Hematocrit | A percentage of the total blood volume that is comprised of RBCs | 37–47% | >33% |
| Mean Corpuscular Volume | A measure of the average volume of a single RBC; used to classify types of anemia | 80–95/cubic micrometer | none |
| Mean Corpuscular Hemoglobin | A measure of the average amount of hemoglobin within a single RBC | 27–31/picogram | none |
| Mean Corpuscular Hemoglobin Concentration | A measure of the average concentration or percentage of hemoglobin within a single RBC | 32–36 g/dL packed RBCs | none |
| WBC Count | A measure of the total number of white blood cells in mm$^3$ of peripheral venous blood; can be used as an indicator of the client's ability to fight infection and react against foreign bodies or tissues | 5,000–10,000/mm$^3$ | 5,000–15,000/mm$^3$ |
| Polymorphonuclear Cells | Sometimes called granulocytes, an increase in these cells can indicate an acute infection, parasitic infestation, or allergic response | 55–70% of WBCs | 60–85% of WBCs |
| Lymphocytes | Sometimes called agranulocytes, an increase can indicate chronic bacterial infection or acute viral infection | 20–40% of WBCs | 15–40% of WBCs |
| Platelet Count | A measure of the number of platelets/mm$^3$ of blood; platelets are essential to blood clotting | 150,000–400,000/mm$^3$ | none until 3–5 days after delivery |

**B. Blood group and Rh typing**

1. Purpose: to determine the client's blood group and Rh status so that the fetus at risk for developing erythroblastosis fetalis or hyperbilirubinemia in the neonatal period may be identified

2. Test procedure: after explaining the procedure to the client, collect 7 to 14 mL of venous blood in red-top tube; avoid hemolysis

3. Interfering factors: none

4. Significant results: Mothers who are type O or Rh negative may require further fetal or infant testing

**C. *TORCH:*** a group of infections caused by viruses and protozoa that cause serious fetal problems when contracted by the mother during pregnancy; each letter represents a different infection including Toxoplasmosis, Other infections (usually hepatitis), Rubella, Cytomegalovirus, and Herpes simplex virus

1. Toxoplasmosis

   a. Cause: Infection with the toxoplasmosis protozoan

   b. Transmission: development of the infection in the mother is associated with consumption of infested undercooked meat and poor hand-washing after handling cat litter; fetal infection occurs if the mother acquires toxoplasmosis after conception and passes it to the fetus via the placenta

   c. Diagnosis: because of the difficulty of growing toxoplasmosis cultures diagnosis is made by serologic testing; the indirect fluorescent antibody test is most commonly used; IgG titers greater than 1:256 suggest a recent infection, whereas IgM titers greater than 1:256 indicate an acute infection

   d. Maternal effects: flu-like symptoms in acute phase

   e. Fetal/neonatal effects: miscarriage is likely in early pregnancy; in neonates central nervous system lesions can result in hydrocephaly, microcephaly, chronic retinitis, and seizures

   f. Test procedure: after explaining the procedure to the client, collect 5 mL of venous blood in a red-top tube; indicate on the lab slip if the client is pregnant or has been exposed to cats

2. Other infections, usually hepatitis virus

   a. Cause: Infection with the hepatitis A (HAV) or B (HBV) virus; hepatitis B is the most common in the fetus

   b. Transmission: HAV is spread by droplets or hands and is associated with poor hand-washing after defecation; transmission to the fetus is rare but can occur; hepatitis B can be transmitted to the fetus via the placenta, but transmission usually occurs when the infant is exposed to blood and genital secretions during labor and delivery

   c. Diagnosis: radioimmunoassay and enzyme-linked immunosorbent assay methods are used to detect HAV antibodies; elevated IgM antibody in the absence of IgG antibody indicates probable acute hepatitis; elevated IgG in the absence of IgM indicates a convalescent or chronic stage of HAV; hepatitis B is detected through the hepatitis B surface antigen (HbsAg)

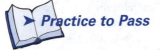

**Practice to Pass**

During the initial interview with the client, the woman tells the nurse that her mother had "that problem with her blood that causes the baby to turn yellow." The client wants to know if she will also have that problem. How should the nurse respond?

  **d.** Maternal effects: fever, malaise, nausea, and abdominal discomfort; may be associated with liver failure

  **e.** Fetal/neonatal effects: preterm birth, hepatitis infection, and intrauterine fetal death

  **f.** Test procedure: after explaining the procedure to the client, collect 5 to 7 mL of venous blood in a red-top tube; handle the blood as though it were capable of transmitting the virus

 **3.** Rubella, sometimes called German measles or 3-day measles

  **a.** Cause: infection with the rubella virus

  **b.** Transmission: the infection is spread by droplet

  **c.** Diagnosis: IgG antibodies to rubella are measured to determine the client's rubella immunity status; a titer of 1:10 or greater indicates that the woman is immune to rubella; a titer of 1:8 or less indicates minimal or no immunity

  **d.** Maternal effects: fever, rash, and mild lymphedema

  **e.** Fetal/neonatal effects: miscarriage, congenital anomalies, and death

  **f.** Test procedure: after explaining the procedure to the client, collect 7 mL of venous blood in a red-top tube

 **4.** Cytomegalovirus (CMV)

  **a.** Cause: exposure to the cytomegalovirus

  **b.** Transmission: cytomegalovirus can be transmitted through respiratory droplet, semen, cervical and vaginal secretions, breast milk, placental tissue, urine, feces, and banked blood; the most common mode of transmission is respiratory droplet; workers in daycare centers, institutions for the mentally retarded, and health settings are especially at risk

  **c.** Diagnosis: a viral culture is the most definitive diagnostic tool; CMV antibodies indicate a recent infection; a fourfold increase in CMV titer in paired sera drawn 10 to 14 days apart is usually indicative of an acute infection

  **d.** Maternal effects: asymptomatic illness, cervical discharge, and mononucleosis-like syndrome

  **e.** Fetal/neonatal effects: fetal death or severe generalized disease with hemolytic anemia and jaundice, hydrocephaly or microcephaly, pneumonitis, hepatosplenomegaly, and deafness

  **f.** Test procedure: After explaining the procedure to the client, a swab specimen is collected from the urine, sputum or mouth for a viral culture; the culture requires 3 to 7 days; if an antibody or antigen titer is desired, collect 4 to 7 mL of venous blood in a red- or gold-top tube; in the client with suspected active CMV, a specimen is collected as soon as possible and repeated in 2 to 4 weeks

 **5.** Herpes simplex virus (HSV)

  **a.** Cause: exposure to the herpes simplex virus

  **b.** Transmission: HSV type II is a sexually transmitted disease transmitted by exposure to vesicular lesions on the penis, scrotum, vulva, perineum,

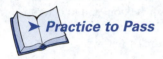

perianal region, vagina, or cervix; the infant is usually infected during exposure to a lesion in the birth canal; the infant is most at risk during a primary infection in the mother

   c. Diagnosis: viral culture is used for definitive diagnosis; serologic tests have a lower accuracy

   d. Maternal effects: blisters, rash, fever, malaise, nausea, and headache

   e. Fetal/neonatal effects: miscarriage, preterm labor, or stillbirth; transplacental infection is rare but can cause skin lesions, intrauterine growth restriction, mental retardation, and microcephaly

   f. Test procedure: after explaining the test to the client, the client is placed in the lithotomy position and the cervix is visualized; a cotton-tipped swab is used to obtain a specimen from the endocervical canal; swab specimens may also be obtained from visible lesions

   g. Significant results: vaginal delivery is recommended if the client has no visible lesions or prodromal symptoms; if visible lesions or prodromal symptoms are present, cesarean delivery is indicated

**D.** *Sexually transmitted infections (STIs):* sometimes called sexually transmitted diseases or venereal diseases; STIs are caused by bacteria, viruses, protozoa, or ectoparasites, and include human papillomavirus (HPV), human immunodeficiency virus (HIV), group B streptococcus (GBS), syphilis, gonorrhea, and chlamydia; all sexual partners of clients with STIs should be contacted and treated, as indicated

   **1.** Human papillomavirus (HPV)

   a. Cause/transmission: sometimes called genital or venereal warts, HPV infection is caused by spread of the human papillomavirus through sexual contact; neonates can acquire the infection during birth

   b. Diagnosis: by direct visualization of the warts and confirmed by biopsy

   c. Maternal effects: symptoms depend on the viral strain causing the infection but can include genital lesions, chronic vaginal discharge, pruritis, and cervical dysplasia; some strains are asymptomatic

   d. Fetal/neonatal effects: juvenile laryngeal papillomata

   e. Test procedure: after explaining the test to the client, colposcopy and direct visualization of the warts, sometimes with biopsy, is completed; vinegar solution may be used to highlight early or flat cervical lesions

   **2.** Human immunodeficiency virus (HIV)

   a. Cause/transmission: transmission of the HIV retrovirus is primarily through exchange of body fluids including semen, blood, or vaginal secretions; in women, now the fastest-growing population of people with HIV, the infection is most commonly spread through heterosexual contact; neonatal transmission can occur transplacentally and is less likely if the mother receives treatment during pregnancy; transmission can also occur by contact at the time of delivery or through breast-milk

   b. Diagnosis: made with a reactive enzyme immunoassay (EIA) and a positive Western blot or immunofluorescence assay; the p24 antigen capture assay can be used as early as 2 to 6 weeks after infection and is used to diagnose neonatal HIV infection, to detect HIV before seroconversion, and to determine the progression of AIDS; viral cultures provide the best diagnostic tool for neonates; however, it is expensive and requires 4 to 6 weeks for results

c. Maternal effects: opportunistic diseases including *Pneumocystis carinii* pneumonia, candida esophagitis and wasting syndrome; HSV and CMV infections are also common; fever, headache, night sweats, malaise, generalized lymphadenopathy, myalgias, nausea, diarrhea, weight loss, sore throat, and rash are associated with seroconversion

d. Fetal/neonatal effects: asymptomatic at birth followed by opportunistic infections, immunodeficiency, failure to thrive, parotitis, lymphadenopathy, hepatosplenomegaly, fever, chronic diarrhea, dermatitis, thrush, and death

e. Test procedure: after explaining the test to the client, an informed consent must be obtained; 7 mL of peripheral venous blood is collected in a red-top tube; clients may remain anonymous through the use of number identification

3. Group B streptococcus (GBS)

a. Cause/transmission: considered normal vaginal flora, it is found in 10 to 30 percent of healthy pregnant women; it is transmitted vertically from the birth canal of the infected mother to the fetus

b. Diagnosis: current recommendations are to screen all women at 36 to 37 weeks gestation with a GBS culture

c. Maternal effects: preterm labor, chorioamnionitis, premature rupture of membranes, urinary tract infections and postpartum infections

d. Fetal/neonatal effects: neonatal meningitis, sepsis, and septic shock; early onset GBS has a significant infant mortality rate

e. Test procedure: after explaining the need for the test to the client, collect GBS cultures from the anorectal and vaginal areas, not the cervix

4. Syphilis

a. Cause/transmission: caused by the *Treponema pallidum,* syphilis is a motile spirochete transmitted through microscopic abrasions in the subcutaneous tissue; it can be transmitted through kissing, biting, or oral-genital sex; transmission to the fetus can occur via the placenta at any time during the pregnancy

b. Diagnosis: can be made by microscopic examination of primary and secondary lesion tissue; serology is used for diagnosis during latency and late infection; women should be screened at the first prenatal visit and possibly again late in the third trimester; screening is done with the VDRL (Venereal Disease Research Laboratories) or the RPR (rapid plasma reagin) test; both tests detect antibodies directed against the *Treponema* organism; if the VDRL or RPR test is positive, the diagnosis is confirmed with a flourescent treponemal antibody absorption test (FTA-ABS)

c. Maternal effects: during the acute stage, a chancre develops on the skin near the infection; the second stage is marked by lymphadenopathy and a

**Practice to Pass**

The client, who has come to the clinic for her first prenatal visit, asks you why she needs to be tested for HIV when only homosexual men are at risk for contracting the infection. How should you respond to the client?

**NCLEX!**

rash located on the palms of the hands and soles of the feet; the third or latent stage, which can last up to 5 years, is asymptomatic; the disease can progress to a tertiary stage that involves central nervous system, cardiovascular, and ocular signs and symptoms; infection can cause miscarriage or premature labor

    **d.** Fetal/neonatal effects: include central nervous system damage, hearing loss, or death

    **e.** Test procedure: after explaining the test to the client, collect 7 mL of venous blood in a red-top tube

  **5.** Gonorrhea

    **a.** Cause/transmission: caused by *Neisseria gonorrhoeae,* an aerobic, gram-negative diplococci bacteria, gonorrhea is transmitted by all types of sexual activity; neonates can acquire the infection by exposure to the bacteria in the birth canal

    **b.** Diagnosis: all pregnant women should be screened at their initial prenatal visit and at-risk women should be screened again at 36 weeks gestation; a Thayer-Martin culture of the endocervix, rectum, or pharynx are completed for diagnosis

    **c.** Maternal effects: sometimes asymptomatic but can cause purulent endocervical discharge, menstrual irregularities, pelvic or lower abdominal pain, and premature rupture of membranes

    **d.** Fetal/neonatal effects: preterm birth, neonatal sepsis, intrauterine growth restriction and ophthalmia neonatorum, which can cause blindness

    **e.** Test procedure: after explaining the procedure to the client, the cervix is cleaned of mucus and a swab specimen is collected from the endocervical canal; the rectum or pharynx may also be swabbed for culture; results may be affected by douching within 24 hours of specimen collection; contamination of the specimen with fecal material, lubricants, disinfectants, or menstrual blood can also affect results

  **6.** Chlamydia

    **a.** Cause/transmission: the *Chlamydia trachomatis* bacteria is spread through sexual contact; the CDC recommends screening of asymptomatic, high-risk women

    **b.** Diagnosis: cultures for chlamydia are expensive, require special transport and storage, and take up to 10 days

    **c.** Maternal effects: although usually asymptomatic, the infection can cause bleeding, mucoid or purulent cervical discharge, pelvic inflammatory disease, or dysuria

    **d.** Fetal/neonatal effects: conjunctivitis, pneumonia, and ophthalmia neonatorum

    **e.** Test procedure: after explaining the test to the client, the cervix is swabbed to remove mucus from the cervical os, and a scraping of endocervical cells is collected; special culture media and proper handling of specimens are important

**E. Urinalysis**

1. Findings

   a. The pH may be decreased with poor glucose metabolism and ketone acids in the urine

   b. Specific gravity may be increased with dehydration caused by excessive vomiting as seen in hyperemesis gravidarium

   c. Color should be pale yellow to amber depending on foods ingested and concentration

   d. Glucose reabsorption is impaired in pregnancy resulting in spilling of glucose in the urine at a blood glucose level of 160 mg/dL

   e. Protein may normally be found in the urine during pregnancy at a level of trace to +1 using the dipstick method; increased protein may indicate pregnancy induced hypertension

   f. WBCs or nitrites can indicate a possible urinary tract infection which can place the client at risk for preterm labor

   g. Casts, which are formed from clumps of materials or cells in the renal distal and collecting tubules, form when the urine is acidic and concentrated; they can be associated with proteinuria and stasis in the renal tubules

   h. Ketones may indicate diabetes and hyperglycemia

   i. Urine culture should be done to identify women with asyptomatic bacteriuria; greater than 10,000 bacteria/mL urine is indicative of a urinary tract infection

   j. Urine toxicology can be used to screen for illicit drug use

2. Test procedure: after explaining the test to the client, collect a fresh urine specimen in a urine container; if a culture is to be done, a midstream, clean-catch specimen is collected

## II. Laboratory and Diagnostic Testing during Follow-up Prenatal Visits

A. **Clean-catch urine specimen:** collected at each visit to assess for glucose, protein, nitrites, and leukocytes, which can indicate diabetes, pregnancy-induced hypertension, or infection

B. **Hemoglobin:** assessed monthly to monitor for iron-deficiency anemia

C. *Glucose tolerance test (GTT):* used to screen pregnant clients for gestational diabetes; it is a standard part of prenatal care for all clients and is generally completed between 24 and 28 weeks gestation

   1. Test procedure: after the test is explained to the client, a 50-g oral glucose load is administered; the time of day or time since the last meal is not a factor; the venous plasma glucose is assessed 1 hour after the glucose load

   2. Findings: a level greater than 140 mg/dL is considered abnormal; abnormal results indicate a need for further testing

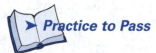

**▶ Practice to Pass**

On her third prenatal visit, the client asks why a urine sample is needed at every visit. What should you tell her?

| Table 6-2 | Time | Abnormal Result |
|---|---|---|
| **Abnormal Oral Glucose Tolerance Test Results** | Fasting | greater than 105 mg/dL |
| | 1 hour | greater than 190 mg/dL |
| | 2 hour | greater than 165 mg/dL |
| | 3 hour | greater than 145 mg/dL |

3. Follow-up: Clients with abnormal GTT results should be assessed with a 3-hour, 100-g **oral glucose tolerance test (OGTT)** used to diagnose gestational diabetes

   a. Test procedure: the client is told to eat a high-carbohydrate diet for 3 days before the test; then, on the day of the test, the woman fasts for 8 hours (overnight) and a fasting serum glucose is obtained; following the fast, 100 g of oral glucose is administered and glucose levels are assessed at 1, 2, and 3 hours

   b. Findings: Gestational diabetes is diagnosed if two or more results are abnormal (see Table 6-2); the results are borderline if one value is abnormal; with borderline results, the OGTT is repeated in 1 month

D. *Alpha-fetoprotein (AFP):* during pregnancy, alpha-fetoprotein leaks from the fetus's body into the amniotic fluid and is absorbed by the mother; peak levels of alpha-fetoprotein are found in maternal serum at around 16 weeks; measurement of alpha-fetoprotein in maternal serum at 16 to 18 weeks is done as a screening test for fetal body wall defects; the **triple-screen test,** an improved screening test for Down syndrome (trisomy 21), trisomy 18, and neural tube defects, includes AFP, human chorionic gonadotropin (hCG), and unconjugated estriol (UE3)

1. Findings: increased maternal serum AFP levels may indicate neural tube defects or other body wall defects, threatened abortion, fetal distress, or death; decreased maternal levels of AFP may indicate trisomy 21 (Down syndrome) or fetal wastage

2. Interfering factors include multiple pregnancy and incorrect estimation of gestational age

3. Test procedure: after explaining the procedure to the client, collect 7 to 10 mL of venous blood in a red-top tube; the gestational age should be indicated on the laboratory slip

4. Follow-up: abnormal levels of AFP may indicate a need for a triple-screen test, ultrasound, or assessment of AFP levels in amniotic fluid

## III. Other Diagnostic Tests

A. *Ultrasound:* sound waves having a frequency higher than 20,000 Hz; can be used to produce a three-dimensional view and pictorial image to identify maternal and fetal tissues, bones, and fluids

1. Transvaginal ultrasound

   a. Purpose: Used primarily during the first trimester to evaluate pelvic anatomy, assess the developing embryo/fetus for number and size, locate the placenta, diagnose intrauterine pregnancy, screen for fetal and placental anomalies, and establish gestational age

    **b.** Advantages: eliminates the need for a full bladder and clearer images in obese clients as the sound waves do not pass through thick abdominal layers

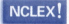

    **c.** Disadvantages: some clients are embarrassed or uncomfortable with vaginal insertion of the probe; vaginal ultrasound is contraindicated in clients with latex allergies as the probe is covered with a latex condom-like sac

    **d.** Test procedure: After explaining the procedure to the client, an informed consent is obtained as the probe is inserted into the body; the client is placed in a supine position and the vaginal probe is inserted; allowing the client to insert the probe herself may promote comfort and decrease embarrassment; fetal structures should be pointed out to the mother during the procedure

**2.** Abdominal ultrasound

    **a.** Purpose: to obtain information on fetal viability; number, position, gestational age, growth pattern, and anomalies; amniotic fluid volume; placental location and maturity; and assessment of fetal well-being

    **b.** Advantages: ultrasound provides a safe, noninvasive fetal assessment; in situations where there is a problem, it allows early diagnosis of many fetal problems allowing the family choices regarding intrauterine surgery or other therapies, termination of pregnancy, or preparation for the birth of an infant with a problem

    **c.** Disadvantages: the procedure is best done when the client's bladder is full; this can result in discomfort

    **d.** Test procedure: clients are instructed to come for the test with a full bladder; the test is explained and transmission gel is applied to the abdomen; the transducer is moved over the abdomen to produce the image; after the examination is completed, the client's abdomen should be cleaned of transmission gel and provisions should be made for her to empty her bladder

**3.** Findings

    **a.** Viability is determined by assessment of fetal heart activity; this is possible at 6 to 7 weeks gestation with real-time echo scan; fetal death can be determined by absence of heart activity as well as scalp edema and maceration

    **b.** Gestational age can best be established during the first 20 weeks gestation as fetal growth rate is fairly consistent during this time; body part to be assessed is based on development; measurement of the gestational sac is done in pregnancies that are about 8 weeks gestation, and the crown-rump measurement is done on fetuses that are 7 to 14 weeks gestation; in the fetus greater than 12 weeks gestation, the biparietal diameter (BPD) and femur length are measured

    **c.** Fetal growth is assessed by serial measurements of BPD and femur length; this information can assist the healthcare provider in distinguishing between intrauterine growth restriction and inaccuracy in dating of the pregnancy

    **d.** **Biophysical profile** is a method of assessing fetal well-being by determining scores on five criteria including fetal breathing movements, body movements, muscle tone, heart rate activity, and amniotic fluid volume; the total score ranges from 0 to 10; if the findings for a criterion are normal, a score of two is given; if the findings are abnormal, a score of zero is given; a total score of 8 to 10 is considered normal, a score of 4 to 6 is interpreted

| Table 6-3 | Biophysical Profile Scoring | |
|---|---|---|
| **Assessment Variable** | **Normal Findings = score of 2** | **Abnormal Findings = score of 0** |
| Fetal breathing movements | At least one episode of breathing movement lasting at least 60 seconds in a 30 minute assessment period | Absence of a 60-second breathing episode during a 30-minute assessment period |
| Fetal body movements | At least three episodes of fetal movement in a 30-minute assessment period | Two or fewer episodes of fetal movement in a 30-minute assessment period |
| Fetal muscle tone | At least one episode of extension and return to flexion during the assessment period | Slow extension with return to only partial flexion during the assessment period |
| Fetal heart rate reactivity | Two or more movement-associated heart rate increases of at least 15 beats per minute above baseline and 15 seconds in duration in a 20-minute assessment period | Fewer than two movement-associated heart rate increases of at least 15 beats per minute above baseline and 15 seconds in duration in a 20-minute assessment period |
| Amniotic fluid volume | At least one pocket of amniotic fluid measuring 1 cm in two perpendicular planes | Either fluid is absent in most areas of the uterine cavity or the largest pocket measures 1 cm or less in the vertical axis |

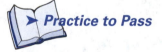

**Practice to Pass**

The client has just had a reactive nonstress test and asks you if this means that her baby will be able to tolerate labor. How will you respond?

as possibly abnormal and a score of less than 4 may indicate a need for delivery; scoring is described in greater detail in Table 6-3

e. **Doppler blood flow analysis** is a noninvasive assessment of fetal blood flow across the placenta; it provides information concerning blood flow and resistance in placental circulation and is useful in detecting intrauterine growth restriction; this assessment can be done as early as 15 weeks; the velocity waveforms from the umbilical and uterine arteries are reported as systolic/diastolic (S/D) ratios; persistently elevated ratios of greater than 3 after 30 weeks gestation are considered abnormal and have been associated with intrauterine growth restriction

B. **Stress and nonstress tests**

1. **Nonstress test (NST)** is an assessment of fetal well-being that analyzes the response of the fetal heart to fetal movement

   a. Advantages: noninvasive, easily interpreted, and can be performed in an outpatient setting at a low cost; the NST is a good indicator of fetal well-being

   b. Disadvantages: a high number of false positive results caused by fetal sleep cycles, medications, and fetal immaturity; the NST is not a good predictor of poor fetal outcomes

   c. Test procedure: the client is placed in a semi-Fowler's position and an ultrasound transducer and tocodynamometer are used to record contractions and fetal heart rate; in some settings, the woman is asked to press a hand-held button when fetal movement is felt which makes a mark on the fetal heart tracing; with this information, episodes of fetal movement can then be compared to changes in the fetal heart rate; acoustical stimulation can be implemented in the absence of fetal movement

   d. Findings: The test is considered normal (reactive) if there are two or more accelerations of 15 beats per minute lasting for 15 seconds over a 20-minute period, the baseline is normal, and long-term variability of 10 or more beats per minute is present; if these criteria are not met within 40 minutes, the test is considered nonreassuring (nonreactive) and further testing is indicated

2. **Contraction stress test (CST)** assesses the ability of the fetus to withstand the stress of uterine contractions and is a means of evaluating placental capacity for oxygen/carbon dioxide exchange; since contractions reduce blood flow to the fetus, the CST can be used to predict a fetus that may not be able to tolerate the stress of labor

  **a.** Indications: factors that place the fetus at risk for asphyxia such as intrauterine growth restriction, diabetes, postdates, nonreactive NST, and biophysical profile score less than 6

  **b.** Contraindications: third-trimester bleeding and previous cesarean birth with classical uterine incision; the advantages of the CST should be weighed against the danger of preterm labor in situations where this is a risk such as premature rupture of membranes or incompetent cervix

  **c.** Test procedure: after the test procedure is explained to the client and informed consent is obtained, electronic monitoring of contractions and fetal heart rate are begun; after a baseline fetal heart tracing is obtained, contractions (if not occurring spontaneously) are initiated with intravenous oxytocin or breast self-stimulation

  **d.** Findings: when a pattern of at least 3 contractions of 40 to 60 second duration in a 10-minute time period is obtained, the fetal heart rate pattern is assessed; the test is reassuring (negative) if no late decelerations occur (see Figure 6-1); the test is not reassuring (positive) if there are late decelerations with at least two of the three contractions; the test is suspicious (equivocal) if there is a late deceleration with one of the three contractions or contractions every 2 minutes for 10 minutes (hyperstimulation pattern)

**C.** *Amniocentesis:* used to assess fetal well-being and maturity; a needle is inserted through the abdominal wall to collect a sample of amniotic fluid, which contains fetal cells (see Figure 6-2); the test can be done after 14 to 16 weeks gestation

  **1.** Purpose: prenatal diagnosis of genetic disorders or congenital anomalies, assessment of pulmonary maturity, and diagnosis of fetal hemolytic disease

**Figure 6-1**    **Contraction stress test.**

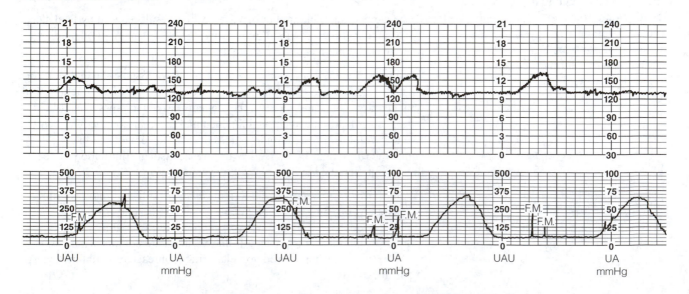

**Figure 6-2**

Amniocentesis.

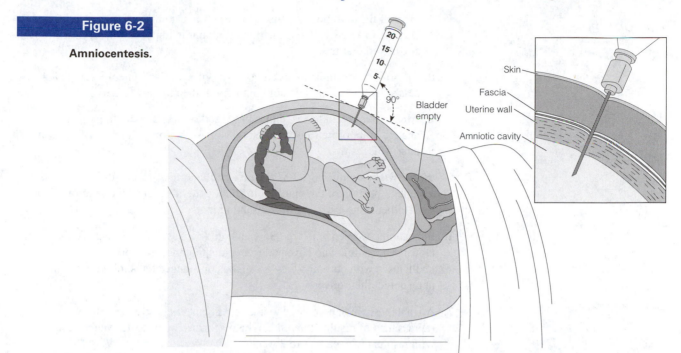

2. Complications occur in less than 1 percent of cases; possible maternal complications include hemorrhage, infection, labor, abruptio placentae, inadvertent damage to the intestines or bladder, and amniotic fluid leakage or embolism; possible fetal complications include death, hemorrhage, infection, and direct injury from the needle

3. Test procedure: after the test is explained to the client, an informed consent is obtained; if the client is greater than 20 weeks gestation, she should be instructed to empty her bladder; with the client in the supine position, the physician, using sterile technique, inserts a needle into the uterus; ultrasound visualization is used to assist the physician in guiding the needle; 15 to 20 mL of fluid are withdrawn and placed in a light-resistant container; fetal heart rate and maternal vital signs should be monitored throughout the procedure and for 30 minutes thereafter; mothers who are Rh-negative should receive RhoGAM following the procedure because of the risk of isoimmunization from fetal blood

4. Follow-up: Instruct the mother to contact the physician if she experiences fluid loss, bleeding, fever, abdominal pain, increased or decreased fetal activity; inform the mother that test results will be available in about 2 weeks

5. Findings

   a. **Lecithin to sphingomyelin (L/S) ratio** is used to assess fetal lung maturity; a ratio of 2:1 or greater indicates probable lung maturity; contamination with meconium or blood may alter the results

   b. **Phosphatidylglycerol (PG)**, a phospholipid found in pulmonary surfactant, in the amniotic fluid is an indicator of fetal lung maturity

   c. Genetic and chromosomal aberrations as well as the gender of the fetus can be determined from cells cultured for **karyotype,** the schematic arrangement of the chromosomes used to assess their number and morphology, and enzymatic activity; determination of gender is important in assessment of sex-linked diseases

    **d.** Rh isoimmunization status and severity of hemolytic anemia can be assessed by measuring bilirubin pigment in the amniotic fluid.

    **e.** Alpha-fetoprotein levels, either increased or decreased, can indicate anatomic abnormalities; fetal blood contamination of amniotic fluid can alter AFP results.

**D.** *Chorionic villus sampling (CVS):* involves collecting a small specimen of tissue from the fetal portion of the placenta for fetal genetic studies; the specimen can be obtained either transcervically or transabdominally

    **1.** Indications: women who are >35 years old (because of their increased risk for Down syndrome), who have had frequent spontaneous abortions, who have had fetuses with chromosomal anomalies or other defects, or who have a genetic defect themselves

    **2.** Advantages: when compared to amniocentesis, include earlier diagnosis and rapid return of results; the test can be performed at 10 to 12 weeks gestation with results returned in 1 to 2 weeks

    **3.** Test procedure: before the procedure, the client should be instructed to come for the procedure with a full bladder; after the procedure is explained to the client, informed consent is obtained; the client is placed in the lithotomy position and, using sterile technique, the physician visualizes the cervix; using ultrasound guidance, a suction cannula is used to collect the specimen; if the sample cannot be obtained transvaginally, the transabdominal route is used; clients who are Rh-negative should be given RhoGAM following the procedure

    **4.** Complications: vaginal spotting or bleeding, miscarriage, rupture of membranes, and chorioamnionitis; limb anomalies have been reported when the procedure is done before 10 weeks gestation; complications are rare

    **5.** Follow-up includes teaching the client signs and symptoms of complications to report to the physician, telling the woman when the results will be available, and arranging genetic counseling as needed

**E. Priority nursing diagnosis:** Health-seeking behaviors; Deficient knowledge; Anxiety; Risk for ineffective sexuality patterns

**F. Planning and implementation**

    **1.** Explain all planned testing including any special pretesting directions and obtain informed consents as needed

    **2.** Answer all client questions including those regarding why tests are needed, what the test entails, when the results will be available, and the significance of the results

    **3.** Protect the client's privacy during testing

    **4.** After specimens are collected, assure accurate labeling, packaging, and storage until tests are completed; use blood and body fluid precautions when handling specimens or diagnostic equipment which may result in exposure

5. Reassure client as to the confidentiality of results and that she will be notified when results are available

6. After results are returned, document results on the client's medical record

7. Contact the client to arrange for follow-up testing, genetic counseling, and education as needed

F. **Evaluation:** follow-up with the client to see that appointments have been kept, results are understood, and sexual partners have been notified of infection or need for treatment, as indicated

**Case Study**

The client is a 38-year-old primigravida who has come to the clinic for confirmation of pregnancy and initial prenatal care. Her last menstrual period was 6 weeks ago. She is married, in good health, and this pregnancy was planned. She is concerned that her age may have an effect on the fetus.

❶ What problem is this fetus at risk for because of maternal age?

❷ In addition to regular prenatal screening, what additional testing should be offered to this client?

❸ What advantages would chorionic villus sampling have over amniocentesis for this client?

❹ The client shares with you that even if the baby has a defect, she would not consider terminating the pregnancy. She wonders if there would be any advantage to knowing before delivery if the baby has a problem. How will you respond?

❺ The client is concerned that prenatal testing might injure the fetus. What will you tell her about possible complication from chorionic villus sampling and amniocentesis?

*For suggested responses, see page 338.*

## Posttest

1 The results have been returned from a complete blood count for a client who came to the clinic for her initial prenatal visit. Which of the following would indicate a possible problem with oxygen-carrying capacity?

(1) Decreased white blood cell count
(2) Decreased red blood cell count
(3) Decreased polymorphonuclear cell count
(4) Decreased platelet count

2 The client, who is 11 weeks gestation, has come to the office complaining of flu-like symptoms. Laboratory work indicates that the woman has contracted toxoplasmosis. From which of the following was the infection probably contracted?

(1) Sexual contact with a heterosexual male
(2) Contact with toxoplasmosis contaminated droplets in the air
(3) Exposure to infected saliva
(4) Poor handwashing after handling infected cat litter

**3** The client's prenatal laboratory findings have been returned. Which of the following would indicate a need for further follow-up related to potential development of erythroblastosis fetalis?

(1) Blood type O
(2) Rh-negative
(3) Blood type A
(4) Rh-positive

**4** During the client's first prenatal visit, the woman denies having had rubella or the rubella vaccine. Which of the following would be an appropriate action based on this information?

(1) Administer the rubella vaccine.
(2) Take a blood sample to assess the rubella titer.
(3) Have the client call her mother to ask if the client had German measles as a child.
(4) Tell the client that since rubella has little affect on the fetus she shouldn't worry about exposure to the disease.

**5** The client, who had an abnormal screening test (GTT) for gestational diabetes, has come to the clinic for a 3-hour oral glucose tolerance test (OGTT). Which of the following statements by the client indicates that she understands how the test is done?

(1) "I have eaten a low-protein diet for the past 3 days."
(2) "I ate breakfast of toast and milk 1 hour ago."
(3) "I have eaten a high-carbohydrate diet for the past 3 days."
(4) "I just had black coffee for breakfast."

**6** The pregnant client is scheduled to have an ultrasound. Which of the following might indicate a need to do the assessment transvaginally?

(1) Client is 5-feet 1-in. tall and weighs 230 pounds.
(2) Client is 15 years old and easily embarrassed.
(3) Client is 32 weeks gestation.
(4) Client is concerned about ultrasound waves hurting the baby.

**7** The client, who is 41 weeks gestation, has just had a biophysical profile with a score of 2. Which of the following nursing interventions would be most appropriate?

(1) Tell the mother that this indicates fetal well-being.
(2) Reschedule the mother for a repeat of the test in one week.
(3) Recognize this as an equivocal test and schedule a repeat of it for the next day.
(4) Consult the physician as this score indicates a probable need for immediate delivery.

**8** The client has come to the clinic for her initial prenatal visit. Based on her menstrual history, the client is 9 weeks gestation and is scheduled to have an ultrasound for estimation of gestation age of the fetus. Which fetal measurement would be the best indicator of gestational age at this time?

(1) Biparietal diameter
(2) Femur length
(3) Abdominal circumference
(4) Crown-rump measurement

**9** The client, who is to have an amniocentesis for genetic testing, asks the nurse if there are any possible complications with this procedure. The nurse's best response would be:

(1) "No, this procedure is completely safe."
(2) "I don't know, you will need to speak with your physician about that."
(3) "Yes, but if you are very still during the procedure they can be avoided."
(4) "Yes, but they occur in less than 1 percent of the cases. Do you have any other questions about the procedure?"

**10** The client, who is at 40 weeks gestation, seems upset and tells the nurse that the physician told her she needs to have a nonstress test. The client asks why she needs the test. The nurse's best response would be:

(1) "This is a test to see if your stress level is affecting your baby's growth and well-being."
(2) "This is a test to see if your baby will be able to withstand the stress of labor."
(3) "This is a test to assess your baby's well-being now that you are due to deliver soon."
(4) "This is a test to let us know if your baby needs to be delivered to avoid a bad outcome."

*See pages 139–140 for Answers and Rationales.*

# Answers and Rationales

## Pretest

1 **Answer: 1** *Rationale:* CVS can be done at 10 to 12 weeks gestation while amniocentesis cannot be done until 14 weeks gestation. CVS has slightly more complications than amniocentesis and provides the same information on genetic makeup of the fetus as amniocentesis. Neither procedure requires anesthesia.
*Cognitive Level:* Analysis
*Nursing Process:* Planning; *Test Plan:* SECE

2 **Answer: 1** *Rationale:* A contraction stress test requires the client to have contractions, a nonstress test (NST) does not. Some testing sites ask the mother to push a button that marks the fetal heart rate strip when she feels the baby move. The NST can be done in an outpatient setting and requires 20 to 30 minutes of testing.
*Cognitive Level:* Application
*Nursing Process:* Evaluation; *Test Plan:* HPM

3 **Answer: 2** *Rationale:* Gestational age is best assessed in the first trimester when growth is fairly consistent among pregnancies. Position, intrauterine growth, and amniotic fluid volume are best assessed later in pregnancy.
*Cognitive Level:* Application
*Nursing Process:* Implementation; *Test Plan:* HPM

4 **Answer: 3** *Rationale:* The test is done at about 24 weeks, as this is when the fetal nutrient requirement rises resulting in increased maternal intake and more sustained levels of blood glucose.
*Cognitive Level:* Analysis
*Nursing Process:* Planning; *Test Plan:* HPM

5 **Answer: 3** *Rationale:* The presence of nitrites, white blood cells, and bacteria are all indicative of a urinary tract infection.
*Cognitive Level:* Analysis
*Nursing Process:* Analysis; *Test Plan:* PHYS

6 **Answer: 3** *Rationale:* When a fetal body wall defect is present, AFP leaks and is absorbed into the maternal circulation causing the woman's serum AFP level to rise. AFP testing has nothing to do with DNA.
*Cognitive Level:* Application
*Nursing Process:* Implementation; *Test Plan:* HPM

7 **Answer: 2** *Rationale:* Transmission occurs through entry of the spirochete into subcutaneous tissue through microscopic abrasions that can occur during sexual contact, kissing, and biting.
*Cognitive Level:* Application
*Nursing Process:* Implementation; *Test Plan:* PHYS

8 **Answer: 2** *Rationale:* Gonorrhea contracted by the infant during the perinatal period can cause sepsis and intrauterine growth restriction. Most neonatal gonorrheal infections occur by the ascending route and result in ophthalmia neonatorum, an eye infection.
*Cognitive Level:* Application
*Nursing Process:* Implementation; *Test Plan:* HPM

9 **Answer: 4** *Rationale:* Rash on the palms of hands and soles of feet as well as chancre sores are associated with syphilis. Crusted ulcers are commonly seen with herpes. A small, soft, papillary swelling is most likely human papillomavirus infection, which can be confirmed by colposcopy and directed biopsy.
*Cognitive Level:* Analysis
*Nursing Process:* Analysis; *Test Plan:* PHYS

10 **Answer: 3** *Rationale:* Early detection and treatment of problems can decrease or eliminate problems for the mother or fetus that may develop or worsen as the pregnancy continues.
*Cognitive Level:* Application
*Nursing Process:* Implementation; *Test Plan:* PHYS

## Posttest

1 **Answer: 2** *Rationale:* The red blood cell (RBC) count is a measure of the number of red blood cells in 1 mm$^3$ of peripheral blood. Within each RBC are molecules of hemoglobin, which are used to carry oxygen.
*Cognitive Level:* Analysis
*Nursing Process:* Analysis; *Test Plan:* PHYS

2 **Answer: 4** *Rationale:* Toxoplasmosis is caused by a protozoan that is spread by ingestion of contaminated raw meat or poor handwashing after contact with cat litter. It is not spread by sexual contact or droplets.
*Cognitive Level:* Analysis
*Nursing Process:* Analysis; *Test Plan:* PHYS

3 **Answer: 2** *Rationale:* Test results indicate that the mother is Rh-negative which means she does not have the Rh antigen. If the fetus is Rh-positive and fetal blood is mixed into the mother's blood, her immune system will make antibodies against the Rh antigen. This could result in erythroblastosis fetalis.
*Cognitive Level:* Analysis
*Nursing Process:* Planning; *Test Plan:* PHYS

4 **Answer: 2** *Rationale:* If the nonimmune client contracts rubella, it can cause miscarriage or serious congenital anomalies. The client should not be

vaccinated during pregnancy as the fetus can contract rubella from the live-virus vaccine. Immunity can be determined by assessing a rubella titer.
*Cognitive Level:* Analysis
*Nursing Process:* Planning; *Test Plan:* HPM

5   **Answer: 3** *Rationale:* The test requires that the client eat a high-carbohydrate diet for 3 days and then fast for at least 8 hours before testing begins. Clients should not consume caffeine as it tends to increase glucose levels.
*Cognitive Level:* Analysis
*Nursing Process:* Evaluation; *Test Plan:* PHYS

6   **Answer: 1** *Rationale:* Transvaginal ultrasound, used most often in the first trimester, avoids the need to scan through thick abdominal layers of obese clients. Some modest clients are embarrassed by the use of vaginal scanning. Neither abdominal nor vaginal ultrasound has been shown to have harmful effects on the fetus.
*Cognitive Level:* Analysis
*Nursing Process:* Planning; *Test Plan:* HPM

7   **Answer: 4** *Rationale:* Scores on the biophysical profile can range from 0 to 10. A score of less than 4

indicates impending fetal death and a need for immediate delivery.
*Cognitive Level:* Analysis
*Nursing Process:* Analysis; *Test Plan:* PHYS

8   **Answer: 4** *Rationale:* Before 12 weeks, length as measured by crown-rump length is the most accurate measure of gestation age. Biparietal diameter and femur length are used to monitor fetal growth later in pregnancy. Abdominal circumference can be used to identify some congenital anomalies.
*Cognitive Level:* Analysis
*Nursing Process:* Planning; *Test Plan:* HPM

9   **Answer: 4** *Rationale:* Complications including hemorrhage, damage to the mother's intestines or bladder, infection, and miscarriage can occur but they are very rare.
*Cognitive Level:* Application
*Nursing Process:* Implementation; *Test Plan:* HPM

10  **Answer: 3** *Rationale:* The nonstress test is a measure of fetal well-being. It is not an accurate predictor of ability to withstand labor or of poor outcome. Test results are not related to the woman's stress level.
*Cognitive Level:* Application
*Nursing Process:* Implementation; *Test Plan:* HPM

# *References*

Dickason, E., Silverman, B., & Kaplan, J. (1998). *Maternal-infant nursing care* (3rd ed.). St. Louis: Mosby.

Lowdermilk, D., Perry, S., & Bobak, I. (2000). *Maternity and women's health care* (7th ed.). St. Louis: Mosby, pp. 154, 158, 169, 397, 798–800, 803, 804, 806–809, 876, 878, 1073.

Olds, S., London, M., & Ladewig, P. (2000). *Maternal newborn nursing: A family and community-based approach* (6th ed). Upper Saddle River, NJ: Prentice Hall Health.

Pagana, K. & Pagana, T. (1999). *Diagnostic testing and nursing implications: A case study approach* (5th ed.). St. Louis: Mosby, pp. 372, 870–872.

Pagana, K. & Pagana, T. (1998). *Manual of diagnostic and laboratory tests*. St. Louis: Mosby.

## CHAPTER 7

# The Complicated Prenatal Experience

Karla L. Luxner, RNC, MSN

## CHAPTER OUTLINE

*Nursing Care of the High-Risk Prenatal Client*

*Pregestational Conditions*

*Gestational Conditions*

## OBJECTIVES

▪ Describe nursing assessments and interventions designed to improve the health of the high-risk prenatal client.

▪ Describe the effect of preexisting conditions on the health of the pregnant woman and her fetus.

▪ Delineate nursing responsibilities in the care of the woman with gestational onset complications of pregnancy.

[ Media Link ]

*Use the CD-ROM enclosed with this text, or log onto the address given to access the free, interactive Companion Website created for this series. The CD-ROM and Companion Website accompanying this book offer additional practice opportunities and information—NCLEX Review, Case Studies, Glossary, In Depth with NCLEX, and more.*

**www.prenhall.com/hogan**

## REVIEW AT A GLANCE

**abortion**  *spontaneous or induced pregnancy loss before 20 weeks gestation*

**abruptio placenta**  *premature separation of the normally implanted placenta away from the uterine wall*

**cerclage**  *looping suture around the cervix to keep it securely closed during pregnancy*

**chorioamnionitis**  *inflammation and infection in the fetal membranes and amniotic fluid*

**Coombs' test**  *lab test to identify antibodies on the RBCs; a direct Coombs' test determines if there are maternal anti-Rh antibodies in the fetal cord blood, while an indirect Coombs' identifies anti-Rh antibodies in the mother's blood*

**ectopic**  *abnormally placed pregnancy outside the uterus*

**erythroblastosis fetalis**  *destruction of fetal red blood cells by maternal anti-Rh antibodies causes production of many immature red blood cells (erythroblasts) in the fetus*

**gestational diabetes**  *a disorder of carbohydrate metabolism caused by inability of the maternal pancreas to produce the additional insulin needed during pregnancy*

**gestational trophoblastic disease (hydatidiform mole)**  *related to the outermost developing layer of the embryo which develops into the fetal membranes and placenta; in GTD cellular differentiation is halted, the embryo does not*

*develop and trophoblastic tissue proliferates*

**hydrops fetalis**  *generalized fetal edema caused by destruction of fetal red blood cells by maternal anti-Rh antibodies*

**kernicterus**  *yellow staining of the basal ganglia and brain from deposit of excessive unbound bilirubin, associated with a poor outcome*

**macrosomia**  *excessively large body as in infants of diabetic mothers who experience high glucose levels in utero*

**placenta previa**  *abnormal implantation of the placenta low in the uterus near or covering the cervical os*

## *Pretest*

**1** A client with Class II heart disease is being seen for her first prenatal visit. Which of the following teaching points would the nurse stress for this client?

(1) Avoid all over the counter (OTC) medications during pregnancy.
(2) Regular exercise will help increase the cardiac capacity during pregnancy.
(3) It's important to take prenatal vitamins and iron as prescribed.
(4) The client's fetus will probably have a similar congenital heart defect.

**2** When an insulin-dependent diabetic client gives birth, the nurse expects the client's insulin requirements in the first 24 hours after delivery to:

(1) Drop significantly.
(2) Gradually return to normal.
(3) Increase slightly.
(4) Stay the same as before.

**3** Which of the following lab tests would the nurse look at to provide the best information about ongoing control of insulin-dependent diabetes in a pregnant adolescent?

(1) Fasting blood glucose
(2) Glycosylated hemoglobin
(3) Oral glucose tolerance test
(4) Post-prandial test

**4** The nurse should be aware that pregnant women who practice substance abuse and present themselves for prenatal care:

(1) Are ready to kick their habit.
(2) Must be reported to the authorities.
(3) Recognize the need for caring interventions.
(4) Will lack appropriate parenting skills.

**5** Which of the following nursing actions would take priority when caring for the woman with a suspected ectopic pregnancy?

(1) Administering oxygen
(2) Monitoring vital signs
(3) Obtaining surgical consent
(4) Providing emotional support

**6** A client is being discharged from the hospital after evacuation of a molar pregnancy. The nurse recognizes that additional discharge teaching is required when the client states:

(1) "I am so sad that I lost this baby."
(2) "I may need to have chemotherapy after this."
(3) "I will need to see the doctor yearly for follow-up. "
(4) "I will use contraception for the next 2 years."

**7** The charge nurse in labor and delivery has become overwhelmed with admissions and births. For which of the following clients can the charge nurse best delegate the needed care to a trusted certified nursing assistant who is currently going to school to become a nurse?

(1) A client in false labor, who needs teaching about true versus false labor signs
(2) A client with PIH who needs to be evaluated for reflexes and clonus
(3) A primigravida in early labor who needs to be helped to the bathroom
(4) An obese laboring client who needs to have her fetal monitor adjusted

**8** A client with a known placenta previa is admitted at 30 weeks with painless vaginal bleeding. The nurse weighs the client's peri-pads to monitor blood loss. An increased weight of 50 g would indicate approximately how much blood loss?

(1) 0.5 mL
(2) 5 mL
(3) 50 mL
(4) 500 mL

**9** A client with hyperemesis gravidarum would most likely benefit from nursing care designed to address which of the following nursing diagnoses?

(1) Imbalanced nutrition: more than body requirements related to pregnancy
(2) Anxiety related to effects of hyperemesis on fetal well-being
(3) Anticipatory grieving related to inevitable pregnancy loss
(4) Ineffective coping related to unwanted pregnancy

**10** The initial laboratory results for a primigravida indicate a hemoglobin of 12 g/dL, hematocrit of 36 percent, and a blood group and type of A, Rh-negative. What would be the priority nursing action to promote a healthy pregnancy for this client and her fetus?

(1) Determine the blood type of the father.
(2) Encourage the client to eat more dark-green leafy vegetables.
(3) Provide information on weight-gain during pregnancy.
(4) Suggest an iron supplement in addition to prenatal vitamins.

*See pages 164–165 for Answers and Rationales.*

## I. Nursing Care of the High-Risk Prenatal Client

**A. Identifying clients at risk:** begins with the first prenatal visit and continues through the puerperium; risk factors are anything that may be associated with a negative pregnancy outcome including physiological, psychological, sociodemographic, or environmental factors

**B. More frequent monitoring of high-risk clients:** important during pregnancy, labor, and birth, and the puerperium to help identify potential complications, ensure early treatment, and improve maternal-fetal outcomes

## II. Pregestational Conditions

**A. Cardiac disease**

1. Description and etiology

a. Hemodynamic changes of pregnancy increase the workload on the heart; cardiac output increases 30 to 50 percent by mid-pregnancy; a compromised heart with inadequate cardiac capacity and decreased reserves may be unable to adapt to the added requirements of pregnancy

b. Treatment options and the likelihood of a positive pregnancy outcome depend on the degree of cardiac compromise; clients with Class I and II cardiac disease have the potential for a good pregnancy outcome whereas those with Class III or IV disease may be at risk for serious maternal and fetal compromise (Table 7-1)

c. Maternal congenital heart defects that have been effectively treated by modern techniques are being seen more often during pregnancy as this population reaches adulthood; there are decreasing numbers of pregnant women with heart damage from rheumatic fever caused by effective treatment of streptococcal infections

2. Assessment: most common complication of heart disease during pregnancy is congestive heart failure (CHF)

a. Edema of varying degree from pedal edema, pitting edema, generalized edema (anasarca), and pulmonary edema

b. Dyspnea on exertion, increasing fatigue, dyspnea at rest, moist cough, basilar rales, cyanosis of nail beds, circumoral cyanosis

c. Tachycardia, irregular pulse, murmurs, chest pain

3. Priority nursing diagnoses: Decreased cardiac output; Fluid volume excess; Activity intolerance; Anxiety; Risk for infection

4. Implementation and collaborative care

a. Monitor client and fetal well-being more frequently during pregnancy; changes in maternal vital signs or signs of fetal compromise may indicate inability to handle the increasing demands on the heart

b. Teach adequate nutrition for pregnancy and provide prenatal vitamins and iron to prevent anemia; monitor for signs of infection

c. Instruct client to avoid excessive weight gain or emotional stress; these conditions all place added stress on cardiac reserves

d. Teach client the signs of infection to report so treatment may begin early

e. Diagnostic procedures may include auscultation, electrocardiogram, echocardiogram, and possible cardiac catheterization

| Table 7-1 | Classification | Functional Capacity |
|---|---|---|
| **Classification of Functional Capacity for Clients with Cardiac Disease (NYHA 1979)** | I | Uncompromised: No limitation on physical activity due to angina or symptoms of cardiac insufficiency |
| | II | Slightly Compromised: Normal activity causes fatigue, palpitation, dyspnea, or angina |
| | III | Markedly Compromised: May be comfortable at rest, but less than usual activity causes fatigue, dyspnea, palpitations, or angina |
| | IV | Severely Compromised: Cannot perform any activity without increasing discomfort; may experience angina and cardiac insufficiency while at rest. |

**f.** Medication therapy in addition to prenatal vitamins and iron may include:

1) Prophylactic antibiotics for any invasive procedures, including dental work and at the time of birth, to prevent bacterial endocarditis; penicillin (PCN) is usually prescribed unless the client is allergic

2) Cardiac glycosides (Digitalis) to increase contractility of the cardiac muscle and slow the heart rate for effective filling

3) Antidysrhythmia agents for cardiac dysrhythmias

4) The diuretic furosemide (Lasix) to decrease fluid excess; care must be taken to ensure adequate circulating volume to maintain uteroplacental perfusion

5) Heparin is considered safe for use in pregnancy if an anticoagulant is indicated (Pregnancy Category C); warfarin (Coumadin) is a Pregnancy Category X drug (Table 7-2)

**g.** Teach the client to avoid exertion and to plan frequent rest periods to maintain cardiac reserves

**h.** Adequate pain relief should be provided during labor to avoid excessive maternal stress; vaginal delivery is preferred with epidural anesthesia, continuous maternal oxygen administration, and a low-forceps delivery to decrease maternal straining

**i.** Observe client carefully for complications from hemodynamic changes immediately after delivery

**5.** Evaluation: client experiences a healthy pregnancy, avoids congestive heart failure or cardiac decompensation, and gives birth to a healthy infant

**B. Diabetes mellitus**

**1.** Description

**a.** An endocrine disorder with major effects on carbohydrate metabolism; it results from insufficient insulin production in the beta cells of the islets of

| Table 7-2 | Category | Risk to the Fetus | Examples of Drugs |
|---|---|---|---|
| **FDA Pregnancy Categories for Prescription Drugs** | A | Controlled studies in women do not demonstrate a risk to the fetus in the first trimester, and the possibility of fetal harm appears remote. | RDA dose of Vitamin C |
| | B | Animal studies have not demonstrated fetal risk but there are no controlled studies in women, or animal studies show an adverse effect not confirmed in controlled studies in women in the first trimester. | Acetaminophen (Tylenol) Penicillins |
| | C | Animal studies show adverse effects and there are no controlled studies in women or studies in women and animals are not available. Drug should be given only if potential benefit justifies the potential risk to the fetus. | Zidovudine (Retrovir) Heparin |
| | D | Positive evidence of fetal risk in humans but the benefits to the mother may be acceptable despite the risk in certain situations. | Phenobarbitol (Luminol) |
| | X | The risks to the fetus clearly outweigh any possible benefit to the mother. The drug is contraindicated in women who may become pregnant. | Warfarin (Coumadin) Diethylstilbestrol (DES) |

Langerhans in the pancreas; insulin facilitates the movement of glucose from the blood into the tissue cells for storage or energy use

   b. **Gestational diabetes** results when the pancreas is unable to meet the increased demands for insulin production during pregnancy

2. Effect of pregnancy on glucose metabolism

   a. During the first half of pregnancy, increasing maternal hormones increase the demand for insulin production to facilitate increased storage of glycogen in maternal tissue

   b. During the last half of pregnancy, human placental lactogen (hPL) from the placenta causes resistance to the action of maternal insulin thereby increasing circulating glucose for fetal use and increasing the demand on the maternal pancreas to produce more insulin

   c. The fetus produces his own insulin but obtains glucose from the mother, across the placenta; the amount of glucose available in maternal circulation stimulates the fetal pancreas to produce insulin

3. Effects of diabetes on pregnancy and the fetus is related to the degree of control of blood glucose levels within a range of 70 mg/dL to 120 mg/dL, and the degree of vascular involvement; complications are more common with insulin-dependent diabetes mellitus and include:

   a. Polyhydraminos

   b. Pregnancy-induced hypertension (PIH)

   c. Stillbirth (usually after 36 weeks)

   d. Neonatal macrosomia, hypoglycemia, hyperbilirubinemia, delayed fetal lung maturity resulting in respiratory distress syndrome (RDS), and increased incidence of congenital anomalies including neural tube defects (NTD)

4. Assessment

   a. Risk factors: family history of diabetes, maternal obesity, previous large-for-gestational age (LGA) infants, previous unexplained stillbirth

   b. Classic symptoms of diabetes mellitus include polyuria, polydipsia, and polyphagia

   c. Client may have more frequent urinary tract infections and vaginal candidiasis (yeast) infections caused by altered pH in the reproductive tract

   d. Urine testing for glycosuria and ketones as part of routine prenatal care

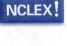

   e. Diabetes screening should be done around 28 weeks gestation with a 50-g oral GTT (glucose tolerance test); if blood glucose is greater than 140 mg/dL at 1 hour, a 3-hour 100-g oral GTT is performed

   f. Long-term glucose control is estimated with the glycosylated hemoglobin (HbA$_{1c}$) blood test which measures the percent of hemoglobin with glucose bound to it (glycohemoglobin); levels depend on the amount of glucose available during the red blood cell's 120-day lifespan

5. Priority nursing diagnoses: Risk for imbalanced nutrition, maternal and fetal: more than body requirements; Risk for injury: maternal and fetal; Anxiety

6. Implementation and collaborative care

   a. Teach client about prescribed ADA diet regulation with no concentrated sweets; dietary regulation usually adequate to control gestational diabetes; excessive weight gain should be avoided; caloric needs will increase as pregnancy progresses

   b. Medications: oral hypoglycemic medications are contraindicated during pregnancy; insulin (human) needs to be carefully regulated and adjusted as pregnancy progresses with as much as a four-fold dose increase needed at term

   c. Instruct client in frequent blood glucose, urine glucose, and ketone testing and keeping a diary of test results and activity levels

   d. Encourage regular nonstrenuous exercise such as walking for weight and blood glucose control

   e. Monitor fetal well-being: maternal serum alpha fetoprotein (MSAFP) at 16 to 18 weeks, ultrasound for anomalies, amniotic fluid volume, and fetal size; fetal movement counts, weekly non-stress test (NST) from 28 to 32 weeks, possible oxytocin challenge test (OCT), bio-physical profile (BPP), and amniocentesis for lung maturity

      1) Lecithin/Sphingomyelin (L/S) ratio needs to be 1:3 (normal is 1:2)

      2) Phosphatidylglycerol (PG) should be present

   f. Monitor client for development of complications: infection, PIH, and diabetic ketoacidosis

   g. Prepare for possible induction of labor at 38 to 39 weeks for clients with IDDM to reduce risk for stillbirth caused by premature placental aging

   h. Insulin requirements drop dramatically after delivery of the placenta and removal of the hormonal influences; client may need no insulin or a very decreased dose; gestational diabetics generally may eat a regular diet

7. Evaluation: client maintains glucose control during pregnancy and delivers healthy fetus without complications; newborn remains normoglycemic

**C. Substance abuse**

1. Description and etiology

   a. As many as 10 percent of pregnant women use tobacco, alcohol, or other drugs, often in combination; clients using illegal drugs may delay seeking care for fear of prosecution; all pregnant women should be screened for substance abuse

   b. Substances frequently used in the United States are tobacco, alcohol, marijuana, cocaine, crack cocaine, and heroin; effects of these substances on pregnancy include spontaneous abortion, intrauterine growth restriction (IUGR), preterm labor, placental abruption, stillbirth, neonatal addiction, and fetal alcohol syndrome (FAS)

2. Assessment

   a. Establish a trusting relationship with the client by remaining open, matter-of-fact, and nonjudgmental; women seeking prenatal care are interested in improving and safeguarding their health and that of the fetus

    **b.** Encourage client to describe all substances used, the amounts, times and triggers to use, and any previous attempts to discontinue use

    **c.** Evaluate client's motivation, support systems, and personal strengths that may be elicited to change behaviors

**3.** Priority nursing diagnoses: Ineffective health maintenance; Ineffective coping; Risk for impaired gas exchange; Risk for delayed growth and development

**4.** Implementation and collaborative care

    **a.** Monitor client for complications: anemia, inadequate nutrition and weight gain, PIH, preterm labor; random urine toxicology screens may be ordered

    **b.** Monitor fetal growth and well-being: fundal height, ultrasound, NST, BPP

    **c.** Teach the client about the potential negative effects of substances used on pregnancy and the fetus/neonate

    **d.** Assist with referrals for the client as indicated: smoking cessation classes, Alcoholics Anonymous, addiction counseling, psychological counseling, and possible hospitalization

    **e.** Reinforce teaching about nutrition and the effects on fetal development; teach client the danger signs of pregnancy including signs of preterm labor and abruption of the placenta

    **f.** Support client's efforts to change negative behaviors

    **g.** The client may need to be followed by a perinatologist during pregnancy; the addicted neonate will require intensive care at birth

    **h.** The client should not go through "cold turkey" drug withdrawal during pregnancy; heroin addicts may be put on methadone hydrochloride (Dolophine)—a narcotic agonist analgesic that blocks the more severe symptoms of heroin withdrawal

**5.** Evaluation: client decreases substance abuse during pregnancy and delivers a healthy term neonate; client develops more effective coping mechanisms

**D. HIV/AIDS**

**1.** Description and etiology

    **a.** The human immunodeficiency virus (HIV) causes the condition known as acquired immunodeficiency syndrome (AIDS); HIV is transmitted through contact with infected blood and body secretions, usually during sexual contact or use of contaminated needles by IV drug users; HIV infection results in AIDS characterized by decreased immunity and overwhelming opportunistic infection

    **b.** Pregnancy doesn't appear to change the course of the illness for the mother; the fetus may contract the virus transplacentally or through breast-milk, but generally fetal infection is considered to occur during vaginal birth

    **c.** Current maternal treatment with antiretroviral drugs including Retrovir (zidovudine) orally during pregnancy and intravenously during labor and delivery has decreased the occurrence of neonatal transmission to less than 7 percent with vaginal birth and less than 1 percent with cesarean birth

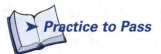

**➤ Practice to Pass**

A client who takes methadone for heroin addiction is in active labor and asking for something for pain. The physician's standing order calls for butorphanol (Stadol), a narcotic agonist-antagonist, to be given IV push. Discuss your concerns about giving this drug to this client.

d. Maternal HIV antibodies cross the placenta so all infants of HIV-positive mothers will test positive at birth and until maternal antibodies are depleted at between 15 to 18 months of age

2. Assessment

a. Antibodies to HIV are detected with the ELISA test and results confirmed by the Western blot test

b. All pregnant women should be offered HIV testing because most clients are asymptomatic for 5 to 10 years before signs of opportunistic infection occur

3. Priority nursing diagnoses: Risk for infection: maternal and fetal; Decisional conflict; Compromised family coping; Anticipatory grieving

4. Implementation and collaborative care

a. Provide emotional support and reproductive counseling to client and family

b. Evaluate client for other sexually transmitted diseases and hepatitis B

c. Review lab results for signs of anemia, thrombocytopenia, leukopenia, and decreased CD-4 T-lymphocyte counts

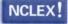

d. Monitor client for signs of opportunistic infection: fever, weight loss, fatigue, candidiasis, cough, skin lesions

e. Administer prophylactic antiretroviral drugs as ordered during pregnancy and labor and delivery

f. Monitor fetal growth and well-being

g. Use universal blood and body fluid precautions with all clients

h. Protect the fetus from maternal secretions

1) Avoid use of fetal scalp electrode or other invasive devices during labor

2) Wash infant's eyes and face at birth before administering prophylactic eye drops or ointment; bathe entire newborn as soon as possible after delivery to remove all maternal secretions

3) Delay any newborn injections or heel-sticks until after the bath

4) Encourage the mother to formula-feed her baby to avoid transmission by breast-milk

5. Evaluation: client's illness remains stable without opportunistic infection during pregnancy and birth; infant is healthy and tests HIV negative at 18 months; client and family develop effective coping mechanisms to plan for the future of the infant

**E. Rh sensitization**

1. Description and etiology

a. Rh-negative women who become pregnant with an Rh-positive embryo/fetus (from an Rh-positive father) may become sensitized to the Rh antigen if there is any accidental contact between maternal and fetal blood; other causes of Rh-sensitization might be blood transfusion of Rh-positive blood to an Rh-negative woman, or fetomaternal blood contact during an amniocentesis or other invasive procedure

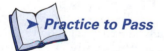

**▶ Practice to Pass**

When caring for a postpartum HIV positive mother, what precautions would you take? What precautions would you teach the mother to take to protect her newborn?

**b.** Sensitized Rh-negative women develop anti-Rh antibodies, which may cross the placenta in subsequent Rh-positive pregnancies and attack and destroy the fetal RBCs

**c.** Fetal effects of Rh incompatibility and sensitization are progressively severe

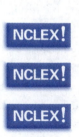

**2.** Hemolysis of fetal erythrocytes leads to greatly increased immature RBC production, termed **erythroblastosis fetalis**

**3.** Continued RBC destruction and anemia results in jaundice and marked fetal edema known as **hydrops fetalis** and may lead to fetal congestive heart failure

**4.** Breakdown of RBCs releases bilirubin, causing jaundice; high levels of circulating bilirubin can cause **kernicterus,** a condition of yellow staining of the basal ganglia and brain from bilirubin deposits and may result in permanent neurological damage

**5.** Assessment

**a.** All pregnant women should be tested for blood group, Rh factor, and routine antibody screening; a history of previous miscarriage, blood transfusions, or infants experiencing jaundice should be noted

**b.** If the client is Rh-negative, the father of the infant is tested to determine his Rh status; an Rh-negative father and mother will only produce Rh-negative offspring who will not be affected by Rh-incompatibility

**c.** An indirect **Coombs' test** on maternal blood is used to determine whether the Rh-negative client has developed antibodies to the Rh antigen; serial antibody screening should continue throughout pregnancy to identify increasing antibody production; a direct Coombs' test is done on the infant's blood after birth to identify maternal antibodies attached to fetal RBCs

**6.** Priority nursing diagnoses: Risk for injury; Deficient knowledge; Anxiety

**7.** Implementation and collaborative care

**a.** Provide support and education to the client and family; the client should carry an Rh-negative identification card and recognize that she may need the medication RhoGAM with future reproductive events

**b.** Unsensitized Rh-negative clients should be given 300 μg of Rh immune globulin (RhoGAM) IM at 28 weeks and also within 72 hours of delivery; the antibodies in the immune globulin bind with any Rh antigens in maternal circulation; this provides passive immunity to the mother so she will not become sensitized to any Rh antigens and produce antibodies of her own

**c.** RhoGAM is not given to mothers who are already sensitized and have antibodies (positive indirect Coombs' test)

**d.** Rh immune globulin is also given after abortion, ectopic pregnancy, amniocentesis, and any other situation that might result in maternal exposure to the fetal Rh antigen

**e.** The Kleihauer-Betke test estimates the amount of fetal blood in the maternal circulation; it is used to determine the dose of Rh immune globulin when a larger fetal-maternal bleed is suspected

NCLEX!

f. Evaluate the fetus for development of complications by serial ultrasound for amniotic fluid volume, fetal size, and the development of edema or an enlarged heart

g. A sinusoidal electronic fetal monitoring pattern indicates severe fetal anemia; biophysical profile (BPP) may be used to identify a compromised fetus

h. Amniocentesis or percutaneous umbilical cord blood sampling (PUBS) may be used to determine fetal Rh; both procedures carry the risk of causing maternal exposure and sensitization, so RhoGAM should be given

i. An early delivery with phototherapy and exchange transfusions may be planned if the fetus is developing anemia close to term

j. Intrauterine exchange transfusion may be performed for the severely affected fetus until viability is reached

8. Evaluation: the Rh-negative client delivers a healthy infant with a negative direct Coombs' test; the client receives prophylactic Rh immune globulin to prevent maternal antibody formation that might complicate future pregnancies

## III. Gestational Conditions

### A. Hyperemesis gravidarum

1. Description and etiology

   a. Hyperemesis gravidarum or pernicious vomiting of pregnancy is characterized by extreme nausea and vomiting during the first half of pregnancy that is associated with dehydration, weight loss, and electrolyte imbalances; the emesis is much more severe than in the common "morning sickness" of early pregnancy and occurs in only 0.1 percent of pregnancies

   b. Theories about the etiology of hyperemesis include psychological as well as physiological factors but the actual cause remains unknown; the condition is rare in developing countries; high levels of hCG, as are found in **gestational trophoblastic disease** (hydatidiform mole, molar pregnancy), are associated with severe nausea and vomiting

   c. The fetus is at risk for **macrosomia** (excessively large body), abnormal development, IUGR, or death from lack of nutrition, hypoxia, and maternal ketoacidosis

2. Assessment

   a. Intractable vomiting during the first 20 weeks of pregnancy

   b. Dehydration with: weight loss of more than 5 percent of prepregnancy weight, poor skin turgor, dry mucous membranes, possible hypotension, tachycardia, and increased lab values for hematocrit and urine specific gravity

   c. Signs and symptoms of electrolyte or acid-base imbalance (acidosis): ketosis, confusion, drowsiness, muscle weakness, cramps, clumsiness, tremors, irregular heartbeat, decreased level of consciousness

   d. Signs and symptoms of starvation: muscle wasting, ketonuria, jaundice, bleeding gums (vitamin deficiency)

3. Priority nursing diagnoses: Deficient fluid volume; Risk for injury; Altered nutrition: less than body requirements; Ineffective coping

4. Implementation and collaborative care

   a. Client may need hospitalization with IV fluid therapy with glucose, electrolytes, and vitamins to begin treatment and then continue at home once stabilized

   b. Monitor daily weight and measure intake and output; assess vital signs as appropriate, hydration, and nutritional status

   c. Administer antiemetic medications such as phenothiazines or antihistamines as ordered to control nausea and vomiting

   d. Encourage six small feedings a day after the acute nausea and vomiting has passed; clear liquids such as lemonade and herbal teas, and salty foods like potato chips are sometimes better tolerated at first

   e. Total parenteral nutrition (TPN) may be required in severe cases when the client is unable to tolerate oral feedings

   f. Monitor fetal growth with serial ultrasounds

   g. Provide emotional support; help client to identify healthy coping mechanisms and support systems she can rely on during pregnancy

   h. Refer for additional counseling and support as indicated

5. Evaluation: client exhibits signs of adequate hydration: moist mucous membranes, good skin turgor, stable vital signs and intake equal to output; client is able to tolerate adequate nutrition for maternal and fetal requirements and gains appropriate weight during pregnancy

**B.** *Ectopic pregnancy*

1. Description and etiology: implantation of a fertilized ovum outside of the uterus; sites may include implantation on the ovary or elsewhere in the abdominal cavity; the most common site is implantation in a fallopian tube that has become narrowed by scarring or adhesions; ascending infections, pelvic inflammatory disease (PID), use of IUD contraception, or tubal surgery are risk factors for tubal damage that may result in an ectopic pregnancy

2. Assessment

   a. Interview reveals last normal menstrual period (LNMP) consistent with possible pregnancy and possible subjective symptoms of pregnancy such as breast tenderness and nausea

   b. Unilateral lower abdominal pain: may be slowly increasing or sudden and severe with abdominal rigidity and referred right shoulder pain

   c. Possible irregular vaginal bleeding or signs of hypovolemic shock if fallopian tube has ruptured; prioritize care accordingly

   d. Laboratory tests: ß-hCG confirms pregnancy

   e. Ultrasound confirms an extrauterine pregnancy

3. Priority nursing diagnoses: Risk for deficient fluid volume; Pain; Fear; Anticipatory grieving

4. Implementation and collaborative care

   a. Monitor blood pressure, pulse, and respiration every 15 minutes or more frequently if indicated by client condition

   b. Start an IV of ordered fluid with at least an 18-gauge needle in case blood products need to be given

   c. Provide oxygen as indicated for shock

   d. Medicate for pain as ordered

   e. Obtain laboratory tests: ß-hCG, CBC, and blood group and type; type and cross-match if hemorrhage is suspected

   f. Prepare the client for surgery; if possible, the pregnancy will be evacuated and the tube preserved for future fertility if desired

   g. Provide routine preoperative care and teaching; offer emotional support to client and family

   h. Provide general postoperative care; facilitate grieving; provide RhoGAM for Rh-negative mothers with an Rh-positive partner

5. Evaluation: client experiences evacuation of ectopic pregnancy; vital signs remain stable without signs of hypovolemic shock; fertility is preserved as desired; client and family begin grieving for their loss

## C. Gestational trophoblastic disease (hydatiform mole)

1. Description and etiology: abnormal growth of trophoblastic tissue including the placenta and chorion; molar pregnancy is more common in Japan and Taiwan for unknown reasons

   a. Complete or partial hydatidiform mole or a molar pregnancy is characterized by abnormal development of the placenta; the chorionic villi grow rapidly into fluid-filled, grape-like clusters; a complete mole develops from an empty ovum that contains no maternal genetic material; a partial mole may have an abnormal embryo that usually spontaneously aborts in the first trimester

   b. Abnormal development of the chorion may result in choriocarcinoma, a rapidly growing malignant neoplasm

   c. Twenty percent of women who have had a complete molar pregnancy will develop malignant trophoblastic disease

2. Assessment

   a. Variable vaginal bleeding usually occurs during the first trimester; may be brown, like prune juice, and may contain some grape-like vesicles

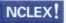

   b. Unusual uterine growth measured by fundal height; no fetal parts can be palpated and no FHT are heard; "snowstorm" pattern seen on ultrasound

   c. Abnormal labs include very high hCG levels and very low MSAFP (maternal serum α-fetoprotein) levels

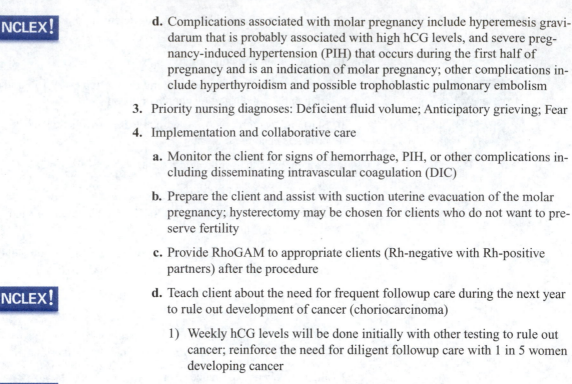

d. Complications associated with molar pregnancy include hyperemesis gravidarum that is probably associated with high hCG levels, and severe pregnancy-induced hypertension (PIH) that occurs during the first half of pregnancy and is an indication of molar pregnancy; other complications include hyperthyroidism and possible trophoblastic pulmonary embolism

3. Priority nursing diagnoses: Deficient fluid volume; Anticipatory grieving; Fear

4. Implementation and collaborative care

   a. Monitor the client for signs of hemorrhage, PIH, or other complications including disseminating intravascular coagulation (DIC)

   b. Prepare the client and assist with suction uterine evacuation of the molar pregnancy; hysterectomy may be chosen for clients who do not want to preserve fertility

   c. Provide RhoGAM to appropriate clients (Rh-negative with Rh-positive partners) after the procedure

   d. Teach client about the need for frequent followup care during the next year to rule out development of cancer (choriocarcinoma)

      1) Weekly hCG levels will be done initially with other testing to rule out cancer; reinforce the need for diligent followup care with 1 in 5 women developing cancer

      2) Client should not become pregnant for 1 year following a molar pregnancy in case chemotherapy is indicated; provide contraceptive counseling

   e. Provide emotional support for the client and family who are grieving the pregnancy loss and living with the fear of developing a malignancy

5. Evaluation: molar pregnancy is identified and evacuated; the client verbalizes the need for follow-up care and uses effective contraception during this period; client remains cancer-free for 1 year

**D. Incompetent cervix**

1. Description and etiology: painless effacement and dilatation of the cervix that is not associated with contractions and usually occurs in the second trimester resulting in spontaneous abortion or very preterm birth; maternal DES (diethylstilbestrol) exposure or congenital uterine anomalies may be associated with incompetent cervix; other possible contributing factors are cervical inflammation or previous cervical trauma

2. Assessment

   a. Previous unexplained second-trimester pregnancy losses may indicate an undiagnosed incompetent cervix

   b. Cervical effacement and dilatation without contractions or pain; client may present for care completely dilated with bulging membranes

3. Priority nursing diagnoses: Risk for injury: fetal; Anticipatory grieving

4. Implementation and collaborative care

   a. Provide emotional support and grief support group referral for the client with pregnancy loss from an incompetent cervix

   **b.** Provide client teaching if the client is to be managed on bedrest at home for a cervix just beginning to efface (shorten)

   **c.** Provide teaching about cervical **cerclage** if this is the treatment method chosen; cerclage is a technique of reinforcing the closure of the cervix with sutures during pregnancy

   **d.** Monitor the cerclage client for signs of preterm labor or infection; client may be placed in Trendelenburg position and be administered tocolytics; provide appropriate nursing assessments and care related to the medication

   **e.** Instruct client to return if contractions begin, as the suture will need to be removed before vaginal birth is accomplished

**5.** Evaluation: the client has cervical cerclage placed without complications; pregnancy is continued until fetal viability is reached

### E. Spontaneous *abortion*

**1.** Description and etiology: spontaneous abortion describes unintended pregnancy loss before 20 weeks gestation; the lay term is "miscarriage"; abortion is the most common cause of bleeding in the first trimester and usually results from chromosomal abnormalities in the embryo; other causes may be teratogen exposure, inadequate implantation, and maternal endocrine disorders or chronic illness; late spontaneous abortion may be the result of incompetent cervix; classification of spontaneous abortion is presented in Box 7-1

**2.** Assessment

   **a.** Vaginal spotting or bleeding is common; client may pass clots and tissue

   **b.** Pelvic cramping or dull backache is usually present

   **c.** Falling hCG levels indicate death of the embryo; ultrasound is used to identify the gestational sac and note whether there is cardiac movement in real-time

**3.** Priority nursing diagnoses: Risk for deficient fluid volume; Anticipatory grieving; Pain

---

**Box 7-1**

**Classification of Spontaneous Abortion**

**Terminology associated with spontaneous abortion helps to classify the clinical condition**

- Threatened abortion: The client experiences vaginal bleeding, but the cervix remains closed. There may be some mild cramping or backache.
- Inevitable abortion: The client experiences cramping and bleeding. The cervix dilates and the membranes may rupture.
- Incomplete abortion: The client experiences bleeding, cramping, and expulsion of part of the products of conception. Tissue remains in the uterus and the cervix is dilated. Hemorrhage is possible.
- Complete abortion: The client experiences bleeding, cramping, and expulsion of all the products of conception. The cervix is closed and the uterus contracts.
- Missed abortion: The client experiences decreasing signs of pregnancy as the fetus has died in utero but not been expelled. The client may be at risk for DIC if the products of conception are not removed.

4. Implementation and collaborative care

   a. Instruct the client with a threatened abortion about bedrest at home and when to return if bleeding or cramping worsen

   b. Assess the amount of bleeding; instruct client to save all clots and tissue that may be passed for further examination

   c. Monitor blood pressure, pulse, and respirations frequently if bleeding is heavy; evaluate client for signs of impending shock

   d. Initiate intravenous therapy with at least an 18-gauge needle as ordered

   e. Assist with dilatation and curettage (D & C) as indicated for an incomplete abortion

   f. Provide emotional support, without false hope, to the client and family; never discount the importance of even a very early pregnancy

   g. Refer to pregnancy-loss or grief support groups

   h. Give RhoGAM to Rh-negative clients with Rh-positive partners within 72 hours of abortion

5. Evaluation: pregnancy is either maintained or products of conception are expelled without further complication; client and family are assisted to mourn the pregnancy loss

### F. *Placenta previa*

1. Description and etiology: the placenta is abnormally implanted near to or over the internal cervical os; as the cervix softens and begins to efface and dilate, placental sinuses are opened causing progressive hemorrhages

   a. May be a low implantation near the cervix (Figure 7-1a), a partial previa covering a part of the os (Figure 7-1b), or a complete placenta previa which covers the entire internal cervical os (Figure 7-1c)

   b. Incidence of placenta previa is higher with multiple gestation and multiparity

   c. Delivery of a client with a complete previa is by cesarean section, usually with a classical uterine incision to avoid the placenta

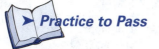

**► Practice to Pass**

A client is admitted with the diagnosis of "threatened spontaneous abortion." What would you teach this client about her condition? The client's symptoms continue and she experiences a complete abortion. What communication techniques would be appropriate at this time?

**NCLEX!**

---

**Figure 7-1**

Placenta previa. A. Low placental implantation, B. Partial placenta previa, C. Complete placenta previa.

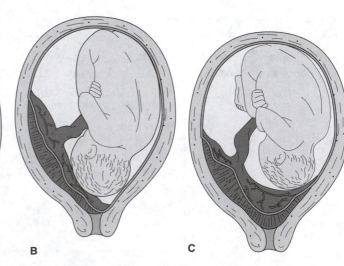

A          B          C

d. Vaginal birth may be possible with a low-lying placenta if the fetal head is down to press against the placenta and occlude the sinuses

2. Assessment

a. Episodic painless vaginal bleeding after the 20th week of pregnancy without contractions; each successive bleeding episode is usually heavier than the last; profuse hemorrhage may occur as the cervix dilates under the placenta

b. Ultrasound identification of placental location

3. Priority nursing diagnoses: Risk for deficient fluid volume; Risk for injury; Fear

4. Implementation and collaborative care

a. Never perform a vaginal exam on a pregnant client presenting with painless vaginal bleeding as this may create profuse hemorrhage

b. Assist with a double setup procedure if indicated: the physician performs a careful vaginal exam in the operating room with equipment and staff ready to perform either a cesarean or a vaginal delivery depending on whether the bleeding is caused by placenta previa or is the increased bloody show of advanced labor

c. Preterm clients should be maintained on bedrest with bathroom privileges until fetal maturity is reached or until hemorrhage is such that cesarean delivery is imperative

d. Monitor maternal vital signs to rule out ascending infection or shock

e. Assess blood loss by weighing peripads and bed pads that are bloody; one gram equals one milliliter (1g = 1 mL)

f. Monitor serial hemoglobin and hematocrit levels; obtain blood group and type, cross-match as needed

g. Monitor fetal well-being with continuous or intermittent monitoring and other testing as indicated

h. Maintain IV access with at least an 18-gauge needle and provide replacement fluids as ordered

i. Provide emotional support to the client on bedrest; facilitate family visits

j. Promote adequate nutrition with prenatal vitamins and iron as needed to prevent maternal anemia

k. Provide routine pre- and post-operative cesarean care if indicated; instruct the client about the location of the uterine incision as it relates to future desire for a vaginal birth after cesarean (VBAC)

5. Evaluation: bleeding does not become excessive; client's vital signs remain stable; client delivers a healthy mature newborn

G. *Abruptio placenta*

1. Description and etiology: premature separation of the placenta away from the uterine wall during pregnancy

a. The placenta may separate only at the margins, causing vaginal bleeding but perhaps little pain (see Figure 7-2a)

**Figure 7-2**

Abruptio placenta.
A. Marginal abruption
with external
hemorrhage, B. Central
abruption with
concealed hemorrhage,
C. Complete separation.

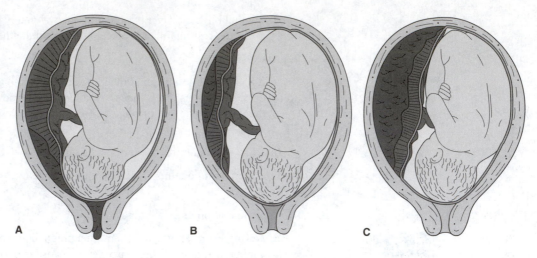

A                                 B                                 C

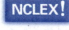

    **b.** A central (concealed) abruption may not result in vaginal bleeding but does cause increasing uterine irritability and tenderness see (Figure 7-2b)

    **c.** A complete (100 percent) separation from the uterine wall results in profuse hemorrhage (Figure 7-2c)

    **d.** Most common identified precipitating factors are maternal hypertension, cocaine abuse, and abdominal trauma

    **e.** The client with an abruptio placenta is at increased risk of depleting clotting factors and developing disseminating intravascular coagulopathy (DIC)

**2.** Assessment

    **a.** A painful, rigid, board-like abdomen with vaginal bleeding is the classic sign of abruptio placenta; the abdomen may increase in size as bleeding continues; ultrasound confirms the diagnosis

    **b.** A central abruption causes severe pain from bleeding behind the placenta distending the uterine muscle but there may be little or no vaginal bleeding; the uterus is very irritable and the fetus shows consistent late decelerations

    **c.** Bleeding behind the placenta is forced into the myometrium and may result in a Couvelaire uterus; the uterus becomes bluish-purple, extremely irritable, distended, and rigid; the uterus does not contract efficiently after delivery leading to postpartum hemorrhage

    **d.** Marginal placental abruption may present with more vaginal bleeding but less pain than a concealed abruption

    **e.** Fetal outcome depends on the degree of placental separation and maturity of the fetus at the time of birth

**3.** Priority nursing diagnoses: Deficient fluid volume; Risk for injury; Risk for impaired gas exchange

**4.** Implementation and collaborative care

    **a.** Monitor maternal blood pressure, pulse, and respiration for signs of impending shock

b. Monitor fetus continuously for signs of distress: increased fetal movement, decreased FHR variability, changes in baseline FHR, late decelerations

c. Assess client for bleeding, uterine activity, and abdominal pain; place on external fetal monitor to evaluate uterine irritability and fetal well-being; palpate uterine tone

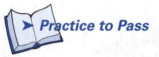

d. Measure client's abdominal girth at the umbilicus for baseline size and repeat periodically to evaluate occult bleeding

e. Review lab values to estimate blood loss (hemoglobin and hematocrit) and monitor for the potential development of disseminating intravascular coagulation (platelets, fibrinogen, fibrin degradation products, PT, and PTT)

f. Monitor client for signs of developing coagulation defects: unusual bleeding from injection sites, gums, development of petechiae

g. Start and maintain IV fluids with at least an 18-gauge needle; monitor intake and output; a Foley catheter may be inserted with expected urine output of 30 mL/hour or greater

h. Provide oxygen as indicated at 8 to 12 L/min via tight face-mask

i. Carefully monitor the client and fetus if vaginal delivery is attempted; prepare for an emergency cesarean delivery if the fetus develops distress

j. Provide ongoing information and emotional support for client and family

5. Evaluation: maternal blood loss is minimized and fetal well-being is maintained; the client delivers a healthy infant without further complications

**H. Premature rupture of the membranes**

1. Description and etiology

a. Premature rupture of membranes refers to amniotic membrane rupture before labor begins; labor will usually begin spontaneously within 24 hours of membrane rupture

b. Preterm rupture of membranes refers to membrane rupture prior to term gestation or before 38 weeks; risk factors for preterm membrane rupture include infection, incompetent cervix, and trauma

c. Prolonged rupture of membranes refers to membranes ruptured more than 12 hours before birth; many caregivers will induce labor rather than risk prolonged rupture with possible ascending infection

2. Assessment

a. Gush of watery, clear, or meconium-stained fluid from the vagina with continued leakage

b. Amniotic fluid turns nitrazine paper blue indicating an alkaline pH; urine is almost always acidic and doesn't change the yellow color of nitrazine paper

c. Amniotic fluid shows characteristic ferning pattern on microscopic examination of a slide with dried fluid on it; urine and vaginal secretions do not display ferning

d. The unengaged fetus is at risk for a prolapsed cord when the membranes rupture

**Practice to Pass**

A client at 37 weeks gestation has been in an automobile accident. She was wearing her seatbelt and is uninjured but complains of shoulder and abdominal pain. What assessments and interventions would you implement for this client?

3. Priority nursing diagnoses: Risk for infection; Anxiety; Risk for injury

4. Implementation and collaborative care

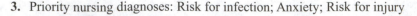

   **a.** Assess FHR when membranes rupture to rule out prolapsed cord; note time, color, and amount of fluid; obtain a baseline maternal temperature

   **b.** Evaluate client's temperature every 2 hours, other vital signs may be routine

   **c.** Avoid vaginal exams to prevent introduction of microorganisms that may cause an ascending infection

   **d.** Monitor for development of uterine contractions and evaluate fetal well-being; decreased amniotic fluid may cause variable decelerations of the FHT

   **e.** Monitor client for signs of **chorioamnionitis** (inflammation and infection of fetal membranes and amniotic fluid): elevated temperature, abdominal tenderness, increased WBCs and erythrocyte sedimentation rate

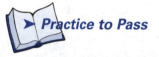
**► Practice to Pass**

   **f.** Obtain vaginal culture for group B streptococcus as ordered

   **g.** Provide client teaching and reassurance that amniotic fluid is continuously produced and that there is no such thing as a "dry birth"

You are caring for a gravida 6 para 5 who calls you into the bathroom where you discover the cord protruding from her vagina. Discuss your nursing actions.

   **h.** Administer antibiotics if ordered; some caregivers prefer to wait and treat the newborn

5. Evaluation: client and fetus remain infection-free; umbilical cord does not prolapse; client delivers a healthy infant without complications associated with prematurity

**I. Pregnancy-induced hypertension (PIH)**

1. Description and etiology: hypertensive disorder that begins during pregnancy; the etiology is unknown, but preeclampsia is associated with vasospasm and vascular endothelial damage; the condition is more common in young primigravidas, women over 35, multiple gestation, diabetes mellitus, and hydatidiform mole; the PIH client is at risk for CVA, DIC, renal failure, and hepatic rupture

   **a.** Gestational hypertension is high blood pressure that occurs during pregnancy and resolves after delivery; it is not associated with proteinuria or edema

   **b.** Preeclampsia is characterized by a triad of symptoms: hypertension of greater than 140/90 or an increase from pre-pregnancy blood pressure greater than 30 mmHg systolic or 15 mmHg diastolic, proteinuria, and edema

   **c.** Eclampsia is the term used to describe preeclampsia that has progressed to include maternal tonic-clonic seizures

   **d.** HELLP syndrome may be associated with PIH; symptoms include hemolysis, elevated liver enzymes, and a low platelet count; the client is at risk for hemorrhage, pulmonary edema, and hepatic rupture

2. Assessment: symptoms usually develop during the third trimester except in cases of gestational trophoblastic disease (hydatidiform mole); the client is at risk for seizures and other complications up to 48 hours after delivery

   a. Mild preeclampsia: hypertension of 140/90 or increase of 30/15 from baseline, proteinuria trace to +1, mild to moderate pretibial edema with weight gain of 2 to 2.5 pounds/week

   b. Severe preeclampsia: hypertension greater than 160/110, proteinuria 3+ to 4+ or more than 5 g in a 24-hour urine specimen, sudden large weight gain with facial edema, pitting pretibial edema and possible signs of central nervous system (CNS) irritation

   c. Systemic responses: CNS irritability causes severe or continuous headache, hyperreflexia (greater than +2, baseline, or clonus), or visual disturbance (blurred vision, seeing spots or flashing lights); renal damage is indicated by oliguria (less than 30 cc/hr); portal hypertension may result in epigastric pain and may precede hepatic rupture

   d. Lab values: increased hematocrit (as fluid moves out of the intravascular space), serum uric acid and BUN; increased liver enzymes (ALT, AST); decreased RBCs and platelets as condition worsens

3. Priority nursing diagnoses: Deficient fluid volume; Risk for injury; Anxiety

4. Implementation and collaborative care: the only cure for PIH is delivery; the goal of care is to deliver a healthy, viable infant while safeguarding the mother's health

   a. Bedrest at home is indicated if preeclampsia is mild; hospitalization if severe until fetus is mature enough to be delivered; bedrest on left side, to facilitate uteroplacental perfusion

   b. A quiet, calm environment is maintained to decrease CNS stimulation; siderails should be up and padded for clients with severe preeclampsia who are at risk of progressing to seizures

   c. A high-protein diet without salt restriction is indicated; restricting salt intake may result in hypovolemia and fetal distress; diuretics should not be used for the same reason

   d. Implement frequent assessments (every 15 minutes to 1 to 4 hours as indicated by client condition) to include blood pressure, pulse, and respirations, edema, deep tendon reflexes, and clonus checks; assess client for headache, visual disturbances, and epigastric pain

   e. Foley catheter is inserted to monitor renal function, strict intake and output; evaluate urine for protein; assess daily weight

   f. Monitor fetal well-being by continuous EFM, serial NSTs, BPP, or amniocentesis as indicated

   g. Administer magnesium sulfate as ordered for seizure prevention; monitor client for signs of magnesium toxicity

      1) Monitor magnesium blood levels: 5 to 8 mg/dL is therapeutic range

      2) Decreased urine output (less than 30 cc/hr) can increase the risk for toxicity as magnesium sulfate is excreted by the kidneys

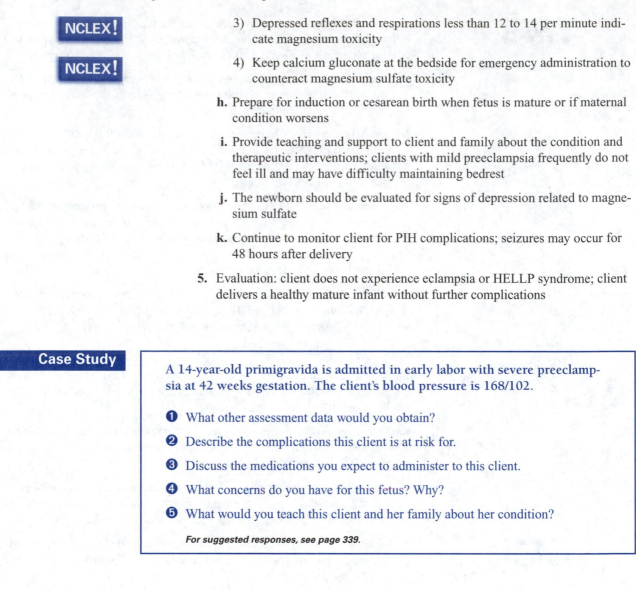

**NCLEX!**

**NCLEX!**

3) Depressed reflexes and respirations less than 12 to 14 per minute indicate magnesium toxicity

4) Keep calcium gluconate at the bedside for emergency administration to counteract magnesium sulfate toxicity

**h.** Prepare for induction or cesarean birth when fetus is mature or if maternal condition worsens

**i.** Provide teaching and support to client and family about the condition and therapeutic interventions; clients with mild preeclampsia frequently do not feel ill and may have difficulty maintaining bedrest

**j.** The newborn should be evaluated for signs of depression related to magnesium sulfate

**k.** Continue to monitor client for PIH complications; seizures may occur for 48 hours after delivery

**5.** Evaluation: client does not experience eclampsia or HELLP syndrome; client delivers a healthy mature infant without further complications

**Case Study**

A 14-year-old primigravida is admitted in early labor with severe preeclampsia at 42 weeks gestation. The client's blood pressure is 168/102.

❶ What other assessment data would you obtain?

❷ Describe the complications this client is at risk for.

❸ Discuss the medications you expect to administer to this client.

❹ What concerns do you have for this fetus? Why?

❺ What would you teach this client and her family about her condition?

*For suggested responses, see page 339.*

# Posttest

**1** A client at 10 weeks gestation, who has recently emigrated from Japan, comes to the prenatal clinic because she is having some dark brown vaginal spotting and is experiencing severe nausea and vomiting. What condition do these symptoms suggest?

(1) Gestational trophoblastic disease
(2) Hyperemesis gravidarum
(3) Placenta previa
(4) Pregnancy-induced psychosis

**2** A client who experienced an incompetent cervix with a previous pregnancy has had a Shirodkar cerclage procedure done at 18 weeks in the current pregnancy. The client calls the clinic at 37 weeks because she is having irregular contractions every 5 to 7 minutes. Which response by the nurse is most appropriate?

(1) "You need to go to the hospital to have the cerclage removed before your baby is born."
(2) "You should wait and come in when the contractions are closer and harder."
(3) "You sound like you are worried about this baby. It must be frightening for you."
(4) "You will need to have a cesarean birth with the Shirodkar cerclage in place."

**3** A client with no prenatal care presents to the labor and delivery unit with a moderate amount of vaginal bleeding and complaints of severe abdominal pain. Fundal height is 34 centimeters. Contractions are every 1.5 minutes lasting 60 seconds and strong with increasing resting tone. The monitor shows consistent late decelerations. What information from the nursing assessment would be most consistent with a risk for placental abruption?

(1) The client admits to using cocaine.
(2) The client has had no prenatal care.
(3) The client is HIV-positive.
(4) The client is poor and uneducated.

**4** A client is hospitalized on the antepartum unit with premature rupture of membranes at 37 weeks gestation. Which of the following routine physician orders would the nurse alter for this client?

(1) Bedrest with bathroom privileges
(2) Diet as tolerated
(3) External fetal monitor prn
(4) Vital signs every shift

**5** Which of the following laboratory tests is least important related to the current condition of a newborn of an HIV-positive mother?

(1) Bilirubin level
(2) Blood glucose level
(3) ELISA testing
(4) Hematocrit

**6** A client with heart disease has been prescribed digoxin (Lanoxin) during her pregnancy. The nurse evaluates that client teaching has been effective when the client states:

(1) "I will avoid eating foods high in potassium while taking this medication."
(2) "I will check my pulse and not take the medication if it is less than 60."
(3) "I will not take antibiotics at the same time as this medication."
(4) "I will take this medication with a full glass of water before breakfast."

**7** A 34-year-old client comes to the emergency room with cramping and vaginal bleeding. She has missed two menstrual periods. Which of the following statements by the nurse is most appropriate when the client is diagnosed with an incomplete abortion?

(1) "I am so sorry. This must be difficult for you."
(2) "The doctor will clean out your womb with a D and C."
(3) "Were you really wanting to be pregnant now?"
(4) "You'll still be able to have children after this is over."

**8** A client with pre-eclampsia is receiving magnesium sulfate and oxytocin (Pitocin) IV to induce labor at 38 weeks. What is the main indication of the magnesium sulfate for this client?

(1) Lower blood pressure
(2) Prevent convulsions
(3) Provide sedation
(4) Soften stools

**9** Which of the following complications of pregnancy would be most consistent with development of a sinusoidal fetal heart rate pattern during labor?

(1) Abruptio placenta
(2) Chorioamnionitis
(3) Pregnancy-induced hypertension
(4) Prolapsed cord

**10** A client who admits to substance abuse during pregnancy tells the nurse, "I know I am just a really weak person, but I will try to cut down while I'm pregnant." Which response by the nurse would be most therapeutic?

(1) "I am concerned about you and your baby. What can I do to help you?"
(2) "I don't believe that you are weak at all. You just need to say no to drugs."
(3) "I have heard that before. You need to get serious now or your baby will suffer."
(4) "That is a very positive plan. Could you tell me more about feeling like a weak person?"

*See pages 165–166 for Answers and Rationales.*

## Answers and Rationales

### Pretest

**1** **Answer: 3** *Rationale:* Anemia increases the cardiac workload and should be avoided by clients with heart disease. The client should discuss medications with her caregiver, but she may be allowed to take acetaminophen or a few other OTC medications. The client with Class II cardiac disease is slightly compromised with ordinary activity levels and would not tolerate exercise. There is a 2 to 4 percent chance that the baby will inherit a congenital defect.
*Cognitive Level:* Analysis
*Nursing Process:* Implementation; *Test Plan:* HPM

**2** **Answer: 1** *Rationale:* The placenta produces human placental lactogen (hPL) and increased amounts of estrogen and progesterone. These hormones interfere with maternal glucose metabolism and require increased insulin production or supplementation. As soon as the placenta is expelled, these hormone levels fall dramatically and the mother may require no insulin at all or a very reduced dose in the first 24 hours.
*Cognitive Level:* Analysis
*Nursing Process:* Planning; *Test Plan:* PHYS

**3** **Answer: 2** *Rationale:* The glycosylated hemoglobin ($HbA_{1c}$) test provides an indication of what glucose levels have been over the last 4 to 8 week lifespan of the red blood cells. Increased blood glucose levels will be reflected in an increased percentage of $HbA_{1c}$. The other tests indicate current blood glucose levels only.
*Cognitive Level:* Application
*Nursing Process:* Analysis; *Test Plan:* HPM

**4** **Answer: 3** *Rationale:* Pregnancy presents an ideal time for nurses to reach out to substance-abusing clients in a caring way since the client herself recognizes that she and her baby will benefit from prenatal care. Option 1 is unrealistic, option 2 is punitive, and option 4 is judgmental.
*Cognitive Level:* Application
*Nursing Process:* Analysis; *Test Plan:* HPM

**5** **Answer: 2** *Rationale:* The client with a suspected ectopic pregnancy may be at risk for the development of hypovolemic shock. Assessment is the first step of the nursing process and airway, breathing, and circulation are the priorities. Options 1 and 4 are possible later interventions, and option 3 is the surgeon's responsibility.
*Cognitive Level:* Application
*Nursing Process:* Implementation; *Test Plan:* PHYS

**6** **Answer: 3** *Rationale:* The client requires frequent monitoring to rule out development of malignancy after experiencing trophoblastic gestational disease. Weekly hCG measurements are done until normal levels are recorded for 3 weeks. Option 2 is a possibility for this client. The client should use contraception for at least 1 year during the follow-up care (option 4), and expressions of sadness are appropriate for any pregnancy loss, even if no fetus developed (option 1).
*Cognitive Level:* Application
*Nursing Process:* Evaluation; *Test Plan:* HPM

**7** **Answer: 3** *Rationale:* The registered nurse is responsible for client assessments (options 2 and 4) and for client teaching (option 1). The intervention of helping the client to the bathroom is within the practice abilities of a nursing assistant if the RN has determined that it is safe for this client to get out of bed.
*Cognitive Level:* Analysis
*Nursing Process:* Implementation; *Test Plan:* SECE

**8** **Answer: 3** *Rationale:* One mL of blood weighs approximately 1 g. The other responses are incorrect.
*Cognitive Level:* Application
*Nursing Process:* Assessment; *Test Plan:* PHYS

**9** **Answer: 2** *Rationale:* The client with hyperemesis gravidarum is anxious or even fearful about the effects of her condition on the fetus. The etiology of hyperemesis is unknown but the incidence is increased in conditions with increased hCG. There may be an

emotional component, but there is no indication that this is an unwanted pregnancy. With appropriate treatment, the prognosis is favorable for the fetus. The client experiences excessive vomiting and would have the diagnosis of Imbalanced nutrition: less than body requirements.
*Cognitive Level:* Application
*Nursing Process:* Planning; *Test Plan:* PSYC

**10  Answer: 1  *Rationale:*** The Rh-negative client whose partner is Rh-positive may carry an Rh-positive fetus and would be at risk for Rh-sensitization which could create risks for future pregnancies. This father of the baby needs to have his blood type assessed. The client is not anemic based on these hemoglobin and hematocrit values so options 2 and 4 are false. There is no relationship between the lab values and the client's weight in this scenario (option 3).
*Cognitive Level:* Analysis
*Nursing Process:* Implementation; *Test Plan:* HPM

## Posttest

**1  Answer: 1  *Rationale:*** The client has three risk factors of molar pregnancy; Japanese background, brownish "prune juice" vaginal bleeding, and the severe nausea and vomiting associated with excessive hCG found in trophoblastic disease. The client has only one symptom of hyperemesis; placenta previa presents with bright red bleeding; and there is no information suggestive of psychosis.
*Cognitive Level:* Analysis
*Nursing Process:* Analysis; *Test Plan:* PHYS

**2  Answer: 1  *Rationale:*** The Shirodkar cerlage is closure of the cervix with suture material to prevent preterm dilatation. When labor ensues, the suture must be cut so the fetus can pass through the birth canal. Waiting for harder contractions will increase the likelihood of cervical damage from the suture. Option 3 does not address the client's risk, which is the priority. Clients who expect to have several future pregnancies may be delivered by cesarean to avoid repeated cerclage, but there is no necessity to this option.
*Cognitive Level:* Application
*Nursing Process:* Implementation; *Test Plan:* PHYS

**3  Answer: 1  *Rationale:*** The risk for placental abruption is increased with cocaine abuse. The other factors make the client high risk for complications of pregnancy but not particularly for abruptio.
*Cognitive Level:* Application
*Nursing Process:* Assessment; *Test Plan:* PHYS

**4  Answer: 4  *Rationale:*** The client with ruptured membranes prior to the beginning of labor is at increased risk for ascending infection (chorioamnionitis.) The client's temperature should be taken every 2 to 4 hours to identify early signs of sepsis.
*Cognitive Level:* Analysis
*Nursing Process:* Implementation; *Test Plan:* SECE

**5  Answer: 3  *Rationale:*** The infant of an HIV positive mother will test positive on an ELISA test for the human immunodeficieny virus because the maternal antibodies cross the placenta during pregnancy. This does not indicate that the newborn has HIV. The diagnosis for the baby is not made until around 15 months when maternal antibodies are degraded. The other tests give information about the infant's current condition.
*Cognitive Level:* Analysis
*Nursing Process:* Analysis; *Test Plan:* PHYS

**6  Answer: 2  *Rationale:*** Digoxin is a cardiac glycoside that increases cardiac output by increasing the strength of contraction of the myocardium and slowing the heart rate. A pulse rate of less than 60 is a serious adverse effect of the medication and the dose should be held. The client needs adequate potassium for myocardial function. Antibiotics are not contraindicated with digoxin. The drug may be given with or without food.
*Cognitive Level:* Analysis
*Nursing Process:* Evaluation; *Test Plan:* PHYS

**7  Answer: 1  *Rationale:*** The nurse should provide emotional support to all clients experiencing perinatal loss. The other answers are insensitive, and option 4 may not be true.
*Cognitive Level:* Analysis
*Nursing Process:* Implementation; *Test Plan:* PSYC

**8  Answer: 2  *Rationale:*** Magnesium sulfate is a CNS depressant used to prevent convulsions in the preeclamptic client. The other options may occur but are not the indication for the drug.
*Cognitive Level:* Analysis
*Nursing Process:* Implementation; *Test Plan:* PHYS

**9  Answer: 1  *Rationale:*** A sinusoidal fetal heart rhythm is associated with fetal anemia, which may be associated with an abruption. The other complications would result in other signs of fetal distress such as tachycardia, loss of variability, and late decelerations.
*Cognitive Level:* Analysis
*Nursing Process:* Assessment; *Test Plan:* PHYS

10   **Answer: 4** *Rationale:*   Option 4 is the only answer that acknowledges the client's intent to cut down on substance abuse while seeking additional information about the client's self-concept. Option 1 places the emphasis on the nurse while options 2 and 3 are demeaning and negative.
*Cognitive Level:* Application
*Nursing Process:* Assessment; *Test Plan:* PSYC

# References

Cunningham, F. G., MacDonald, P. C., Gant, N. F., Loveno, K. J., Gilstrap, L. C., III., Hankins, G. D.V., & Clark, S. L. (1997). *Williams obstetrics* (20th ed.). Stamford, CT: Appleton & Lange.

Kozier, B., Erb, G., Berman, A., & Burke, K. (2000). *Fundamentals of nursing: Concepts, process, and practice* (6th ed.). Upper Saddle River, NJ: Prentice-Hall, Inc.

Luxner, K. (1999). *Maternal-infant nursing care plans.* Englewood, CO: Skidmore-Roth.

Murray, M. (1997). *Antepartal and intrapartal fetal monitoring* (2nd ed.). Albuquerque, NM: Learning Resources International, Inc.

Olds, S. B., London, M. L., & Ladewig, P. A. W. (2000). *Maternal-newborn nursing: A family and community-based approach* (6th ed.). Upper Saddle River, NJ: Prentice-Hall, Inc., pp. 351–420, 526, 634, 640.

Sherwen, L. N., Scoloveno, M. A., & Weingarten, C. T. (1999). *Maternity nursing:Care of the childbearing family* (3rd ed.). Stamford, CT: Appleton & Lange, p. 597.

Smith, S. F., Duell, D. J., & Martin, B. C. (2000). *Clinical nursing skills: Basic to advanced skills* (5th ed.). Upper Saddle River, NJ: Prentice-Hall, Inc., pp. 40–41.

Wilkerson. J. M. (2000). *Nursing diagnosis handbook with NIC interventions and NOC outcomes.* Upper Saddle River, NJ: Prentice-Hall, Inc.

Wilson, B. A., Shannon, M. T., & Stang, C. L (2001). *Prentice Hall nursing drug guide 2001.* Upper Saddle River, NJ: Prentice-Hall, Inc.

Wong, D. L. & Perry, S. E. (1998). *Maternal child nursing care.* St Louis: Mosby, Inc.

## CHAPTER 8

# The Normal Labor and Delivery Experience

Pamela Hamre, RN, CNM, MS

## CHAPTER OUTLINE

*Nursing Care of the Labor and*
*Delivery Client*

*The Labor Process*
*The Stages of Labor*

*Pain Management during Birth*

## OBJECTIVES

▌ Describe the nursing care needed during each of the four stages of labor.

▌ Describe the process of labor in terms of the passenger, passageway, powers, and psyche.

▌ Explain the cardinal movements of the fetus during delivery.

▌ Identify nursing responsibilities during the administration of analgesia and anesthesia.

[ *Media Link* ]

*Use the CD-ROM enclosed with this text, or log onto the address given to access the free, interactive Companion Website created for this series. The CD-ROM and Companion Website accompanying this book offer additional practice opportunities and information—NCLEX Review, Case Studies, Glossary, In Depth with NCLEX, and more.*

**www.prenhall.com/hogan**

## REVIEW AT A GLANCE

**accelerations** *transient increases in the fetal heart rate accompanying contractions or fetal movement*

**Apgar score** *assessment of the fetal response to extrauterine life; 0 to 2 points given in each of five areas: color, muscle tone, reflex irritability, respiratory effort, and heart rate*

**attitude** *relationship of the fetal parts to one another*

**baseline fetal heart rate** *average heart rate between contractions; measured in beats per minute (bpm)*

**cardinal movements** *individual adaptations that the fetus undertakes to maneuver through the pelvis during labor and birth*

**crowning** *outward bulging and thinning of the perineal body and opening of the vagina that occurs as the fetal head presses downward onto the perineum*

**dilatation** *opening of the cervix from 1 to 10 centimeters*

**early deceleration** *gradual deceleration in FHR beginning at the onset of a contraction with the return to baseline by the end of the contraction; inversely mirrors contractions; caused by fetal head compression*

**engagement** *the widest diameter of the presenting part has passed through the pelvic inlet*

**effacement** *thinning and shortening of the cervix from 0 to 100 percent*

**epidural block** *very small diameter catheter is inserted into the potential space between the layers of the dura of the lumbar spine and local anesthetic agent is injected to produce labor analgesia or anesthesia*

**episiotomy** *surgical incision into the perineum to enlarge the vaginal opening*

**internal fetal scalp electrode** *fine-spiral wire that is attached to the epidermis of the presenting part to provide a direct ECG of the fetal heart rate*

**intrauterine pressure catheter** *pressure-sensitive device that is inserted through the cervix and past the presenting part into the amniotic fluid in the uterus to measure the intensity of contractions in mm of Hg*

**late deceleration** *deceleration of the FHR that begins after the contraction starts, with the nadir occurring after the peak of the contraction, and returns to baseline after the end of the contraction; caused by utero-placental insufficiency*

**lie** *relationship of the longitudinal axis of the fetus to the longitudinal axis of the mother*

**long-term variability** *cyclical and rhythmic fluctuations in the FHR that occur 2 to 6 times per minute*

**paracervical block** *local anesthetic agent injected into the lateral aspects of the cervix for labor analgesia*

**position** *relationship of the fetal presenting part to the maternal pelvis*

**presentation** *fetal part entering the pelvis first*

**pudendal block** *local anesthetic agent injected near the ischial spines and pudendal nerve for delivery anesthesia*

**short-term variability** *change in rate between one fetal heart beat and the next*

**station** *relationship between the widest diameter of the presenting part and the ischial spines of the maternal pelvis*

**variable deceleration** *decelerations that occur suddenly, have steep sidewalls, return rapidly to baseline and are variable in relationship to contractions; caused by compression of the umbilical cord*

## *Pretest*

**1** The nurse performs a vaginal examination and determines that the fetus is in a sacrum anterior position. This means:

(1) The fetal sacrum is toward the maternal symphysis pubis.
(2) The fetal sacrum is toward the maternal sacrum.
(3) The fetal face is toward the maternal sacrum.
(4) The fetal face is toward the maternal symphysis pubis.

**2** The client has been having contractions every 5 minutes for 7 hours. Which factor is used to determine if this is true or false labor?

(1) The cervix is effacing and dilating.
(2) This is the client's second baby.
(3) The contractions are becoming more intense and lasting longer.
(4) The membranes have ruptured.

**3** The highest priority in nursing care of the laboring client is:

(1) Pain relief measures are offered that are acceptable to the client.
(2) The client's partner is involved with the labor and delivery.
(3) Appropriate fluid intake is monitored.
(4) Fetal response to the labor is assessed.

**4**  As labor progresses, the nurse expects to find contractions becoming:

(1) More intense, less frequent, and of longer duration.
(2) More intense, more frequent, and of longer duration.
(3) Constant in intensity, more frequent, and of shorter duration.
(4) Constant in intensity and frequency, but of shorter duration.

**5**  The neonate is crying, pink except for blue extremities, has flexed arms with clenched hands, a heart rate of 154, and gags when the bulb suction is used. The Apgar score would be:

(1) 10.
(2) 9.
(3) 8.
(4) 7.

**6**  Which of the following nursing observations would indicate a sign of impending placental separation and expulsion?

(1) Steady trickle of blood with an unchanged cord length
(2) No bleeding with lengthening of the cord
(3) Small gush of blood with lengthening of the cord
(4) Small gush of blood with an unchanged cord length

**7**  The nurse determines a laboring client is anxious and recognizes that this may result in:

(1) Rapid progression of labor.
(2) Increased pain during labor.
(3) No reliance on support person.
(4) Need for episiotomy.

**8**  Earlier in the day, the fetal heart rate baseline was 140. It is now 170. One explanation for this could be:

(1) Maternal fever.
(2) Narcotic administration.
(3) Fetal movement.
(4) Utero-placental insufficiency.

**9**  The nurse determines teaching has been effective when a laboring client responds:

(1) "Effacement is the opening of the cervix."
(2) "My cervix will probably efface before it dilates because this is my first pregnancy."
(3) "Effacement is measured from 0 to 10 centimeters."
(4) "My cervix will probably efface and dilate simultaneously because this is my first pregnancy."

**10**  The client's vaginal examination reveals: 3 centimeters dilated, 80 percent effaced, vertex at a −1 station. The woman is talkative and appears excited. The nurse determines the client to be in which stage and phase of labor?

(1) First stage, latent phase
(2) First stage, active phase
(3) Second stage, latent phase
(4) Third stage, transition phase

*See pages 184–185 for Answers and Rationales.*

## I. Nursing Care of the Labor and Delivery Client

**A. Physiologic safety:** the laboring client is actually two clients—the mother and the newborn; nursing care focuses on the physiologic safety of both

**B. Psychological safety:** nursing care also focuses on the pyschological safety of the mother and includes consideration of fear, comfort, partner involvement, parental attachment to the newborn, and past experiences; primigravida women experience fear of the unknown and often have longer labors, while multigravida women can expect a shorter labor with subsequent pregnancies but may have memories of perceived bad experiences from previous births

**C. Maternal history:** must be assessed for abuse, assault, and violence, as these past experiences will often manifest as extreme fear and tension during the labor process or vaginal examinations

**D. Cultural background:** must be assessed and understood in order to provide a safe and acceptable birthing environment for the childbearing family; some common nursing actions may be cultural taboos for a particular client and affect the parents' view of the child throughout life

**E. Preparation for labor by the client and her support person(s):** can vary from formal prenatal education classes to information passed from generation to generation; misconceptions of the birthing process and expectations of the sensations during birth can occur, and should be addressed in a nonjudgmental manner that informs and supports the birthing family

**F. Electronic fetal monitoring:** provides computer-assisted auditory and visual assessment of the fetal heart rate (FHR) and uterine contractions (UC)

1. Fetal heart rate monitoring continuously records the fetal heart rate on the upper portion of the monitor strip

   a. **External monitoring:** an ultrasound transducer is placed over the fetal back and detects movements of the fetal heart; fetal or maternal movement and maternal obesity may interfere with obtaining a continuous reading

   b. **Internal monitoring:** an **internal fetal scalp electrode** is inserted through the cervix (which must be at least 2 cm dilated with ruptured membranes) and attached to the epidermis of the presenting part providing a direct ECG of the fetal heart; unaffected by maternal obesity, maternal or fetal movement; thick fetal hair may prevent adequate insertion on a cephalic presentation

   c. **Baseline fetal heart rate** (FHR) is the average heart rate between contractions; measured in beats per minute (bpm); normal range: 120 to 160, bradycardia: <120, tachycardia: >160.

   d. **Short-term variability:** change in rate between one fetal heart beat and the next; creates a jaggedness or zigzag appearance in the baseline FHR; determined by interplay between the fetal sympathetic and parasympathetic nervous systems; decreased by fetal tachycardia, prematurity, fetal heart and CNS anomalies, and fetal sleep; normal: 2 to 3 bpm; classified as present or absent and can only be evaluated by internal monitoring

   e. **Long-term variability:** rhythmic fluctuations that occur 2 to 6 times per minute; determined by interplay between the fetal sympathetic and parasympathetic nervous systems; increased by fetal movement and decreased by fetal sleep or hypoxia and subsequent acidosis; average or moderate: 6 to 25 bpm

   f. Periodic changes in the FHR are deviations from the baseline separate from the variability which occur in relationship to or independent of contractions.

      1) **Accelerations:** transient increases in the FHR

         a) Non-periodic (spontaneous): symmetric, uniform, not related to contractions, occur in response to fetal movement and indicate fetal well-being

         b) Periodic: occur with contractions and may indicate decreased amniotic fluid or mild umbilical cord compression

2) Decelerations are categorized as early, late, or variable

    a) **Early decelerations:** decrease in FHR beginning at the onset of a contraction and return to baseline by the end of the contraction with the nadir at the acme

        (1) Uniform shape inversely mirrors contraction

        (2) Caused by fetal head compression; usually benign

        (3) Nursing interventions include performing a vaginal examination to determine if the fetus is descending in the pelvis, and if the fetus is not descending, notify the healthcare provider

    b) **Late decelerations** begin after the contraction starts with the nadir occurring after the peak of the contraction and return to baseline after the end of the contraction

        (1) Smooth, uniform shape that inversely mirrors contractions but late in onset and recovery

        (2) Caused by utero-placental insufficiency; always considered ominous

        (3) Nursing interventions focus on maintaining oxygenation and include repositioning the client to left lateral, administering oxygen by mask at 7 to 10 L/min, correcting hypotension through increased IV fluid rate or administration of medications, discontinuing oxytocin if being administered, and reporting to the healthcare provider

    c) **Variable decelerations** occur suddenly, vary in duration and intensity, vary in relation to contractions, and resolve abruptly

        (1) Variable shape, usually "U" or "V," with steep sides; may or may not be associated with contractions

        (2) Caused by compression of the umbilical cord

        (3) Categorized as mild, moderate or severe based on the lowest FHR reading and duration of the deceleration; repetitive, prolonged, or more severe decelerations with a slow return or overshoot to baseline are ominous and indicate fetal asphyxia

        (4) Nursing interventions focus on relieving cord compression through repositioning the client until improvement occurs, vaginal examination to detect prolapsed cord, and oxygen if decelerations are severe or uncorrectable

        (5) Amnio-infusion, the instillation of warmed normal saline through an intrauterine pressure catheter, may be used to recreate the cushioning effect of the umbilical cord during contractions that is normally provided by amniotic fluid

2. Uterine contraction monitoring documents contraction frequency, duration, and intensity; contractions are documented on the lower half of the monitor strip

    a. External monitoring: pressure-sensitive tocodynamometer is placed on the maternal abdomen near the fundus; accurate only for documenting contraction frequency and duration; affected by fetal or maternal movement,

► **Practice to Pass**

The fetal heart rate baseline was 155 bpm prior to the onset of the contraction, decreases to 120 bpm during the contraction, and returns to the baseline 40 seconds after the contraction ends. Describe the nursing interventions the nurse should implement.

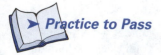

transverse or oblique lie, and maternal abdominal fat: a thin woman's mild contractions may look strong on the monitor strip, while an obese woman's strong contractions may not be detected at all

b. Internal monitoring is accomplished through an **intrauterine pressure catheter** (IUPC), a wire with pressure gauge on one end or a saline-filled tube, which is inserted through the cervix and past the presenting part into the amniotic fluid in the uterus; the increase in intrauterine pressure is detected by the IUPC, and measured in mm of Hg; cervix must be at least 2 to 3 cm dilated with ruptured membranes before an IUPC can be inserted

## II. The Labor Process

**A. Initiation of labor:** comes about from an interplay of factors including the distension of the uterus causing irritability and contractility, and the hormonal influence of prostaglandins, oxytocin, fetal cortisol, estrogen, and progesterone

**B. True versus false labor:** differentiated by cervical change: effacement and dilatation

**C. Factors of labor:** the passageway, passenger, powers, and psyche

1. Passageway refers to the maternal bony pelvis comprised of the two innominate bones (ilium, ischium and pubis), the sacrum and coccyx

   a. The false pelvis lies above the pelvic brim, supports the increasing weight of the enlarging pregnant uterus and directs the presenting part into the true pelvis below

   b. The true pelvis consists of the inlet, the midpelvis, and the outlet and represents the bony limits of the birth canal; the adequacy of each part, measured as transverse and anterior-posterior diameters, must be sufficient to allow passage of the fetus through the passageway

   c. The four pelvic types are gynecoid, android, anthropoid, and platypelloid (see Table 8-1); the type of pelvis and its diameters influence the descent of the fetus, the progression of labor, and the type of delivery

2. Passenger refers to the fetus

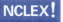

   a. **Attitude** is the relationship of the fetal parts to one another; the normal attitude is flexion of the neck, arms, and legs

| Table 8-1 | | Pelvic Types | | | |
|-----------|-----------|-------|-----------|--------|-----------------------|
| **Pelvic Type** | **Incidence** | **Inlet** | **Midpelvis** | **Outlet** | **Implications for Birth** |
| **Gynecoid** | 50% | Round, adequate diameters | Round, adequate diameters | Wide transverse and long anterior-posterior diameters | Occiput anterior most common, NSVD favorable |
| **Android** | 20% | Heart-shaped, angulated | Short anterior-posterior diameter | Short anterior-posterior diameter | Slow descent, arrest of labor, operative birth more common |
| **Anthropoid** | 25% | Ovoid, long anterior-posterior diameter | Rounded, adequate diameters | Narrow transverse | Occiput anterior or posterior, NSVD favorable |
| **Platypelloid** | 5% | Ovoid, wide transverse diameter | Rounded, wide transverse diameter | Wide transverse, short anterior-posterior diameter | Occiput posterior more common, NSVD not favorable |

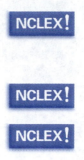

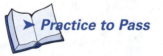

**Practice to Pass**

Describe the attitude, lie, presentation, and position of a fetus listed as frank breech, RSA.

b. **Lie** is the relationship of the longitudinal axis of the fetus to the longitudinal axis of the mother; vertex (head first) is most common, but breech (buttocks first), transverse (laterally across the uterus), and oblique (diagonally across the uterus) lies are possible

c. **Presentation** refers to the fetal part entering the pelvis first; the most common presentation is cephalic, but breech and shoulder can also occur

d. **Position** is the relationship of the fetal presenting part to the maternal pelvis; a three-letter notation is used to describe fetal position

1) R for right or L for left is the first letter, indicating which side of the maternal pelvis the presenting part is toward

2) The second letter indicates the landmark of the fetal presenting part: O = occiput, M = mentum, S = sacrum, or A = acromion process.

3) The third letter indicates the relationship of the landmark of the presenting part to the front, back or side of the pelvis: A = anterior P = posterior, T = transverse; the most common positions at delivery are ROA or LOA

e. **Engagement** occurs when the largest diameter of the presenting part reaches the pelvic inlet and can be detected by vaginal examination

1) If the presenting part is directed toward the pelvis but can easily be moved out of the inlet, it is floating

2) When the presenting part dips into the inlet but can be displaced with upward pressure from the examiner's fingers, it is ballotable

3) If the presenting part is fixed in the pelvic inlet and cannot be displaced, it is engaged

f. **Station** is the relationship of the presenting part to the ischial spines of the pelvis; measured in centimeters above (−1 to −5 station), at (0 station), or below (+1 to +4 station) the ischial spines (see Figure 8-1)

3. Powers include the primary and secondary forces of labor

a. Primary forces consist of the involuntary contractions of the uterine muscle fibers, which are stimulated by a pacemaker located in the upper uterine segment

1) Contractions consist of the increment (building-up phase), acme (peak), and the decrement (letting-up phase) and are followed by a resting phase (nadir) to facilitate utero-placental-fetal reoxygenation

2) Frequency of contractions is the time in seconds or minutes from the onset of one contraction to the onset of the next contraction

3) Intensity is the strength of the contraction at the acme, which can be palpated as mild, moderate, or strong, or detected with a fetal monitor externally or measured internally in mm Hg

4) Duration is the length of the contraction measured in seconds from the beginning of the increment to the end of the decrement

5) With each contraction the muscles of the upper uterine segment shorten and exert longitudinal traction on the cervix causing **effacement,**

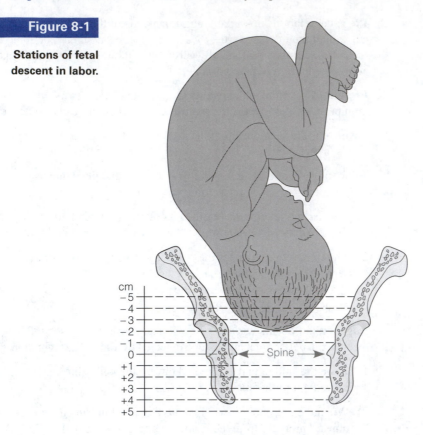

**Figure 8-1**

**Stations of fetal descent in labor.**

cm
−5
−4
−3
−2
−1
0 ← Spine →
+1
+2
+3
+4
+5

the thinning and drawing up of the internal os and cervical canal into the uterine side walls; measured from 0 to 100 percent; in primigravidas effacement usually precedes dilatation; in multigravidas effacement and dilatation normally occur simultaneously

6) As the uterus elongates with contractions, the fetal body straightens and exerts pressure against the lower uterine segment and cervix; **dilatation,** or opening of the cervix, results, is measured from 0 to 10 cm, and allows for the birth of the fetus

b) Secondary powers consist of the voluntary use of abdominal muscles during the second stage of labor to facilitate the descent and delivery of the fetus

4. Psyche represents the psychological component of childbearing; excitement, fear, perceived loss of control, and anxiety are common emotions during the labor and birth process

a. Extreme emotions such as fear will result in muscular tension, which can create more pain from friction between the working uterus and tense abdominal muscles, or impede the descent of the fetus when pelvic and perineal muscles are tense rather than relaxed when pushing

b. The psyche can also be manifested physiologically as changes in maternal vital signs; increased blood pressure, pulse, and respiratory rates occur with fear, excitement, and anxiety

c. Lack of knowledge and preparation for childbirth can negatively affect the psyche

### III. The Stages of Labor

**A. First stage:** extends from the onset of true labor to complete dilatation of the cervix (0 to 10 cm) and is divided into three phases

1. Latent phase: 0 to 3 centimeters dilated, little descent occurs; contractions usually begin irregularly and become more regular, with frequency becoming closer, duration increasing, and intensity increasing from mild to moderate; the woman is usually relieved labor has started, able to recognize and express anxiety, happy, excited, and talkative, and changes position without reminder; average length for nullipara is 8.6 hours and 5.3 hours for multiparas

2. Active phase: 4 to 7 centimeters dilated, effacement and descent are progressive, contractions usually every 2 to 3 minutes, 60 seconds in duration, and moderate to strong intensity; the woman is usually serious, intense, has a need for increased concentration, and will answer questions in short phrases only between contractions; fatigue increases and the woman becomes more dependent; pain increases, relaxation becomes more difficult, and the woman may need reminders to change positions; average length for nulliparas is 4.6 hours and 2.4 hours for multiparas

3. Transition phase: 8 to 10 centimeters dilated, effacement is completed, and descent increases; contractions every 1½ to 2 minutes, lasting 60 to 90 seconds, strong intensity; the woman is working hard with intense concentration and will give one-word answers to questions only between contractions; anxiety increases, fears loss of control and abandonment, senses helplessness and may state "I can't do this anymore"; relaxation is difficult as contraction time exceeds the resting phase between contractions; may experience intense low abdominal, pelvic, and rectal discomfort from descent of the fetus; nausea and vomiting are common; may need reminders to empty bladder and change position; average length for nulliparas is 3.6 hours and 30 minutes for multiparas

4. Assessment

   a. Upon admission: review of medical, obstetric and prenatal history; labor status (contractions, vaginal examination if indicated), fetal status (heart rate, variability, periodic changes), status of membranes (intact or if ruptured, length of time and amount, color, odor), maternal vital signs, laboratory testing if ordered (Hgb and UA), desired birth plan including cultural considerations, preparation for childbirth, level of comfort and coping, and support system

   b. First stage of labor

      1) Latent phase: blood pressure, pulse, respirations q1h if normal; temperature q4h if normal or membranes intact, if abnormal or membranes ruptured q2h; contractions q30 min; FHR q1hr for low-risk women or q30min if high-risk or non-reassuring pattern

      2) Active phase: blood pressure, pulse, respirations, temperature, contractions same as latent phase; FHR q30min for low-risk women or q15min for high-risk women or non-reassuring pattern

      3) Transition phase: blood pressure, pulse, respirations q30min; temperature same as latent phase; contractions q15min, FHR q15min

5.  Priority nursing diagnoses: Anxiety; Fear; Deficient knowledge; Pain; Compromised family coping

6.  Implementation and collaborative care

    a.  Orient to environment, expected assessments, and procedures

    b.  Encourage ambulation (if presenting part is engaged) unless contraindicated

    c.  Provide comfort through frequent position change, effluerage, focal point, hydrotherapy, caregiver presence, therapeutic touch, sacral pressure, back rub, or administration of analgesia as requested by client and ordered by healthcare provider

    d.  Encourage voiding q2h

    e.  Monitor labor progress and fetal well-being

    f.  Provide ice chips and clear liquids to prevent dehydration

    g.  Teach, reinforce, or support use of relaxation, visualization, or breathing patterns

    h.  Encourage rest between contractions

    i.  Document in the client record and provide continuing status reports to healthcare provider

7.  Evaluation: client states she is able to cope with contractions; maternal and fetal well-being is maintained throughout labor

B.  **Second stage:** extends from complete dilatation of the cervix to delivery of the fetus; accompanied by involuntary efforts to expel the fetus characterized by low-pitched, guttural, grunting sounds; many women initially feel renewed energy because they can voluntarily work with the contractions to push out the fetus; over time can be exhaustingly hard work; normal length for nulliparas is up to 3 hours and up to 30 minutes for multiparas

1.  **Cardinal movements** are the adaptations that the fetus undertakes to maneuver through the pelvis during labor and birth; a mnemonic phrase to assist in remembering these movements is created by using the first letter (shown in boldface type) of each cardinal movement (shown in italics) to begin a word, these words are used to create a phrase: ***Every darn fool in Rotterdam eats rotten egg rolls everyday;*** in the most common presentation, occiput, the movements occur in the following order:

    a.  *Engagement* of the presenting part occurs

    b.  *Descent* of the fetus into the pelvis

    c.  *Flexion* of the fetal head; (descent and flexion often occur simultaneously)

    d.  *Internal rotation* of the fetal head must take place to accommodate the maternal pelvis and occurs so that the anterior-posterior diameter of the fetal head, the largest diameter of the fetus, aligns with the anterior-posterior dimension of the maternal pelvis

    e.  *Extension* of the fetal head occurs as it comes under the maternal symphysis pubis and emerges from the vagina

**f.** *Restitution* occurs as the fetal head turns 45 degrees to untwist the neck after the head has delivered

**g.** *External rotation* is viewed as the head turns an additional 45 degrees as the second-largest fetal diameter, the lateral diameter of the fetal shoulders, rotates into alignment with the anterior-posterior dimension of the maternal pelvis

**h.** *Expulsion* occurs as the anterior shoulder slips beneath the symphysis pubis which facilitates delivery of the body

**2.** **Crowning** is the outward bulging and thinning of the perineum and opening of the vagina that occurs as the fetal presenting part presses downward onto the perineum and becomes visible prior to delivery; this process is slower in the nulliparous client than the multiparous client

**3.** Assessment

   **a.** Blood pressure, pulse, and respirations q5–15min

   **b.** Contractions palpated continuously

   **c.** Fetal heart rate q15min if low risk, q5min if high risk, and if non-reassuring pattern, monitor continuously

   **d.** Monitor fetal descent, cardinal fetal movements and crowning

**4.** Priority nursing diagnoses: Pain; Fear; Deficient knowledge; Ineffective coping

**5.** Implementation and collaborative care

   **a.** Position comfortably for pushing and birth; encourage rest and relaxation between contractions

   **b.** Comfort measures: cool cloth to forehead, support legs while pushing, provide encouragement to push

   **c.** Ice chips and clear fluids to prevent dehydration

   **d.** Empty bladder, straight catheter if bladder distended or unable to void

   **e.** Local infiltration of anesthetic agent for birth by healthcare provider

   **f.** **Episiotomy** is a surgical incision into the perineum to enlarge the vaginal opening (see Figure 8-2); it is usually done during or just prior to crowning; medically indicated in the presence of fetal distress, but often performed to prevent tearing of the perineal tissues because lacerations have irregular edges and are more difficult to repair

      1) Midline episiotomy: 1- to 3-centimeter incision is made straight back from vagina toward the rectum; advantage: muscle fibers are split lengthwise allowing faster and less painful healing; disadvantage: 30 percent will extend into 3rd- or 4th-degree lacerations

      2) Mediolateral episiotomy: 4- to 5-centimeter incision is made from vagina obliquely toward one buttock; advantage: larger episiotomy possible and rectal structures avoided; disadvantage: muscle fibers are cut across causing more pain during healing

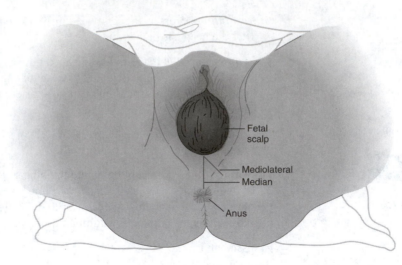

**Figure 8-2**

Locations for episiotomy.

Fetal scalp

Mediolateral

Median

Anus

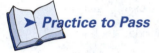

**► *Practice to Pass***

The laboring client asks the nurse if she will need an episiotomy or have a laceration. How should the nurse respond?

**g.** Lacerations to the perineum or surrounding tissues may occur during childbirth; 3rd- and 4th-degree lacerations most commonly occur after midline episiotomy is performed

   1) 1st degree: involves only the epidermal layers, if no bleeding may not need repair

   2) 2nd degree: epidermal and muscle/fascia involvement which requires suturing

   3) 3rd degree: extends into the rectal sphincter

   4) 4th degree: extends through the rectal mucosa

**h.** Document in the client record: time of birth, gender, position, nuchal cord, if present, and medications administered

**6.** Evaluation: client states is able to cope with contractions and pushing; Maternal and fetal well-being is maintained through delivery

**C. Third stage:** extends from the birth of the newborn to delivery of the placenta; average length is 30 minutes for nulliparas and multiparas

**1.** Maternal assessment

   **a.** Blood pressure, pulse and respirations q5min

   **b.** Uterine fundus maintains tone and contraction pattern to deliver placenta by decreasing the surface volume of the uterus and shearing the placenta from the uterine wall

   **c.** Monitor for signs of placental separation: uterus rises up in the abdomen, uterine volume shrinks as a result of the contractions creating a gush of blood vaginally as the contents of the uterus are expelled, and as the placenta is separating and beginning to be expelled, the umbilical cord protrudes further from the vagina and appears to lengthen

**2.** Fetal assessment

   **a. Apgar score** is a quick method to assess fetal adaptation to extrauterine life (see Table 8-2); Five criteria are scored at 1 and 5 minutes after birth with

NCLEX!

| Table 8-2 | | Color (Appearance) | Heart Rate (Pulse) | Reflex Irritability (Grimace) | Muscle Tone (Activity) | Respiratory Effort (Respirations) |
|---|---|---|---|---|---|---|
| **Apgar Scoring** | **0 Points** | Blue, pale | Absent | Absent | Absent | Absent |
| | **1 Point** | Blue extremities, pink body | < 100 | Grimace | Some flexion of extremities | Slow, irregular |
| | **2 Points** | Completely pink | ≥100 | Vigorous cry | Active motion | Good cry |

0, 1, or 2 points given for each criteria; the five criteria include color, heart rate, reflex irritability, muscle tone, and respiratory effort; Apgar scores of 8 or greater indicate the newborn needs minimal intervention (nasopharyngeal suction and oxygen near face); scores of 4 to 7 indicate a need for intervention through oropharyngeal suctioning, tactile stimulation, and oxygen administration; and scores of 3 or less indicate a need for resuscitation

**b.** Respirations: normally 30 to 60, may be irregular

**c.** Apical pulse: 120 to 160, may be irregular

**d.** Temperature: skin temperature above 97.8°F (36.5°C)

**e.** Umbilical cord: normally two arteries and one vein

**f.** Gestational age assessment: consistent with expected date of delivery

**g.** Physical assessment: abbreviated examination is conducted to detect the presence of visible congenital anomalies

**3.** Priority nursing diagnoses: Pain; Fear; Deficient knowledge; Ineffective coping

**4.** Implementation and collaborative care

**a.** Encourage mother to rest and relax while awaiting delivery of placenta

**b.** Immediate care of newborn includes placing in a modified Trendelenburg position, suctioning the nose and oropharynx (bulb syringe or DeLee mucus trap), providing and maintaining warmth (dry immediately with warm blankets, skin-to-skin contact with mother covered with warm blankets, radiant heat source, cap)

**c.** Assist parents to see and hold the newborn to begin attachment

**d.** Document time of placental delivery, appearance and intactness of placenta, mechanism of placental expulsion and estimated delivery blood loss (averages 250 to 500 cc)

1) If the placenta separates from the edge progressing toward the center and the rough maternal side of the placenta is visible, it is called a dirty Duncan mechanism of delivery

2) If the placenta separates from the center progressing outward and the membrane-covered fetal side of the placenta is visible, it is called a shiny Schultze mechanism of delivery

  **e.** Administer oxytocic agent as ordered

  **f.** Consider cultural practices in the disposal of the placenta

5. Evaluation: Mother and newborn experience a safe labor and birth.

**D. Fourth stage (immediate recovery phase):** includes the first 1 to 4 hours after delivery; the term is misleading because labor and birth are completed with the delivery of the placenta; this stage is actually part of the postpartal period but the client usually remains in the birthing suite for nursing care

1. Assessment: blood pressure, pulse, respirations, fundus, lochia and perineum per agency protocol; usually q15min for 1 hour; q30min for 2 hours; q60min for 1 hour

2. Priority nursing diagnoses: Pain; Deficient knowledge; Interrupted family processes

3. Implementation and collaborative care

  **a.** Episiotomy or lacerations are repaired

  **b.** Provide comfort: clean gown, warm blanket, position of comfort, ice to perineum if sutures or edema present, analgesia as requested and ordered

  **c.** Assist parents to explore their newborn and initiate breast-feeding, if desired and mother and baby are stable

  **d.** Provide fluids and regular diet as tolerated; consider cultural preferences

4. Evaluation: maternal and newborn well-being are maintained; the family unit is supported and participates in the birth process as desired

## IV. Pain Management during Birth

**A. Analgesia and anesthesia:** can be given to decrease or eliminate pain during the birthing process when nonpharmacologic methods of pain relief are ineffective

**B. Type of analgesia or anesthesia:** determined by the obstetric history of the client, the stage and phase of labor, the rate of progression in labor, and the preferences of the client and healthcare provider; regional differences in the use of particular methods or medications exist

**C. Nonpharmacologic methods of pain relief**

1. Position changes to decrease the weight of the fetus from the area of most intense pain

2. Hydrotherapy by standing or sitting in a warm shower or reclining in a tub

3. Breathing techniques to prevent breath-holding and to facilitate oxygen and carbon dioxide exchange; use of a focal point for concentration

4. Relaxation through verbal instruction, massage, soft music, or therapeutic touch

**D. Pharmacologic methods of pain relief**

1. Analgesic agents decrease the amount of pain perceived; goal is maximum pain relief with minimal risk for woman and fetus; must consider the effect on the woman, fetus and contractions; all systemic drugs cross the placental barrier in varying amounts; analgesia given too early may prolong labor and

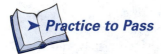

**► Practice to Pass**

The nulliparous client is experiencing a normal progression of labor. She is currently 4 centimeters, 100 percent effaced, vertex, at a 0 station, with contractions of moderate intensity every 4 minutes lasting 60 seconds. She asks what she can do for pain relief. How should the nurse respond?

depress the fetus; analgesia given too late may cause neonatal respiratory depression with no benefit to the woman

a. Intravenous narcotics: nalbuphine hydrochloride (Nubain) and butorphanol tartrate (Stadol) most commonly used in active phase of first stage of labor

1) Advantages: RN administration, rapid onset of pain relief, ease of administration, relatively short duration

2) Disadvantages: may decrease contraction frequency and intensity, crosses the placenta resulting in neonatal respiratory depression, short duration may not give adequate pain control during nulliparous or prolonged labor

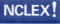

3) Nursing implications: Nubain is a narcotic agonist-antagonist and should never be given to a client with narcotic dependency or abuse as immediate withdrawal will occur that can stimulate seizures

b. Intrathecal narcotics: morphine sulphate (Morphine) or fentanyl citrate (Fentanyl) injected into the L4–L5 or L5–S1 subarachnoid space

1) Advantages: Excellent pain control that occurs within several minutes, lasts several hours, rarely results in neonatal respiratory depression, easier and faster injection method for both provider and client than epidural

2) Disadvantages: time involved with setting up needed supplies and administration make it undesirable for rapidly progressing labors or transition phase; may eliminate the urge to push; must be injected by anesthesia personnel; injection is uncomfortable; laboring client must hold very still during injections even if having contractions; spinal headache may occur from leakage of CSF through the dura at the injection site

3) Nursing implications: monitor for common side effects including nausea, pruritus, urinary retention, muscle spasms at the site of injection

2. Regional analgesia and anesthesia provides temporary and reversible loss of sensation by injection of an agent into an area with direct contact to nervous tissue

a. Lumbar **epidural block:** a needle is placed into the epidural space at the L4–L5 or L5–S1 level, a very small diameter catheter is threaded into the space, and local anesthetic agents such as bupivacaine hydrochloride (Marcaine) or lidocaine hydrochloride (Xylocaine) are injected; depending on the dose injected, can provide either analgesia or anesthesia

1) Advantages: excellent pain relief, re-dosing of medication into the epidural catheter is possible, no neonatal respiratory depression results, may provide a few hours of postpartum pain relief as well as during labor and delivery

2) Disadvantage: time involved with setting up needed supplies and administration make it undesirable for rapidly progressing labors or in transition phase, must be inserted by anesthesia personnel, usually causes numbness of lower extremities limiting mobility, decreases contraction frequency and intensity thus requiring pharmacologic augmentation, contraction intensity difficult to detect and may require

use of IUPC, little or no urge to push is felt, relaxation of musculature below the site of injection often results in failure of the fetus to accomplish internal rotation necessitating an operative birth

3) Nursing implications: monitor urinary output as retention requiring indwelling urinary catheter may result; monitor blood pressure as maternal hypotension commonly results from vasodilation; avoid supine position

b. **Paracervical block:** local anesthetic agent is injected into the lateral aspects of the cervix during active or transition phases

1) Advantages: rapid onset of pain relief, no neonatal respiratory depression, can be administered during transition, relative ease of administration

2) Disadvantages: systemic absorption of the medication through the vascular cervix can occur, excessive bleeding from the cervix may result, or the woman may experience a decreased or absent urge to push

3) Nursing implications: monitor fetal heart as bradycardia can result from systemic absorption

c. **Pudendal block:** local anesthetic agent is injected into the lateral vaginal walls near the ischial spines to anesthetize the pudendal nerve; administered during the second stage in preparation for cutting and repairing an episiotomy

1) Advantages: excellent anesthesia of the perineum, rarely need readministration, provides a few hours of postpartum pain relief

2) Disadvantages: must inject along the presenting part creating increased vaginal pressure and discomfort for the client, eliminates the urge to push

3) Nursing implications: monitor patient safety as decreased sensation in the lower extremities affects mobility

d. Local infiltration: local anesthetic agents are injected into the tissues of the perineum to provide anesthesia for episiotomy incision or repair and suturing of lacerations

1) Advantage: ease of administration, provides a few hours of postpartum pain relief

2) Disadvantages: reinjection may be needed to obtain complete anesthesia with extensive lacerations or large episiotomies

3) Nursing implications: loss of sensation may decrease urge or ability to urinate

**Case Study**

The client is a nullipara at 5 centimeters dilation, 100 percent effacement, 0 station, vertex presentation, LOP position, with intact membranes. Contractions are occurring every 3 minutes lasting 60 seconds with strong intensity. The healthcare provider orders continuous external electronic fetal monitoring.

❶ How often should the nurse assess maternal vital signs and fetal well-being?

❷ Where might the client be feeling discomfort and why?

❸ What interventions should the nurse use to promote the client's comfort at this stage and phase of labor?

❹ When the client asks what to expect as labor progresses, how should the nurse respond?

❺ The client states she has experienced a healthy pregnancy and asks why continuous fetal monitoring is necessary. How should the nurse respond?

*For suggested responses, see page 339.*

## Posttest

1  A nurse determines that a vaginal delivery of a vertex presentation is more likely to occur if the passenger (fetus) adapts to the passageway (pelvis) in which sequence of movements?

(1) Flexion, internal rotation, external rotation, extension
(2) Extension, flexion, descent, external rotation
(3) Descent, internal rotation, extension, external rotation
(4) Internal rotation, descent, flexion, extension

2  Which statement would indicate that the laboring client needs further education?

(1) "Because this is my first labor, I will need an epidural."
(2) "Labor can be long and difficult sometimes."
(3) "I should keep taking at least ice chips throughout labor."
(4) "My partner can help me stay relaxed and focused."

3  Assessment of a normal episiotomy immediately postdelivery is most likely to reveal:

(1) Gaping between the sutures.
(2) Slight bruising.
(3) Pus coming from the sutures.
(4) Edema that makes the tissue look shiny.

4  Fourth-stage nursing care for a client with an episiotomy includes whichof the following?

(1) Application of ice beginning 4 hours after delivery
(2) Ice pack to the perineum for up to 60 minutes per application
(3) Inspection every 15 minutes during the first hour after childbirth
(4) Instructions to avoid intercourse for at least 12 weeks

5  The nurse's goal in teaching childbirth education classes is to:

(1) Provide education for all pregnant clients.
(2) Ensure a normal spontaneous vaginal delivery.
(3) Help clients know what to expect during labor.
(4) Prepare the couple for all possible complications.

**6** You know that your teaching has been effective when the laboring client's partner shouts, "She's crowning!" as:

(1) You first start to see a little of the baby's head.
(2) The baby's head recedes upward between pushing contractions.
(3) The perineum is thin and stretching around the occiput.
(4) The mouth and nose are being suctioned.

**7** The nurse note on the antepartal history that the client has an android pelvis and recognizes an increaded risk for:

(1) A prolonged labor.
(2) Occiput posterior position.
(3) Precipitous delivery.
(4) Developing postpartum complications.

**8** The nurse determines teaching has been effective when a client with a fetus in a frank breech position says, "My baby's hips are:

(1) Flexed and the knees are flexed."
(2) Extended and the knees are flexed."
(3) Flexed and the knees are extended."
(4) Extended and the knees are extended."

**9** If the fetal head is determined to be presenting in a position of complete extension, the nurse should anticipate a:

(1) Precipitous labor and delivery.
(2) Prolonged labor and possible cesarean delivery.
(3) Normal labor and spontaneous vaginal delivery.
(4) Forceps-assisted vaginal delivery.

**10** The pregnant client is 7 centimeters, 100 percent effaced, and at a +1 station. The fetus is in a face presentation. You know your teaching has been effective when the client's husband states:

(1) "Our baby will come out face first."
(2) "Our baby will come out facing one hip. "
(3) "Our baby will come out buttocks first."
(4) "Our baby will come out with the back of the head first."

*See pages 185–186 for Answers and Rationales.*

## Answers and Rationales

### Pretest

**1 Answer: 1** *Rationale:* The presenting part is given first when describing fetal position. The second half of the fetal position description refers to the maternal pelvis. In this example, it is the sacrum presenting, and the fetal sacrum is toward the maternal anterior pelvis.
*Cognitive Level:* Application
*Nursing Process:* Analysis; *Test Plan:* HPM

**2 Answer: 1** *Rationale:* A change in the cervix is the only indicator of true labor.
*Cognitive Level:* Application
*Nursing Process:* Assessment; *Test Plan:* HPM

**3 Answer: 4** *Rationale:* The fetal heart rate response to contractions is a physiologic assessment that indicates the presence or absence of fetal well-being. The other options are appropriate for the laboring client, but safety of the fetus is the first priority.
*Cognitive Level:* Application
*Nursing Process:* Analysis; *Test Plan:* SECE

**4 Answer: 2** *Rationale:* As labor progresses, contractions will become more intense, occur more frequently (shorter resting phase between contractions), and have an increasing duration. Less frequent or shorter contractions can impede labor progress.
*Cognitive Level:* Application
*Nursing Process:* Assessment; *Test Plan:* HPM

**5 Answer: 2** *Rationale:* Apgar scores are based on 0, 1, or 2 points in each of the five categories: respiratory effort, color, muscle tone, heart rate, and reflexes. This neonate would score 2 points in each category except color, where the presence of acrocyanosis would warrant a score of 1 point.
*Cognitive Level:* Application
*Nursing Process:* Assessment; *Test Plan:* HPM

**6 Answer: 3** *Rationale:* As the uterus contracts and the placenta begins to shear off the uterine wall and be expelled, you will see a small gush of blood resulting from the uterine contractions emptying the uterus. In addition, the cord will lengthen as the placenta is

released from the uterine wall and moves toward the cervix prior to expulsion.
*Cognitive Level:* Analysis
*Nursing Process:* Analysis; *Test Plan:* HPM

**7  Answer: 2  Rationale:**  Anxiety commonly increases the perception of pain, and childbearing is no exception to this. Decreasing anxiety through education and support will facilitate the birthing process.
*Cognitive Level:* Application
*Nursing Process:* Analysis; *Test Plan:* HPM

**8  Answer: 1  Rationale:**  An increase in fetal heart rate baseline can be an indication of fetal distress, as well as maternal fever. Narcotics may decrease the short-term variability but do not affect the baseline. Fetal movement will create an acceleration of the fetal heart rate. Utero-placental insufficiency causes late decelerations.
*Cognitive Level:* Application
*Nursing Process:* Analysis; *Test Plan:* HPM

**9  Answer: 2  Rationale:**  Effacement is the thinning of the cervix from 0 to 100 percent. The opening of the cervix from 0 to 10 centimeters is called dilatation. In primigravidas effacement usually precedes dilatation while in multigravidas these processes usually occur concurrently.
*Cognitive Level:* Analysis
*Nursing Process:* Evaluation; *Test Plan:* HPM

**10  Answer: 1  Rationale:**  The first stage of labor is from the onset of labor to complete dilatation, and is divided into latent (0 to 3 centimeters), active (4 to 7 centimeters), and transition (8 to 10 centimeters) phases. The second stage of labor has no phases and is from complete dilatation until delivery of the newborn. The third stage has no phases and extends from delivery of the newborn to delivery of the placenta.
*Cognitive Level:* Application
*Nursing Process:* Analysis; *Test Plan:* HPM

## Posttest

**1  Answer: 3  Rationale:**  The cardinal movements of the fetus occur in the order of engagement, descent, flexion, internal rotation, extension, restitution, external rotation, and expulsion. These movements represent the normal adaptation of the fetus to the maternal pelvis and facilitate vaginal birth.
*Cognitive Level:* Application
*Nursing Process:* Assessment; *Test Plan:* HPM

**2  Answer: 1  Rationale:**  Analgesia and anesthesia methods are used for pain relief during labor as indicated by the client's response to pain, what phase and stage of labor the woman is in, how fast labor is progressing, and the fetal response to contractions. Parity alone does not determine what analgesia or anesthesia is indicated.
*Cognitive Level:* Application
*Nursing Process:* Evaluation; *Test Plan:* HPM

**3  Answer: 2  Rationale:**  Moderate ecchymosis and edema are a normal response to the trauma of childbirth, as well as to the presence of sutures. Sutures should be closely aligned without gaps and there should be no pus-like drainage indicating infection. Edema severe enough to cause the tissue to look shiny or taut is abnormal.
*Cognitive Level:* Application
*Nursing Process:* Analysis; *Test Plan:* HPM

**4  Answer: 3  Rationale:**  Frequent inspection for redness, swelling, tenderness, and hematoma is essential to fourth stage nursing care. Pain relief begins with immediate application of ice. Ice packs should be applied for 20 to 30 minutes and removed for a least 20 minutes. If ice is applied for more than 30 minutes, vasodilation and edema may occur. Clients are usually advised to wait until bleeding stops and stitches are healed (about 3 weeks) before resuming sexual activity, but this teaching would be part of the client's discharge instructions, and is not appropriate during the fourth stage of labor.
*Cognitive Level:* Application
*Nursing Process:* Implementation; *Test Plan:* HPM

**5  Answer: 3  Rationale:**  The goal of childbirth education classes is to teach pregnant women and their support person(s): the birth process, strategies to cope with the pain of labor and to facilitate an easier labor, what to expect during childbirth, an understanding of operative delivery (use of forceps, vacuum extraction, and cesarean birth), and common procedures that may be performed throughout the birthing process. Many pregnant families get the information they need about the childbearing process by reading or from friends or extended family members. Childbirth preparation cannot prevent complications and thus cannot ensure vaginal deliveries for all clients.
*Cognitive Level:* Application
*Nursing Process:* Analysis; *Test Plan:* HPM

**6  Answer: 3  Rationale:**  Crowning is the point in time when the perineum is thin and stretching around the fetal head both between and during contractions. Delivery is imminent when crowning occurs.
*Cognitive Level:* Application
*Nursing Process:* Evaluation; *Test Plan:* HPM

**7** **Answer: 1** *Rationale:* An android pelvic structure is narrow in both the anterior-posterior diameter and the lateral diameter, and can cause a prolonged labor with a large fetus or a malpositioned fetus.
*Cognitive Level:* Application
*Nursing Process:* Analysis; *Test Plan:* HPM

**8** **Answer: 3** *Rationale:* Frank breech position is when the sacrum of the baby is presenting, the hips are flexed, and the feet are extended upward toward the fetal head. Option 1 describes a complete breech; option 2 is characteristic of a kneeling breech; and option 4 represents a double footling breech.
*Cognitive Level:* Application
*Nursing Process:* Evaluation; *Test Plan:* HPM

**9** **Answer: 2** *Rationale:* The normal attitude of the fetal head is one of moderate flexion. Changes in fetal attitude, particularly the position of the head, present larger diameters to the maternal pelvis, which contributes to a prolonged and difficult labor and increases the likelihood of cesarean delivery.
*Cognitive Level:* Analysis
*Nursing Process:* Analysis; *Test Plan:* HPM

**10** **Answer: 1** *Rationale:* Presentation refers to the part of the fetus that is coming through the cervix and birth canal first. Thus a face presentation occurs when the face is coming through first.
*Cognitive Level:* Application
*Nursing Process:* Evaluation; *Test Plan:* HPM

# References

Dickason, E., Silverman, B., & Kaplan, J. (1998). *Maternal-infant nursing care* (3rd ed.). St. Louis: Mosby, Inc.

Hoerst, B., & Fairman, J. (2000). Social and professional influences on the technology of electronic fetal monitoring on obstetrical nursing. *Western Journal of Nursing Research, 22*(4): 475–491.

Hofmeyr, G. J. (2001) Amnioinfusion for meconium-stained liquor in labour (Cochrane Review). In *The Cochrane Library,* Issue 1. Oxford: Update Software.

Kozier, B., Erb, K., Wilkinson, J., & Van Leuven, K. (1998). *Fundamentals of nursing* (Updated 5th ed.). Menlo Park, CA.: Addison Wesley Longman, Inc.

Lowdermilk, D., Perry, S., & Boback, I. (2000) *Maternity and women's health care* (7th ed.). St. Louis: Mosby, Inc., pp. 307, 393, 459–460.

McKinney, E., Ashwill, J., Murray, S., James, S., Gorrie, T., & Droske, S. (2000). *Maternal-child nursing.* Philadelphia: W.B. Saunders Company.

Olds, S., London, M., & Ladewig, P. (2000) *Maternal new-born nursing* (6th ed.). Upper Saddle River, NJ: Prentice Hall Health, pp. 221, 473–489, 500–511, 560, 571, 665–667.

Pilliteri, A. (1999). *Maternal and child health nursing* (3rd ed.). Philadelphia: Lippincott, pp. 487–488.

Robinson, J., Norwitz, E., Cohen, A., & Lieberman, E. (2000). Predictors of episiotomy use at first spontaneous vaginal delivery. *Obstetrics and Gynecology, 96*(2): 214–218.

Sherwen, L., Scoloveno, M., & Weingarten, C. (1999). *Maternity nursing: Care of the childbearing family* (3rd ed.). Stamford, CT: Appleton & Lange, pp. 671–678, 694, 702–722.

Thacker, S. B., & Stroup, D. F. (2001). Continuous electronic heart rate monitoring for fetal assessment during labor (Cochrane Review) In *The Cochrane Library,* Issue 1. Oxford: Update Software.

## CHAPTER 9

# The Complicated Labor and Delivery Experience

Molly Meighan, RNC, PhD

## CHAPTER OUTLINE

*Nursing Care of the High-Risk Labor and Delivery Client and Her Family*

*Problems with the Passenger*
*Problems with the Passageway*
*Problems with the Powers*

*Problems with the Psyche*
*Cesarean Delivery*

## OBJECTIVES

▌ Discuss nursing assessments that lead to early recognition of complications during labor and delivery.

▌ Describe nursing interventions to promote maternal and fetal well-being during a complicated labor and delivery.

▌ Summarize nursing care needed by the client experiencing a cesarean delivery.

[ **Media Link** ]

*Use the CD-ROM enclosed with this text, or log onto the address given to access the free, interactive Companion Website created for this series. The CD-ROM and Companion Website accompanying this book offer additional practice opportunities and information—NCLEX Review, Case Studies, Glossary, In Depth with NCLEX, and more.*

**www.prenhall.com/hogan**

## REVIEW AT A GLANCE

**amnioinfusion** *infusion of warmed, sterile saline solution into the uterine cavity to replace amniotic fluid and prevent fetal distress*

**amniotomy** *artificial breaking of the amniotic sac to hasten labor*

**augmentation of labor** *stimulating uterine contractions by pharmacologic means to hasten labor and delivery*

**Bishop score** *a means of measuring the readiness of the cervix for induction of labor*

**cephalopelvic disproportion (CPD)** *pelvic size is too small to allow the descent and passage of the fetal head*

**cesarean section** *delivery of the fetus through an abdominal incision*

**dystocia** *difficult labor caused by factors of the pelvis, fetus, or abnormal or uncoordinated uterine contractions*

**external cephalic version** *external manipulation of the fetus from a breech or to a vertex presentation*

**hypertonic uterine dysfunction** *frequent, painful uterine contractions that are uncoordinated and do not efface or dilate the cervix; often occurs in latent phase of labor*

**hypotonic uterine dysfunction** *weak ineffective uterine contractions; often occurs in active phase of labor and is associated with cephalopelvic disproportion (CPD)*

**induction of labor** *the process of causing the onset of labor through the administration of pharmacologic agents or amniotomy*

**intrauterine resuscitation** *an emergency procedure instituted during labor to treat fetal distress by stopping uterine contractions with a tocolytic agent and allowing the restoration of maternal-fetal circulation so that the fetus can recover from distress.*

**labor graph (Friedman's curve)** *plotting cervical dilatation and descent of the fetal head over time and comparing to normal labor progress (curve) as determined by research of Friedman (1978); a partogram*

**malpresentation** *abnormal presentation occurring when any other fetal part besides the flexed head enters the pelvis*

**malposition** *abnormal position of the presenting part of the fetus in relation to the maternal pelvis occurring when any other position besides the flexed fetal head in an occiput anterior position presents*

**precipitate labor and birth** *rapid labor and delivery of less than 3 hours from the beginning of dilatation to birth of the infant; often results in unattended or nurse attended delivery*

**premature labor** *the onset of regular contractions between 20 to 37 weeks gestation with or without cervical change*

**tocolytic agents** *pharmacologic agents that suppress or stop uterine contractions*

**trial of labor (TOL)** *observation period to determine if a laboring woman with a borderline or small pelvis can progress to a vaginal birth*

**uterine inversion** *prolapse of the uterine fundus through the cervix and vagina during or following the third stage of labor; associated with massive bleeding and shock and requires emergency intervention*

**uterine rupture** *tearing open or separation of the uterine wall; associated with severe hemorrhage and shock necessitating hysterectomy*

**vaginal birth after cesarean (VBAC)** *vaginal birth of an infant to a woman who has had at least one previous cesarean delivery*

## *Pretest*

**1** Following amniotomy, the most important nursing action is to:

(1) Reposition the mother on her left side.
(2) Place a clean underpad on the bed.
(3) Listen to fetal heart tones.
(4) Observe the color and consistency of the amniotic fluid.

**2** The nurse may help a client with a fetus in the right occiput posterior (ROP) position by avoiding which of the following actions?

(1) Positioning her on her left side
(2) Positioning her on her right side
(3) Helping her walk around the room
(4) Assisting her to a knee-chest position

**3** A nulliparous client has not made any progress in cervical dilatation or station since she was 7 centimeters and 0 station over 2 hours ago. According to the Friedman curve, this is termed:

(1) Prolonged deceleration phase.
(2) Protracted active phase.
(3) Arrest of descent.
(4) Secondary arrest of dilatation.

**4** A client's amniotic fluid is greenish-tinged. The fetal presentation is vertex. Fetal heart rate (FHR) and uterine activity have remained within normal limits. At the time of delivery, the nurse should anticipate the need for:

(1) An infant laryngoscope and suction catheters.
(2) Forceps.
(3) A transport isolette.
(4) Emergency cesarean set-up.

**5** A client who is 34 weeks gestation has been having contractions every 10 minutes regularly. In addition to instructing her to lie down and rest while continuing to time contractions, the nurse should also tell her to:

(1) Refrain from eating or drinking anything.
(2) Take slow deep breathes with each contraction.
(3) Go to the hospital if contractions continue for more than 1 hour.
(4) Drink 3 to 4 cups of water.

**6** The client who has had a previous cesarean birth asks about vaginal birth after cesarean (VBAC). Which of the following factors from her history is a contraindication for VBAC?

(1) Previous cesarean was for breech presentation
(2) Client had a classical uterine incision
(3) The abdominal incision was vertical rather than transverse
(4) An induction of labor is planned for this delivery

**7** Which of the following statements by the nurse is most therapeutic in talking with a client and her family following emergency cesarean birth?

(1) "I'm sorry that you couldn't have a normal delivery."
(2) "Your baby was really in danger. I think he is doing better now."
(3) "You did so well throughout the delivery. I'm sorry I didn't have more time to explain things."
(4) "I know you never expected this to happen. Maybe things will work out better next time."

**8** A client is undergoing induction of labor with oxytocin (Pitocin). An important observation by the nurse that requires stopping or slowing the infusion is:

(1) Contractions lasting longer than 60 seconds.
(2) Resting phase interval less than 60 seconds.
(3) Maternal blood pressure 90/50.
(4) Nausea and vomiting.

**9** In addition to routine assessment and care, nursing care of the client who is receiving terbutaline (Brethine) to prevent premature labor should include assessing:

(1) Oral temperature every 2 hours.
(2) Fetal heart tones every 30 minutes.
(3) Breathe sounds every 4 hours.
(4) Deep tendon reflexes every 4 hours.

**10** The greatest risk of vaginal delivery of a breech infant is:

(1) Umbilical cord prolapse.
(2) Intracranial hemorrhage.
(3) Meconium aspiration.
(4) Fracture of the clavicle.

*See pages 213–214 for Answers and Rationales.*

## I. Nursing Care of the High-Risk Labor and Delivery Client and Her Family

**A. High-risk factors:** may develop at any time during the course of labor in a client who has been otherwise healthy throughout her pregnancy and may be related to:

1. The passenger or fetus

2. The passageway or pelvic bones and other pelvic structures

3. The powers or uterine contractions

4. The client's psyche or psychological state

**B. Client response to the onset of high-risk factors in labor**

1. Stress, fear, and anxiety brought about by unexpected complications during labor may have profound effects on maternal and fetal outcome

2. Maternal anxiety can increase tension, produce higher pain perception, and may make labor contractions less effective

3. Catecholamines released during stress produce vasoconstriction that may negatively affect uterine blood flow

**C. Family members:** may be overwhelmed with concern and less capable of providing needed emotional support for the client

**D. Nursing care:** in addition to basic intrapartal care, nursing care during complicated labor requires special knowledge and skill in assessment and care of the mother and fetus

## II. Problems with the Passenger

**A. Fetal *malposition:*** the ideal fetal position is flexed with occiput in the right or left anterior quadrant of the maternal pelvis

1. Types of malpositions

   **a.** Occiput posterior (OP) position

   1) Right or left OP position occurs in about 25 percent of all term pregnancies but usually rotates to occiput anterior (OA) as labor progresses

   2) Failure to rotate is termed persistent occiput posterior

   3) Maternal risks include prolonged labor, potential for operative delivery, extension of the episiotomy, or 3rd- or 4th-degree laceration of the perineum

   4) Maternal symptoms include intense back pain in labor, dysfunctional labor pattern, prolonged active phase, secondary arrest of dilatation, and/or arrest of descent

   **b.** Occiput transverse (OT) position

   1) Incomplete rotation of OP position to OA results in the fetal head being in a horizontal or transverse position (OT)

   2) Persistent occiput transverse position occurs as a result of ineffective contractions or a flattened bony pelvis

   3) In the absence of abnormal pelvic structure, vaginal delivery can be accomplished by stimulating contractions with oxytocin (Pitocin) and application of forceps for delivery

2. Nursing care

   **a.** Nursing diagnoses: Pain; Ineffective coping

   **b.** Planning and implementation

   1) Encourage the mother to lie on her side opposite from the fetal back, which may help with rotation

   2) Knee-chest position may facilitate rotation

   3) Pelvic rocking may help with rotation

   4) Apply sacral counter-pressure with heel of the hand to relieve back pain

5) Continue support and encouragement

   a) Keep client and family informed of progress

   b) Encourage relaxation with contractions

   c) Praise client's efforts to maintain control

6) Anticipate forceps rotation and forceps-assisted birth

**c.** Evaluation

   1) The client's discomfort is decreased

   2) The woman's coping abilities are strengthened

**3.** Medical management

**a.** Forceps: metal instruments applied to the fetal head to facilitate delivery

   1) Provides traction or a means of rotating the fetal head

   2) Risks are fetal ecchymosis or edema of the face, transient facial paralysis, maternal lacerations, or episiotomy extensions

**b.** Vacuum extraction: a suction cup applied to the fetal head to facilitate delivery

   1) Provides traction to shorten the second stage of labor

   2) Risks are newborn cephalohematoma, retinal hemorrhage, and intracranial hemorrhage

**B. Fetal *malpresentation***

**1.** Vertex malpresentations are caused by failure of the fetus to assume a flexed attitude

**a.** Brow presentation

   1) Fetal forehead is presenting part

   2) 50 percent convert to vertex or face presentation

**b.** Face presentation

   1) Increased risk of prolonged labor and operative delivery

   2) Anticipate vaginal delivery if pelvis is adequate and the chin (mentum) is in the anterior position

   3) Anticipate cesarean delivery if mentum is posterior or signs of fetal distress occur

   4) Fetal monitor electrode should not be placed on the presenting part (the infant's face); requires external fetal heart rate (FHR) monitoring

   5) Edema and bruising of the face, eyes, and lips are common occurrences—clients should be prepared for this possibility before seeing the infant for the first time

**c.** Sincipital presentation (military attitude)

   1) Larger diameter of the fetal head is presented

   2) Labor progress is slowed with slower descent of the fetal head

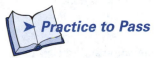

**▶ *Practice to Pass***

A client asks you if forceps will leave a mark on her baby's head or face. How will you answer this question?

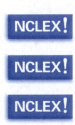

NCLEX!

NCLEX!

NCLEX!

2. Breech presentations

   a. Three types (see Figure 9-1)

      1) Complete breech: sacrum is the presenting part, knees flexed

      2) Frank breech: sacrum is the presenting part, legs are extended

      3) Incomplete (footling) breech: one or both feet are presenting, increasing the risk of umbilical cord prolapse

   b. Maternal risks

      1) Prolonged labor due to decreased pressure exerted by the breech on the cervix

      2) Premature rupture of membranes may expose client to infection

      3) Cesarean or forceps delivery

      4) Trauma to birth canal during delivery from manipulation and forceps to free the fetal head

      5) Intrapartum or postpartum hemorrhage

### Figure 9-1

**Breech presentation. A. Frank breech, B. Incomplete footling breech, C. Complete breech in left sacral anterior (LSA) position, D. On vaginal examination, the nurse may feel the anal sphincter. The tissue of the fetal buttocks feels soft.**

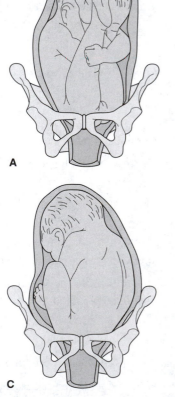

A

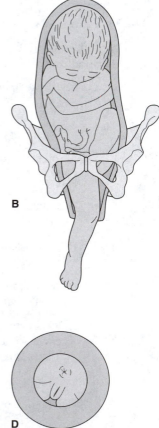

B

C

D

**c.** Fetal risks

   1) Compression or prolapse of the umbilical cord

   2) Entrapment of the fetal head in incompletely dilated cervix

   3) Aspiration and asphyxia at birth

   4) Birth trauma from manipulation and forceps to free the fetal head

**d.** Vaginal delivery of breech

   1) Fetal body may pass through an incompletely dilated cervix entrapping the larger fetal head that follows

   2) Delivery of fetal head must be done quickly to avoid hypoxia

   3) Piper (long handle) forceps may be applied to the after-coming fetal head

**e. Cesarean section:** increased morbidity and mortality of the fetus has convinced most physicians that vaginal delivery should not be attempted; most breech presentations are delivered by cesarean section, or abdominal delivery

**f. External cephalic version:** manipulation of the fetus through the abdominal wall from a breech or shoulder to a vertex presentation

   1) Client is placed on external fetal monitor

   2) IV fluids are started

   3) Terbutaline (Brethine) is administered via a piggybacked IV line to relax the uterine muscle

   4) FHR is closely monitored during version attempt

   5) Version is discontinued if undue maternal or fetal distress is noted

**3.** Shoulder presentation (transverse lie): acromium process is the presenting the part (see Figure 9-2)

   **a.** Vaginal delivery is not considered possible in term infant

   **b.** Cesarean birth is preferred method of delivery

**Figure 9-2**

Shoulder presentation.
A. Frontal view,
B. Vaginal view.

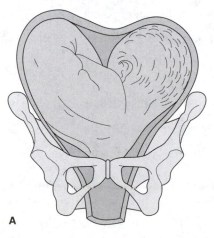

Scapula

Ribs

Humerus

Acromion process

A

B

4. Compound presentations: more than one part of the fetus presents

   **a.** Most common type is a hand or arm prolapsing beside the head

   **b.** Risk of cord compression and prolapse is increased

   **c.** Vaginal versus cesarean delivery depends on size of the fetus, presence of fetal distress, and the progress in labor

5. Nursing care of clients with malpresentations

   **a.** Assessment and nursing diagnoses

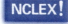

      1) Leopold's maneuvers may help detect abnormal presentation

      2) Priority nursing diagnoses: Risk for injury; Anxiety; Fear; Deficient knowledge; Ineffective individual coping; Ineffective family coping

   **b.** Planning and implementation

      1) Observe closely for abnormal labor patterns

      2) Monitor fetal heart rate and contractions continuously

      3) Provide client and family teaching

      4) Provide client support and encouragement

      5) Anticipate forceps-assisted birth

      6) Anticipate cesarean birth for incomplete breech or shoulder presentation

      7) Be prepared for childbirth emergencies such as cesarean section, forceps-assisted delivery, and neonatal resuscitation

   **c.** Evaluation

      1) The client and fetus have a safe labor and delivery

      2) The client verbalizes understanding of the implications of the malpresentation

  **C. Fetal distress:** insufficient oxygen supply to meet the demands of the fetus

   1. Causes

     **a.** Compression of the umbilical cord

     **b.** Uteroplacental insufficiency caused by placental abnormalities or maternal condition

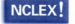

   2. Signs and symptoms

     **a.** Meconium-stained amniotic fluid (excluding breech presentation)

     **b.** Changes in fetal heart rate baseline

       1) Tachycardia (above 160): early sign of distress

       2) Bradycardia (below 110): late sign of distress

     **c.** Decreased or absence of variability of heart rate

       1) Heart rate varies less than 2 to 5 beats per minute causing a flattened appearance to the heart rate

> ➤ *Practice to Pass*
>
> In doing Leopold's maneuvers, what findings would make you suspect that the fetus is in a breech presentation?

      2) Indicates depression of the autonomic nervous system that controls heart rate

      3) Fetal sleep, sedation, and hypoxia may affect variability

  **d.** Late deceleration pattern

      1) Fetal heart rate slows following the peak of a contraction and slowly returns to baseline rate during the resting phase

      2) Indicates fetal response to hypoxia from uteroplacental insufficiency

      3) Considered an omnious pattern regardless of the depth of the deceleration of the FHR and requires immediate intervention

  **e.** Severe variable deceleration pattern

      1) Fetal heart rate repeatedly decelerates below 90 beats per minute for over 60 seconds before returning to baseline

      2) Indicates interference of fetal blood flow from cord compression

      3) Leads to fetal hypoxia and low APGAR scores unless steps are taken to correct it

**3.** Nursing care

  **a.** Assessment and nursing diagnoses

      1) Assess FHR baseline, variability, and pattern of periodic changes

      2) Assess contraction pattern and maternal response to labor

      3) Priority nursing diagnoses: Decreased cardiac output (fetal), Impaired gas exchange (fetal), Anxiety (maternal)

  **b.** Planning and implementation

**NCLEX!**

      1) Institute emergency measures to correct fetal hypoxia based on FHR pattern (see Box 9-1); for late deceleration, take steps to improve

---

**Box 9-1**

**Nursing Management of Fetal Distress**

**Late decelerations (uteroplacental insufficiency)**
The goal is to improve maternal blood flow to the placenta

- Reposition the mother on her left side
- Administer $O_2$ by face-mask at 8–10 L/min
- Increase IV fluids
- Discontinue oxytocin infusion, if labor is being induced
- Notify the health care provider immediately

**Severe variable decelerations or prolonged bradycardia (cord compression)**
The goal is to relieve pressure on the umbilical cord

- Reposition the mother on either side
- If not corrected, reposition to opposite side
- Administer $O_2$ by face-mask at 8–10 L/min
- Trendelenburg or knee-chest position, if not corrected
- Perform vaginal examination and apply upward digital pressure on the presenting part to relieve pressure on the umbilical cord

uteroplacental blood flow and for severe variable deceleration, initiate actions to relieve cord compression

2) Provide appropriate information and emotional support to the client and family

3) Maintain continuous monitoring of FHR and uterine activity, and labor progress

c. Evaluation

1) The fetal heart rate remains in normal range with adequate variability and absence of ominous periodic changes

2) The client verbalizes that anxiety is decreased

3) Family coping strategies are strengthened

4. Medical management

a. **Amnioinfusion:** amniotic fluid may be replaced with warmed sterile saline through an intrauterine catheter when signs of cord compression are present during labor

1) FHR monitoring is continued

2) Intrauterine catheter is inserted

3) Warmed sterile saline is delivered via the catheter using an infusion pump

4) Infusion is continued until signs of cord compression disappear

b. **Intrauterine resuscitation:** administration of terbutaline (Brethine), a tocolytic agent, to stop uterine contractions and provide an opportunity for uteroplacental circulation to improve when fetal distress is present during the first stage of labor

c. Prevention of meconium aspiration

1) If meconium is present during labor (green-tinged amniotic fluid), steps to prevent aspiration at the time of delivery should be taken

2) The nasopharynx of the infant is suctioned prior to delivery of the chest and abdomen

3) Visualization of the larynx and vocal cords with deep suction is performed immediately after delivery and before the first breath is taken

**D. Prolapsed umbilical cord**

1. Cause: fetus is not firmly engaged, allowing room for the cord to move beyond (prolapse) or alongside the presenting part (occult prolapse)

2. Contributing factors

a. Rupture of membranes before engagement of the presenting part

b. Small fetus

c. Breech presentation

d. Multifetal pregnancy

e. Transverse lie (shoulder presentation)

NCLEX!

NCLEX!

NCLEX!

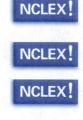

**➤ Practice to Pass**

Following several late decelerations, a client asks you why she needs to lie on her left side. How will you answer her?

3. Assessment and nursing diagnoses

   a. Identify the client at risk for prolapsed umbilical cord

   b. Priority nursing diagnoses: Risk for impaired gas exchange; Risk for injury; Fear

4. Planning and implementation: actions to relieve pressure on the cord and restore fetal oxygenation

   a. Place mother's hips higher than her head

      1) Knee-chest position

      2) Trendelenburg position

   b. Perform sterile vaginal exam pushing fetal presenting part upward with the fingers to relieve pressure on the cord

   c. Administer $O_2$ by face mask at 8 to 10 L/min

   d. Maintain continuous electronic fetal monitoring

   e. Prepare for rapid delivery vaginally or by cesarean section

   f. If cord protrudes through the vagina, determine that pulsation is present and apply sterile saline soaked dressing to prevent drying

5. Evaluation

   a. The fetal heart rate remains within normal range and without ominous signs

   b. The fetus is safely delivered

   c. The client and family verbalize understanding of the implications of prolapsed umbilical cord and the need for emergency management

## III. Problems with the Passageway

### A. Abnormal size or shape of the pelvis

1. Contracted pelvic inlet: anterior-posterior diameter less than 10 centimeters; transverse diameter less than 12 centimeters

   a. Makes engagement difficult

   b. Influences fetal position and presentation

2. Contracted mid-pelvic plane: interspinous diameter less than 9.5 centimeters

   a. Hampers internal rotation of fetal head

   b. Secondary arrest of dilatation or arrest of descent of the fetal head occurs

3. Contracted pelvic outlet: interischial tuberous diameter less than 8 centimeters

4. **Trial of labor (TOL):** the physician may allow labor to continue or even stimulate labor with oxytocin when pelvic measurements are borderline to see if the fetal head will descend making vaginal delivery possible; if progressive changes in dilatation and station do not occur, a cesarean delivery is performed

### B. *Cephalopelvic disproportion (CPD)*

1. Fetal head is too large to pass through the bony pelvis

2. Signs and symptoms: fetal head does not descend even though there are strong contractions

3. Maternal risks include prolonged labor, exhaustion, hemorrhage, and infection

4. Fetal risks include hypoxia and birth trauma

5. Cesarean birth is necessary

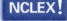

C. **Shoulder dystocia:** an obstetric emergency resulting from difficulty or inability to deliver the shoulders

1. Fetal macrosomia increases the risk of shoulder dystocia

2. Inability to deliver shoulders leads to fetal hypoxia and death

3. Maternal risks

   a. Lacerations and tears of birth canal

   b. Postpartum hemorrhage

4. Neonatal risks

   a. Hypoxia

   b. Fractures of clavicle

   c. Injury to neck and head

D. **Nursing care**

1. Assessment and identification of the client at risk for shoulder dystocia

   a. Obesity

   b. Increased fundal height

   c. History of macrosomia

   d. Maternal diabetes or gestational diabetes

   e. Prolonged second-stage labor

2. Priority nursing diagnoses: Risk for injury; Fear; Deficient knowledge

3. Planning and implementation

   a. Assist with positioning during delivery: **McRoberts maneuver** (see Figure 9-3)

      1) Woman flexes thighs on her abdomen

      2) Position changes the angle of the pelvis, increases pelvic diameters, and facilitates delivery of the shoulders

   b. Assess for maternal and newborn injury following delivery

4. Evaluation

   a. Client and fetus experience a safe delivery without injury

   b. The client indicates that fear is diminished

   c. Client is able to verbalize increased understanding of pelvic disproportion and dystocia, its causes, and implications for delivery

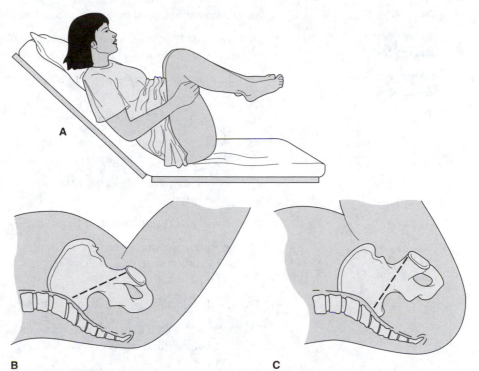

**Figure 9-3**

McRoberts maneuver. A. Thighs flexed onto abdomen, B. Angle of maternal pelvis prior to maneuver, C. Angle of pelvis with maneuver.

## IV.  Problems with the Powers

**A.** ***Induction of labor:*** pharmacologic (see Table 9-1) and nonpharmacologic measures to initiate contractions and cervical change

    **1.** Methods of induction

        **a.** Cervical ripening

            1)  Prostaglandins ($PGE_2$) gel

            2)  Laminaria (hydrophilic agent): when inserted into the cervix, it absorbs water from cervical mucus, expands, and dilates the cervix

**Table 9-1**

**Drugs Used for Induction of Labor**

| Drug | Route/Action | Side Effects and Potential Complications |
|---|---|---|
| Prostaglandins Prostaglandin gel (Cervidil; Prepidil) | Intravaginally close to cervix; Causes softening and effacement or cervical ripening | Abdominal cramping, nausea, vomiting, diarrhea |
| Misoprostol (Cytotec) | Synthetic prostaglandin administered orally or intravaginally to produce contractions | Sudden onset of hypertonic contractions and elevated resting tone of the uterus which may lead to fetal distress |
| Oxytocin (Pitocin) | Synthetic oxytocin administered IV in small amounts and titrated to produce contractions that mimic normal labor | Uterine tetany and fetal distress are major concerns; can lead to water intoxication, hyponatremia and hypochloremia |

**b. Amniotomy** or artificial rupture of membranes (AROM)

       1) Auscultate FHR prior to and immediately after AROM to detect prolapse of the umbilical cord or fetal distress

       2) Take maternal temperature q 1 to 2 hours following AROM to detect signs of infection

    **c.** Misoprostol (Cytotec) administration

       1) A synthetic prostaglandin agent administered intravaginally and/or orally at doses of 25 to 50 mg to stimulate the onset of contractions

       2) Continuous monitoring of the FHR, uterine activity, and maternal vital signs is essential

    **d.** Oxytocin (Pitocin) administration (see Box 9-2)

       1) The **Bishop score** may be used to assess maternal readiness for induction by determining dilatation, effacement, station, cervical consistency, and position of the cervix

       2) Prior to induction, begin external fetal monitoring

       3) Assess and record maternal vital signs, intake and output, and contraction frequency and intensity

       4) Begin primary intravenous infusion

       5) Mix oxytocin in 500 to 1000 cc of IV balanced-saline fluid such as lactated Ringer's and piggyback into the primary IV at a site as close to the client as possible

       6) Control and titrate the oxytocin solution using an infusion pump

---

**Box 9-2**

**Oxytocin (Pitocin) Administration**

Hospital protocols for mixing Pitocin with IV fluids vary. Therefore, the nurse should be familiar with the institution's policies and procedures regarding induction of labor. Pitocin is administered IV beginning with 0.5 to 2 milliunits (mU)/min and is increased by 1 to 2 mU every 15 to 60 min to a maximum of 32 to 40 mU/min (per protocol) or until contractions are regular and effective.

Pitocin 10 U in 1000 cc = Pitocin 10,000 milliunits in 1000 cc or 10 mU in 1 cc

Set infusion pump to deliver:

  3cc/hour = 0.5mU/min

  6cc/hour = 1.0mU/min

  12cc/hour = 2.0mU/min

Increase in increments of 3 to 6 cc to a maximum of 32 to 40 mU/min

- Pitocin infusion is stopped and the physician notified if:

    Contractions are closer than 2 min or last longer than 90 sec

    There signs of fetal distress (late decelerations, severe variable decelerations, or bradycardia)

- Pitocin given in an electrolyte-free solution or at a rate exceeding 20mU/min increases the risk of water intoxication

    Signs include: nausea, vomiting, hypotension, tachycardia, and cardiac arrhythmia

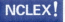

7) Begin at 0.5 to 2 milliunits (mU) per minute, increasing at increments of 1 to 2 mU every 15 to 60 minutes up to a maximum of 40 mU according to hospital protocol and until contractions occur regularly

8) Continue to monitor contractions and FHR closely and stop the infusion immediately if contractions are closer than 2 minutes, last longer than 90 seconds, or if there is any indication of fetal distress

2. Absolute contraindications to induction of labor

   a. Placenta previa

   b. Transverse lie and other fetal malpresentations

   c. Prior classic uterine incision

   d. Pelvic structure abnormality

   e. Prolapsed umbilical cord

   f. Active genital herpes

   g. Invasive cervical cancer

B. *Dystocia* **or difficult labor**

1. **Hypertonic uterine dysfunction:** frequent contractions with decreased intensity and increased uterine tone

   a. Maternal risks are prolonged or nonprogressive labor, pain, and fatigue

   b. Fetal risks include hypoxia caused by decreased uteroplacental blood flow

   c. Medical treatment includes sedation aimed at stopping contractions, promoting rest, and allowing a normal labor pattern to develop

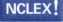

   d. Hydration, monitoring of intake and output, and steps to promote relaxation are important nursing interventions

2. **Hypotonic uterine dysfunction:** infrequent contractions with decreased intensity

   a. Maternal and fetal risks are related to nonprogressive labor, which is often associated with prolonged rupture of membranes, and frequent vaginal examinations leading to infection

   b. More commonly occurs in the active phase of labor

   c. Medical treatment includes ruling out CPD and **augmentation of labor,** or stimulation of contractions, with oxytocin

3. Abnormal progress in labor: the **labor graph,** or **Friedman's curve,** is used to identify deviations from normal progress in labor by plotting cervical dilatation and descent of the fetal head over time

   a. Prolonged latent phase: > 20 hours in a nulliparous patient or > 14 hours in a multiparous client

      1) May indicate CPD

      2) May be caused by false labor

      3) Medical treatment is sedation and rest

      **b.** Protracted active phase: dilatation < 1.2 centimeters in a nulliparous client or < 1.5 centimeters in a multiparous client

         1) May be caused by malposition

         2) CPD and fetal presentation and position is assessed

      **c.** Protracted descent: < 1 centimeter per hour change in station in the nulliparous client or < 2 centimeters per hour in the multiparous client

         1) CPD is ruled out

         2) Contraction intensity and duration are assessed

         3) Labor may be augmented with oxytocin

      **d.** Secondary arrest of dilatation: cessation of dilatation for > 2 hours in a nulliparous client or > than 1 hour in a multiparous client

         1) CPD is ruled out

         2) If no CPD, labor is augmented with oxytocin

      **e.** Arrest of descent: no progress in fetal station for >1 hour

         1) CPD is assessed

         2) Labor is augmented, if no CPD

   **4.** Retraction rings

      **a.** Physiologic retraction ring: boundary between upper uterine segment and lower uterine segment that normally forms during labor

         1) Upper segment contracts and becomes thicker as muscle fibers shorten

         2) Lower segment distends and becomes thinner

      **b.** Bandl's ring: a pathological retraction ring that forms when labor is obstructed caused by CPD or other complications

         1) Upper segment continues to thicken

         2) Lower segment continues to distend

         3) Risk of uterine rupture increases if contractions continue

         4) Cesarean delivery is indicated

      **c.** Constriction ring

         1) Retraction ring forms and impedes fetal descent

         2) Relaxation of the constriction ring with analgesics, anesthetics, or both allows vaginal delivery

**C. *Premature labor:*** contractions occurring between 20 to 37 weeks gestation

   **1.** Client teaching for every woman about signs and symptoms of premature labor

      **a.** Contractions occurring q 10 minutes or less with or without pain

      **b.** Low abdominal cramping with or without diarrhea

      **c.** Intermittent sensation of pelvic pressure, urinary frequency

    **d.** Low backache (constant or intermittent)

    **e.** Increased vaginal discharge, may be pink-tinged

    **f.** Leaking amniotic fluid

2. Immediate actions to be taken by clients experiencing suspected premature labor

    **a.** Empty bladder

    **b.** Assume a side-lying position, left preferred

    **c.** Drink 3 to 4 cups of water

    **d.** Palpate abdomen for uterine contractions; if 10 minutes apart or closer, contact healthcare provider

    **e.** Rest for 30 minutes and slowly resume activity, if symptoms disappear

    **f.** If symptoms do not subside within 1 hour, contact healthcare provider

3. Medical management

    **a.** Bedrest

    **b.** Continued monitoring of uterine activity and FHR

    **c.** Administration of **tocolytic agents,** drugs to stop contractions, if labor continues (see Table 9-2)

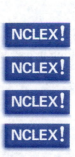

        1) Ritodrine (Yutopar)

        2) Terbutaline (Brethine)

        3) Magnesium sulfate

    **d.** Administration of betamethasone (Celestone) or dexamethasone to stimulate fetal lung maturity

| Table 9-2 | Drugs Used in Premature Labor | | |
|---|---|---|---|
| **Drug** | **Type/Purpose** | **Major Side Effects** | **Nursing Concerns** |
| Ritodrine (Yutopar) | Beta adrenergic/Tocolysis | Maternal or fetal tachycardia, shortness of breath, pulmonary edema, nervousness, tremors, nausea and vomiting, hyperglycemia, hypokalemia | Assess vital signs, breath sounds, fetal heart rate, contractions, and maternal response (not widely used because of cardiac effects) |
| Terbutaline (Brethine) | Beta adrenergic/Tocolysis | Nervousness, palpitations, maternal or fetal tachycardia, nausea and vomiting, pulmonary edema | Assess vital signs, breath sounds, fetal heart rate, contractions, and maternal response |
| Magnesium Sulfate | CNS depressant/Tocolysis | Lethargy, heat sensation, respiratory depression, depressed reflexes and cardiac arrest, if high serum level (> 10 to 12 mg/dL) | Assess respiratory rate, deep tendon reflexes, and hourly urinary output; monitor serum magnesium levels |
| Betamethasone (Celestone) or Dexamethasone | Corticosteroid/Stimulates fetal lung maturation by stimulating surfactant production | Increased risk of infection and poor wound healing, produces hypoglycemia, increased risk of pulmonary edema when given with a beta adrenergic agent | Must be given 24 to 48 hours before delivery to be effective; commonly used between 24 to 34 weeks gestation unless fetal lung maturity can be documented |

**4.** Nursing assessment and diagnoses

    **a.** Identify clients at risk for premature labor

    **b.** Priority nursing diagnoses: Deficient knowledge; Fear; Ineffective coping

**5.** Planning and implementation

    **a.** Provide client and family teaching regarding signs and management of premature labor

    **b.** Promote bedrest encouraging left lateral position

    **c.** Monitor uterine activity and FHR

    **d.** Administer tocolytics and monitor for adverse reactions

    **e.** Provide emotional support encouraging client and family to express feelings and concerns

**6.** Evaluation

    **a.** The client can identify signs and symptoms of premature labor that need to be reported to the healthcare provider

    **b.** The client can identify self-care measures to initiate, if premature labor is suspected

    **c.** The client's coping strategies are strengthened

    **d.** Client and fetus are delivered safely

**D.** *Precipitate labor and birth:* rapid labor (< 3 hours) resulting in precipitous (unattended or nurse attended) birth

**1.** Maternal risks

    **a.** Cervical, vaginal, or rectal lacerations

    **b.** Hemorrhage

**2.** Fetal risks

    **a.** Hypoxia caused by decreased perfusion to intervillous spaces

    **b.** Intracranial hemorrhage due to rapid passage through the birth canal

    **c.** Injury at birth

**3.** Nursing assessment and diagnoses

    **a.** Identify the client at risk for precipitous labor and birth

    **b.** Priority nursing diagnoses: Risk for injury; Anxiety; Fear

**4.** Planning and implementation

    **a.** Do not leave the client; send someone or call for help

    **b.** Don sterile gloves, if time allows

    **c.** Instruct the client to pant or blow to decrease the urge to push

    **d.** Support the perineum with a sterile towel as crowning occurs

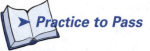

**➤ *Practice to Pass***

A client who is at 34 weeks gestation asks you why it is necessary to stop her labor instead of just letting the baby be born. What explanation would you give her?

e. Apply gentle pressure on the fetal head to prevent rapid delivery

   1) Lacerations of the perineum can occur

   2) Subdural or dural tears may occur with sudden expulsion of the infant's head

f. After delivery of the head, suction the infant's mouth then nose with bulb syringe

g. Check around the infant's neck for a possible tight umbilical cord; if present, cord must be clamped and cut before delivery

h. Place hands on each side of the infant's head and instruct client to push

i. Gentle downward pressure facilitates birth of the anterior shoulder

j. Gentle upward traction facilitates birth of the posterior shoulder

k. Support the infant's body with a towel as it is expelled from the birth canal

l. Suction and dry the infant thoroughly

m. Place infant on the mother's abdomen as soon as stable

n. Clamp and cut the umbilical cord

o. Observe for signs of placental separation

   1) Gush of bright blood

   2) Lengthening of the cord

p. Gently pull the cord while massaging the fundus to deliver the placenta

q. Continue to massage the fundus to prevent hemorrhage or put the infant to breast

r. Inspect the perineum for lacerations or tears

5. Evaluation

   a. Client's fear and anxiety are reduced

   b. Client and fetus are safely delivered

E. **Uterine prolapse**

1. Vigorous massage of the fundus and pulling on the umbilical cord to speed placental separation may cause prolapse of the cervix and lower uterine segment through the introitus

2. **Uterine inversion:** turning inside out of the uterus

   a. Complete inversion

      1) Inverted uterus is visible outside the introitus

      2) Life-threatening because of severe hemorrhage and shock

      3) Uterus must be immediately replaced manually to stop blood loss

   b. Partial inversion

      1) Is not visible but can be palpated

      2) Uterine fundus is partially inverted hampering contraction and control of hemorrhage

      3) Corrected by the physician using a bimanual technique

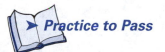

**➤ *Practice to Pass***

A client is about to deliver a breech infant. As the nurse in attendance, what steps should you take, how would these differ from a vertex presentation, and what are your major concerns?

**F.** *Uterine rupture:* tearing open or separation of uterine wall

1. Rare but serious complication, occurring in 1 in 1,500 to 2,000 births

2. Most common causes

    **a.** Separation of scar from previous classical cesarean

    **b.** Uterine trauma

    **c.** Intense uterine contractions

    **d.** Overstimulation of labor with oxytocin

    **e.** Difficult forceps-assisted birth

    **f.** External cephalic or internal version

3. Risk factors for uterine rupture

    **a.** Multiparity

    **b.** Overdistension of the uterus (multifetal pregnancy)

    **c.** Malpresentation

    **d.** Previous uterine surgery

4. Types

    **a.** Complete extends through the uterine wall into the peritoneal cavity

    **b.** Incomplete extends into the peritoneum but not into the peritoneal cavity

        1) Partial separation of cesarean scar

        2) May go unnoticed until repeat cesarean is performed

5. Medical management depends on type of rupture

    **a.** Complete rupture requires management of shock, replacement of blood, and hysterectomy

    **b.** Incomplete rupture may require laparotomy, repair, and blood transfusion

6. Nursing assessment: signs and symptoms may be silent or dramatic

    **a.** Sudden, sharp, lower abdominal pain

    **b.** Tearing sensation

    **c.** Signs of shock

    **d.** Cessation of contractions

    **e.** FHR ceases

    **f.** Blood loss is often concealed

    **g.** Fetal parts may be easily palpated through abdominal wall

7. Priority nursing diagnoses: Risk for injury; Impaired gas exchange; Deficient fluid volume

8. Planning and implementation

    **a.** Prevention is best

        1) Identify clients at risk

        2) Avoid hyperstimulation of the uterus during induction

NCLEX!

NCLEX!

      **9.** Evaluation

        **a.** Client and infant are delivered without injury

        **b.** Client's fluid volume is restored to normal

## V. Problems with the Psyche

### A. Factors influencing the psyche of the client in labor

    **1.** Fear and anxiety

    **2.** Perception of the problem

    **3.** Self-image

    **4.** Preparation for childbirth

    **5.** Support systems

    **6.** Coping ability

### B. The effect of fear and anxiety on labor progress

    **1.** Epinephrine secretion in response to stress

    **2.** Vascular changes divert blood from the uterus to skeletal muscles

    **3.** Decrease in oxygen and glucose supply with accumulation of lactic acid in uterine muscle

    **4.** Higher perception of pain

    **5.** Decrease in available energy supply to support effective contractions

    **6.** Labor progress is slowed

### C. Nursing assessment

    **1.** Determine client's past experiences with, preparation for, and expectations of labor and birth

    **2.** Determine client's current coping behaviors and their effectiveness with the current situation

### D. Priority nursing diagnoses: Ineffective coping; Fear; Anxiety; Deficient knowledge

### E. Planning and implementation

    **1.** Establish a trusting relationship with the client and family

    **2.** Remain at the bedside with the client and family during labor

    **3.** Encourage relaxation

    **4.** Keep the client and family informed about progress and procedures

    **5.** Encourage positive coping behaviors and discourage negative behaviors

    **6.** Promote self-image by praising efforts

### F. Evaluation

    **1.** Client coping strategies are strengthened

    **2.** Client's fear and anxiety are reduced

    **3.** Client verbalizes increased understanding of the labor and birth process

## VI.  Cesarean Section

**A. Delivery of the infant by an abdominal incision:** purpose is to facilitate delivery to preserve the health of the mother and fetus

1. Number of cesarean births has increased dramatically beginning in the late 1970s and early 1980s

2. National goal of Healthy People 2010 is to reduce the incidence from the current rate of 25 percent to 30 percent to 15 percent of all deliveries

**B. Major indications for cesarean delivery**

1. Dystocia or CPD

2. Fetal distress

3. Breech presentation

4. Previous cesarean birth

**C. Maternal risks**

1. Aspiration

2. Hemorrhage

3. Infections

4. Injury to bowel or bladder

5. Thrombophlebitis

6. Pulmonary embolism

**D. Fetal/neonatal risks**

1. Prematurity

2. Injury at birth

3. Respiratory problems related to delayed absorption of fetal lung fluid

**E. Surgical techniques**

1. Skin incisions

    a. Vertical

    b. Pfannenstiel's (transverse lower abdominal incision)

2. Uterine incisions

    a. Classical: through the upper uterine segment

    b. Low cervical transverse: lower uterine segment

    c. Lower uterine segment vertical

**F. Nursing assessment**

1. Determine the reason for the cesarean delivery

2. Determine the client's understanding of the indication, procedure, and implications for recovery from abdominal delivery

**G. Priority nursing diagnoses:** Deficient knowledge; Fear; Anxiety; Self-concept, disturbance in self-esteem/body image

**H. Planning and implementation**

1. Discuss cesarean birth in childbirth preparation classes

   **a.** Clients and families cope better if they have time to learn about cesarean birth

   **b.** Emergency cesarean birth increases anxiety and alters the couple's expectations about childbirth

2. Preoperative care

   **a.** Assess NPO status (mother should have had nothing by mouth, if possible, to prevent aspiration)

   **b.** Explain procedure so that client and family will know what to expect

   **c.** Obtain client signature on consent form

   **d.** Perform abdominal prep

   **e.** Insert Foley catheter to prevent bladder trauma during surgery

   **f.** Start intravenous fluids using a large bore catheter

   **g.** Administer an antacid either IV or PO to decrease risk of lung damage from aspirating acidic gastric contents during surgery

   **h.** Administer antibiotics, as ordered

   **i.** Assist with positioning and administration of regional anesthesia, if used

3. Intraoperative care

   **a.** Provide heated crib and supplies to receive the newborn

   **b.** Provide immediate care to the newborn or assist nursery personnel as needed

   **c.** Provide assistance to surgical team and immediate care for the mother

4. Postoperative care

   **a.** Begin postanesthesia (recovery room) monitoring of vital signs, pulse oximetry, and cardiac monitoring; monitor vitals signs q 15 minutes for first hour and until stable

   **b.** Assess fundus for firmness and location (if boggy, massage until firm)

   **c.** Assess vaginal bleeding

   **d.** Assess abdominal dressing

   **e.** Assess catheter and urine output

   **f.** Turn, cough, and deep breathe hourly

   **g.** Administer medications for pain, as needed

   **h.** Promote maternal-infant contact and bonding

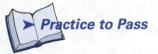

➤ *Practice to Pass*

As the childbirth education instructor, you are discussing emergency cesarean delivery. A client asks what she can do to avoid having an emergency cesarean section. How will you answer her?

**H. Evaluation**

1. Client experiences a safe and satisfying delivery of a healthy infant

2. Client's fear and anxiety are decreased

3. Client's coping strategies are strengthened

4. Client is able to express feelings regarding delivery

5. Client verbalizes understanding of the indication for and plan of care following cesarean delivery

**I. Vaginal birth after cesarean (VBAC)**

1. Labor and vaginal birth after a previous cesarean is considered a safe option, if the indication for cesarean delivery is not likely to be repeated

2. Contraindications

   a. Previous classical incision into the uterus

   b. Large infant (> 4000 g)

   c. Malpresentation

   d. Pelvic measurements inadequate

   e. Any fetal or placental problem that may require cesarean section

   f. Delivery in an alternative birth setting: access to a facility where emergency cesarean may be performed is necessary

3. Assessment of risks versus benefits

   a. Risks

      1) Possible uterine rupture and hemorrhage: less likely to occur if the previous uterine incision was in the lower uterine segment; risk of rupture is approximately 1 percent

      2) Failure of trial of labor requiring a repeat cesarean

   b. Benefits

      1) Ability to experience labor and vaginal delivery, which is desired by some clients; success rates are approximately 70 percent

      2) Vaginal delivery is less costly than cesarean delivery with faster, easier recovery period and less risk of complications

      3) VBAC does not preclude induction or augmentation of labor

4. Priority nursing diagnoses: Potential for injury; Anxiety; Fear; Knowledge deficit

5. Planning and implementation

   a. Monitor uterine activity and progress in labor; identifying deviations from normal progress in labor and reporting to the physician is essential

   b. Monitor fetal heart rate and response to contractions, identifying and reporting indications of fetal distress quickly

**c.** Provide teaching before onset of labor that the early period of labor carries the greatest risk of uterine rupture for VBAC clients

**d.** Observe for indications of uterine rupture

1) Signs of shock or hemorrhage

2) Report of "ripping or tearing" sensation or sharp uterine pain

3) Abrupt cessation of contractions

4) Abrupt onset of fetal distress

5) Fetus, lying outside the uterus may be palpated more easily than before

**e.** Be alert and prepared for possible emergency cesarean delivery

**f.** Provide support and encouragement for client attempting VBAC

6. Evaluation

**a.** Client and fetus are delivered safely

**b.** Client's anxiety and fear are decreased

**c.** Client is able to verbalize risks and benefits of VBAC and signs and symptoms to be reported immediately to the nurse or health care provider

**Case Study**

A nulliparous client was admitted to the birthing unit 9 hours ago. She progressed from 3 centimeters and 0 station to 6 centimeters and +1 station, but has not made any additional progress for almost 2 hours. FHR is in the normal baseline range with moderate variability. There are no decelerations. Contractions are presently q 3 minutes, 40 seconds duration, and of strong intensity.

❶ Following the vaginal examination, what other assessments will you make at this time?

❷ During the vaginal examination, you determine that the small triangular fontanel is toward the mother's back on the right side. What is the fetal position?

❸ The client's husband asks you why labor has not progressed very much. How will you answer him?

❹ What nursing interventions will be most helpful to this client at this time?

❺ Should you notify her physician at this time? If so, what information will you give and what medical interventions do you anticipate?

*For suggested responses, see pages 339–340.*

## Posttest

1 A multiparous client who has been in labor for almost 3 hours suddenly announces that the baby is coming. The nurse sees the infant crowning. Which of the following actions should the nurse do first?

(1) Ask the woman to pant while preparing to place gentle counter pressure on the infant's head as it is delivered.
(2) Quickly obtain sterile gloves and a towel.
(3) Retrieve the precipitous delivery tray from the nursing station.
(4) Telephone the physician using the bedside phone.

2 The nurse determines that a client does not understand what to expect during cesarean delivery, when the client states:

(1) "An indwelling (Foley) catheter will be inserted before surgery."
(2) "My husband can be present during birth."
(3) "I may be given an antacid before surgery."
(4) "I will receive a blood transfusion during surgery."

3 The nurse concludes that deceleration of the fetal heart rate from 130 to 70 beats per minute with contractions followed by a rapid return to a normal baseline rate is most likely a client's response to:

(1) Umbilical cord compression.
(2) Fetal head compression.
(3) Severe fetal hypoxia.
(4) Uteroplacental insufficiency.

4 The nurse determines that fetal distress is occurring after noting which of the following signs?

(1) Moderate amount of bloody show
(2) Pink-tinged amniotic fluid
(3) Meconium-stained amniotic fluid
(4) Acceleration of fetal heart rate with each contraction

5 On performing Leopold's maneuvers on a multiparous client in early labor, the nurse finds no fetal parts in the fundus or above the symphysis. The fetal head is palpated in the right mid quadrant. The nurse notifies the admitting physician and anticipates:

(1) An external version.
(2) An internal version.
(3) A cesarean delivery.
(4) Prolonged labor.

6 The nurse discovers a loop of the umbilical cord protruding through the vagina when preparing to perform a vaginal examination. The most appropriate intervention is to:

(1) Call the physician immediately.
(2) Place a moist clean towel over the cord to prevent drying.
(3) Immediately turn the client on her side and listen to the fetal heart rate.
(4) Perform the vaginal examination and apply upward digital pressure to the presenting part while having the mother assume a knee-chest position.

7 The client has refused sedation ordered by the physician for hypertonic contractions and prolonged latent phase labor for fear that her labor will stop. The nurse may help by explaining:

(1) Sedation helps to provide needed rest and allows time for the uterine contractions to become coordinated so that labor is progressive.
(2) If the woman is experiencing true labor, contractions will not stop even with sedation.
(3) If contractions continue without cervical effacement and dilatation, the fetus is at risk for hypoxia.
(4) Sedation will stop contractions that are uncoordinated and provide more time to determine if a cesarean delivery is needed.

**8** The client is receiving intravenous magnesium sulfate at 2 g/h to stop premature labor. The most important nursing assessments of this client include:

(1) Intake and output, level of consciousness, and blood pressure.
(2) Blood pressure, pulse, and uterine activity.
(3) Deep tendon reflexes, hourly urine output, and respiratory rate
(4) Intake and output, blood pressure, and reflexes.

**9** During augmentation of labor with intravenous oxytocin (Pitocin), a multiparous client becomes pale and diaphoretic and complains of severe lower abdominal pain with a tearing sensation. Fetal distress is noted on the monitor. The nurse should suspect:

(1) Precipitate labor.
(2) Amniotic fluid embolus.
(3) Rupture of the uterus.
(4) Uterine prolapse.

**10** During the vaginal examination, the nurse palpates the fetal head and a large diamond-shaped fontanel. The fetal presentation is:

(1) Face.
(2) Transverse.
(3) Vertex.
(4) Brow.

*See pages 214–215 for Answers and Rationales.*

## Answers and Rationales

### Pretest

**1** **Answer: 3** *Rationale:* The risk of umbilical cord compression or prolapse increases when amniotic fluid is released. Listening to fetal heart tones after amniotomy will quickly detect the presence of cord compression. Observing color and consistency of the fluid should be done next. Placing a clean under pad on the bed and repositioning the mother is important in providing comfort but is not the first priority.
*Cognitive Level:* Analysis
*Nursing Process:* Implementation; *Test Plan:* PHYS

**2** **Answer: 2** *Rationale:* Gravity may help the fetus rotate to an anterior position for vaginal delivery. The positions in options 1, 3, and 4 enlist the aid of gravity. Option 2 should be avoided because it will not help the fetus to rotate.
*Cognitive Level:* Application
*Nursing Process:* Implementation; *Test Plan:* HPM

**3** **Answer: 4** *Rationale:* Dilatation has stopped (arrested) after considerable progress. Causes may be hypotonic uterine contractions, malposition, or cephalo-pelvic disproportion. Options 1 and 2 are not correct because, prolonged and protracted mean that progress occurs at a very slow rate. Arrest of descent (option 3) occurs when the station rather than cervical dilatation does not change.
*Cognitive Level:* Application
*Nursing Process:* Assessment; *Test Plan:* HPM

**4** **Answer: 1** *Rationale:* Meconium released by the fetus causes amniotic fluid to be greenish-tinged. Although the presence of meconium is associated with fetal distress, there is no evidence of immediate danger to the fetus during labor in this case. However, the infant is at risk for aspirating meconium at the time of delivery. Steps to prevent aspiration include thorough suctioning of the nasopharynx including visualization of the vocal cords to remove meconium particles before the first breath.
*Cognitive Level:* Application
*Nursing Process:* Planning; *Test Plan:* HPM

**5** **Answer: 4** *Rationale:* Hydration has been shown to decrease premature labor contractions. Therefore, drinking water or other noncaffeinated beverage is recommended. If contractions continue at 10 minutes apart or less for an hour with rest, the client should call her healthcare provider.
*Cognitive Level:* Application
*Nursing Process:* Implementation; *Test Plan:* HPM

**6** **Answer: 2** *Rationale:* A classical incision involves the upper uterine segment and is more likely to separate or rupture with subsequent uterine contractions. Induction is not a contraindication if managed judiciously. The type of abdominal incision is not a concern, since it is not affected by uterine contractions.
*Cognitive Level:* Analysis
*Nursing Process:* Assessment; *Test Plan:* PHYS

**7** **Answer: 3** *Rationale:* Promoting a positive feeling about how well she was able to cope with an emergency cesarean delivery will have an influence on self-image and the client's feelings about her ability to handle future pregnancies and births. In addition, providing an opportunity for the client and her family to ask questions and to express feelings helps in dealing with any disappointment, anger, or guilt they may feel. Other options indicate that the birth was not normal and can promote negative feelings about the infant or the experience.
*Cognitive Level:* Application
*Nursing Process:* Implementation; *Test Plan:* PSYC

**8** **Answer: 2** *Rationale:* Each contraction exerts pressure that interrupts uteroplacental blood flow. The resting phase (between contractions) allows uteroplacental circulation to resume, transporting oxygen and nutrients to the fetus and the uterine muscle as well as removing waste products. A resting phase of < 60 seconds does not allow enough time for this to take place. The duration of contractions may be longer than 60 seconds especially in later phases of labor without causing fetal distress.
*Cognitive Level:* Analysis
*Nursing Process:* Assessment; *Test Plan:* PHYS

**9** **Answer: 3** *Rationale:* Terbutaline, a beta-adrenergic agent has many maternal and fetal side effects including tachycardia, cardiac arrythmias, and pulmonary edema. In addition to taking vital signs, the nurse should assess for pulmonary edema. The frequency of assessment of fetal heart tones and oral temperature depends on the intensity and length of the drug therapy, as well as surrounding circumstances. Deep tendon reflex assessment is not indicated.
*Cognitive Level:* Application
*Nursing Process:* Assessment; *Test Plan:* PHYS

**10** **Answer: 1** *Rationale:* With breech presentation, fetal parts do not completely fill the lower uterine segment allowing more opportunity for the umbilical cord to proceed through the cervix or become compressed by the fetus, especially following rupture of membranes. The incidence of the other options is no higher in breech than it is with vertex presentation.
*Cognitive Level:* Knowledge
*Nursing Process:* Analysis; *Test Plan:* PHYS

## Posttest

**1** **Answer: 1** *Rationale:* Nursing action should be directed toward preventing a rapid and uncontrolled delivery of the infant's head. Directing the client to pant prevents pushing. If time allows, the nurse may don gloves or obtain a towel or blanket to support the fetal head. Delivery is imminent, so there may not be time to obtain sterile gloves or contact the physician. The client should not be left alone, so going to the nursing station to get the precipitous delivery tray is not an option.
*Cognitive Level:* Application
*Nursing Process:* Implementation; *Test Plan:* PHYS

**2** **Answer: 4** *Rationale:* Blood transfusions are not routinely given during cesarean section. Although blood typing and screening is often ordered prior to surgery, it is seldom necessary for a client to receive a blood transfusion. A Foley catheter is inserted to prevent bladder damage during surgery and an antacid is administered to prevent aspiration of acidic gastric contents, thus reducing the risk of lung damage. The client's husband or primary support person is usually present at the birth except in extreme emergencies.
*Cognitive Level:* Analysis
*Nursing Process:* Evaluation; *Test Plan:* HPM

**3** **Answer: 1** *Rationale:* The pattern described is a variable deceleration, which is associated with umbilical cord compression. During variable decelerations, the FHR drops below 90 beats a minute very quickly as fetal blood flow through the umbilical cord is interrupted. FHR returns rapidly to baseline as soon as the cord compression is relieved. FHR patterns associated with fetal head compression (early deceleration) and uteroplacental insufficiency (late deceleration) have a shallower appearance since they do not drop as precipitously. Variable deceleration, unless severe (lasting longer than 60 seconds) does not indicate severe hypoxia.
*Cognitive Level:* Analysis
*Nursing Process:* Analysis; *Test Plan:* PHYS

**4** **Answer: 3** *Rationale:* Meconium passage prior to birth occurs in response to a stressful event for the fetus. Moderate bloody show often occurs late in labor. Pink-tinged amniotic fluid occurs because of a small amount of blood usually from the cervix. Accelerations of FHR are considered a normal response and do not indicate fetal distress.
*Cognitive Level:* Analysis
*Nursing Process:* Assessment; *Test Plan:* PHYS

**5** **Answer: 3** *Rationale:* Findings on palpation are consistent with shoulder presentation or transverse lie. Vaginal delivery is not possible, so the nurse

should anticipate cesarean section. Since the client is in labor, version is contraindicated.
*Cognitive Level:* Analysis
*Nursing Process:* Planning; *Test Plan:* HPM

6 **Answer: 4** *Rationale:* Pressure on the cord must be relieved to save the life of the fetus. Applying upward manual pressure to the presenting part and having the mother assume a knee-chest position are appropriate emergency actions, followed by starting oxygen and calling the physician. Options 2 and 3 do nothing to relieve cord occlusion.
*Cognitive Level:* Application
*Nursing Process:* Implementation; *Test Plan:* PHYS

7 **Answer: 1** *Rationale:* Prolonged latent phase labor is associated with uncoordinated, hypertonic, and painful contractions that do little to dilate or efface the cervix. Maternal exhaustion and dehydration are concerns. Medical management is directed toward providing rest and hydration and allowing time for contractions to become coordinated. Often clients awaken from sedation in progressive labor. While option 2 is correct, this does little to explain the rationale for sedation. Option 3 is incorrect. There is very little risk to the fetus unless contractions are intense and < 2 minutes apart. Option 4 is not correct, because it is too soon to anticipate the need for cesarean delivery.
*Cognitive Level:* Application
*Nursing Process:* Implementation; *Test Plan:* HPM

8 **Answer: 3** *Rationale:* Early signs of magnesium toxicity that may lead to respiratory arrest are loss of patellar reflexes and decreased respiratory rate (< 12/min). Since magnesium is excreted from the body through the renal system, hourly urine output should be assessed. Although blood pressure is a standard assessment for most antepartum clients, there is minimal blood pressure change, if any, associated with administration of magnesium sulfate.
*Cognitive Level:* Application
*Nursing Process:* Assessment; *Test Plan:* PHYS

9 **Answer: 3** *Rationale:* Although rupture of uterus is rare, there is an increased risk for multiparas and clients undergoing induction or augmentation of labor. Early signs include pain and a tearing sensation, signs of shock, and fetal distress. Blood loss is usually severe but may not be visible. Amniotic fluid embolus is frequently associated with cardiac and respiratory distress. Symptoms of precipitate labor and uterine prolapse do not include pallor, diaphoresis, or fetal distress.
*Cognitive Level:* Analysis
*Nursing Process:* Assessment; *Test Plan:* PHYS

10 **Answer: 4** *Rationale:* In a brow presentation, the fetal forehead and the large, diamond-shaped, anterior fontanelle is palpated during vaginal exam. In vertex presentation, the back of the fetal head (occiput) and small, triangular fontanelle is palpated. In breech and shoulder presentations, fetal parts would feel soft and irregular.
*Cognitive Level:* Analysis
*Nursing Process:* Assessment; *Test Plan:* HPM

## References

American College of Obstetricians and Gynecologists. (1999). *Induction of labor* (Practice Bulletin # 10). Washington, DC: ACOG.

Association of Women's Health, Obstetric and Neonatal Nurses (1998). *Standards and guidelines for professional nursing practice in the care of women and newborns* (5th ed.). Washington, DC: AWHONN.

Braden, P. S. (1998). *Nurses clinical guide: Maternity care* (2nd ed.). Springhouse, PA: Springhouse Corp.

Brown, C. (1998). Intrapartal tocolysis: An option for acute intrapartal fetal crisis. *JOGNN, 27*(3): 257–261.

Burroughs, A. & Leifer, G. (2001). *Maternity nursing: An introductory text* (8th ed.). Philadelphia: W. B. Saunders Co.

Clayworth, S. (2000). The nurses role during oxytocin administration. *Maternal Child Nursing, 25*(2): 80–84.

Creasy, R. K. (1997). *Management of labor and delivery.* Malden, MA: Blackwell Science, Inc.

Davis, L. J., Okuboye, S, & Ferguson, S. L. ( 2000). Healthy people 2010: Examining a decade of maternal & infant health. *AWHONN Lifelines, 4*(3): 26–33.

Eisenhauer, L. A., Nichols, L. W., Spencer, R. T., & Bergan, F. W. (1998). *Clinical pharmacology & nursing management* (5th ed.). Philadelphia: Lippincott.

Friedman, E. (1978). *Labor: Evaluation and management* (2nd ed.). New York: Appleton-Century-Crofts.

Gagnon, A. J. & Waghorn, K. (1999). One-to-one nurse labor support of nulliparous women stimulated with oxytocin. *JOGNN 28*(4): 372–376.

Harmon, J. H. & Andrew, K. (1999). Current trends in cervical ripening and labor induction. *American Family Physician 60* (2): 477–483.

Lowdermilk, D. L., Perry, S. E.,& Bobak, I. M. (2000). *Maternity and women's health care* (7th ed.). St. Louis: Mosby, pp. 498–499, 1004–1005.

Olds, S. B., London, M. L., & Ladewig, P. A. (2000). *Maternal newborn nursing: A family and community-based approach* (6th ed.). Upper Saddle River, NJ: Prentice-Hall, Inc., pp. 398–405, 576–577, 618, 620–624, 630, 644, 878.

Parer, J. T. (1997). *Handbook of fetal heart rate monitoring* (2nd ed.). Philadelphia: W. B. Saunders.

Payton, R. G., & Brucker, M. C. (1999). Drugs and uterine motility. *JOGNN  28*(6): 628–638.

Sherwen, L. N., Scoloveno, M. A., & Weingarten, C. T. (1999). *Maternity nursing: Care of the childbearing family* (3rd ed.). Stamford, CT: Appleton & Lange, pp. 609–626, 735–810, 972–973.

Simpson, K. R. & Poole, J. H. (1998). Labor induction & augmentation: Knowing when, and how, to assist women in labor. *AWHONN Lifelines 2*(6): 39–42.

Sweha, A., Hacker, T.W., & Nuovo, J. (1999). Interpretation of the electronic fetal heart rate during labor. *American Family Physician 59*(9): 2487–2500.

Wilson, C. (2000). The nurse's role in Misoprostol induction: A proposed protocol. *JOGNN 29*(6): 574–583.

## CHAPTER 10

# The Normal Postpartal Experience

Deborah Bartnick, RN, MSN

## CHAPTER OUTLINE

*Physical Changes during the Postpartal Period*

*Psychosocial Changes during the Postpartal Period*

*Nursing Care of the Postpartal Client*

## OBJECTIVES

- Describe the physical changes that occur in the woman during the postpartal period.

- Discuss the psychological changes that occur in the new mother.

- Describe nursing care designed to promote safety and self-care during the postpartal experience of the maternity client.

[ Media Link ]

*Use the CD-ROM enclosed with this text, or log onto the address given to access the free, interactive Companion Website created for this series. The CD-ROM and Companion Website accompanying this book offer additional practice opportunities and information—NCLEX Review, Case Studies, Glossary, In Depth with NCLEX, and more.*

**www.prenhall.com/hogan**

## REVIEW AT A GLANCE

**afterpains** *uncomfortable uterine cramps that occur intermittently during the first 2 to 3 days postpartum, more common in the multiparous woman*

**boggy uterus** *uterus that is not well-contracted and feels soft when palpated*

**bonding** *a process by which parents form an emotional relationship with their infant over time*

**colostrum** *fluid in the breast during pregnancy and into early postpartal period; rich in antibodies, high in protein, and acts as a laxative for the newborn*

**diastisis recti** *separation of the two rectus muscles along the median line of the abdominal wall*

**en face** *face-to-face position in which the parent's and the infant's faces are approximately 20 centimeters apart and on the same plane*

**engorgement** *swelling of the breast tissue; primary engorgement typically lasts 48 hours and reaches a peak between the 3rd and 5th days postpartum*

**engrossment** *a father's absorption, pre-occupation, and interest in his infant*

**fundus** *dome-shaped upper portion of the uterus between the points of insertion of the fallopian tubes*

**Homan's sign** *client complains of sharp calf pain when the leg is extended and the foot is dorsiflexed; can be an early sign of thrombophlebitis*

**involution** *reduction in size of the uterus after delivery to its pre-pregnant state*

**let-down reflex** *release of breast milk caused by contraction of the milk glands in response to natural release of oxytocin; also known as milk ejection reflex*

**lochia alba** *thin, clear, yellow-to-white vaginal discharge that follows lochia serosa, from approximately 11 days to 3 to 6 weeks postpartum*

**lochia rubra** *red, menstrual-like vaginal discharge, from birth to 3 days postpartum*

**lochia serosa** *serous, pinkish-brown vaginal discharge that follows lochia rubra until approximately 10 days postpartum*

**postpartum blues** *a maternal adjustment reaction accompanied by irritability, anxiety, and a mild let-down feeling usually occurring between the 2nd to 3rd postpartum day through the 1st to 2nd week postpartum*

**puerperium** *period starting after the third stage of labor and ending with return of the uterus to the pre-pregnant state at 6 weeks postpartum*

## *Pretest*

**1** The nurse is assessing a client 24 hours after delivery and finds the fundus to be slightly boggy and 2 centimeters above the umbilicus. What should the priority nursing intervention be?

(1) Document this expected finding.
(2) Assess the mother's vital signs.
(3) Gently massage the fundus until firm.
(4) Notify the physician.

**2** A new mother complains of "afterpains." The nurse's first action should be to:

(1) Administer an analgesic.
(2) Advise her to stop breast-feeding until the pain stops.
(3) Encourage her to empty her bladder.
(4) Assess her vital signs.

**3** The nurse is caring for a woman who gave birth to a daughter yesterday but greatly desired a son. Today she seems withdrawn, staying in bed and staring at the wall. What is the most appropriate intervention?

(1) Monitor this normal response after delivery.
(2) Refer the client for a psychiatric consultation.
(3) Tell the client she should be thankful her baby is healthy.
(4) Encourage the mother to verbalize her disappointment.

**4** The nurse is preparing to instruct a new mother on resuming sexual intercourse postpartum. The nurse should include which of the following in the teaching plan?

(1) Use petroleum jelly for vaginal lubrication.
(2) An IUD is an appropriate method of birth control in the early postpartum period.
(3) Wait until the episiotomy has healed and the lochia has stopped before resuming intercourse.
(4) Refrain from intercourse until the first menstrual period after delivery is completed.

**5** The nurse is caring for a client who has decided not to breast-feed. Client teaching to promote lactation suppression should include which of the following?

(1) Applying warm compresses
(2) Pumping the breasts
(3) Applying ice bags
(4) Using medication to suppress lactation

**6** A client has a temperature of 100.2°F 4 hours after delivery. What is the appropriate action for the nurse to take?

(1) Encourage increased fluid intake.
(2) Do nothing since this is an expected finding at this time.
(3) Check the physician's orders for an antibiotic to treat the client's infection.
(4) Medicate the client for pain.

**7** A client delivered 90 minutes ago. She is alert and physically active in bed. She states that she needs to go to the bathroom. The nurse's most appropriate response is:

(1) "I'll walk you to the bathroom and stay with you."
(2) "I'll get a bedpan for you."
(3) "It's important that you wipe yourself from front to back after urinating."
(4) "Wipe the stitches back and forth to increase circulation."

**8** Which laboratory finding should the nurse assess further on a client 24 hours after delivery?

(1) Hemoglobin 7.2 g/dL
(2) White blood cell count 20,000/mm$^3$
(3) Trace to 1+ proteinuria
(4) Hematocrit 35%

**9** A client is to be discharged 12 hours after delivery. The nurse should delay the discharge and notify the physician if which of the following is observed?

(1) Moderate lochia rubra
(2) Fundus firm at umbilicus
(3) Pulse 62 beats per minute
(4) Three voidings totaling 240 cc in 12 hours

**10** A client had an episiotomy and complains of perineal discomfort. She is also afraid to have a bowel movement. Which of the following nursing diagnoses is the highest priority for this client at this time?

(1) Activity intolerance
(2) Deficient knowledge
(3) Pain
(4) Risk for constipation

*See page 232 for Answers and Rationales.*

## I. Physical Changes during the Postpartal Period (*Puerperium*)

### A. Reproductive

**NCLEX!**

1. **Involution:** the reduction in the size of the uterus after delivery to the pre-pregnant size caused by uterine contractions that constrict and occlude underlying blood vessels at the placental site; Table 10-1 presents factors that slow or hasten this process during the puerperium, the 6-week period after delivery

**NCLEX!**

2. **Fundus:** the top portion of the uterus; a palpable indicator of involution, as shown in Figure 10-1; if contractions of the uterine muscle are interrupted, a **boggy uterus,** one that is soft, relaxed, and likely to cause hemorrhage results

| Table 10-1 Factors that Influence Involution | Factors that Enhance Involution | Factors that Slow Involution |
|---|---|---|
| | Uncomplicated labor and delivery | Prolonged labor and difficult delivery |
| | Breastfeeding | Anesthesia |
| | Early ambulation | Grand multiparity |
| | Complete expulsion of placenta and membranes | Retained placental fragments or membranes |
| | | Full urinary bladder |
| | | Infection |
| | | Overdistention of the uterus |

**Figure 10-1**

**Involution of the uterus.**

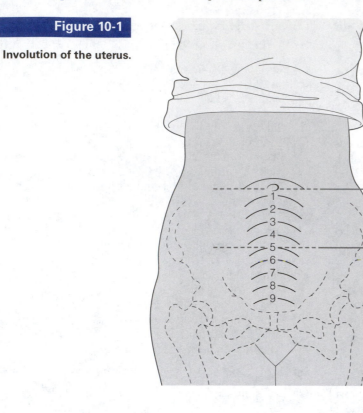

3. Lochia is the discharge of blood and debris following delivery; types include **lochia rubra, lochia serosa,** and **lochia alba;** characteristics of lochia are shown in Table 10-2

   **a.** Should not contain large clots

   **b.** Total volume is 240 to 270 mL, and daily volume gradually decreases

   **c.** Amount may be increased by exertion or breast-feeding

   **d.** Pooling in the uterus or vagina may occur while reclining with increased bleeding upon arising

   **e.** Unexplained increase in amount or reappearance of lochia rubra is abnormal

**Table 10-2**

**Characteristics of Lochia**

| Type | Occurrence | Appearance | Composition |
|------|-----------|-----------|-------------|
| Lochia rubra | 1–3 days | Dark red, bloody; fleshy, musty, stale odor that is non-offensive; may have clots smaller than a nickel | Blood with small amounts of mucus, shreds of decidua, epithelial cells, leukocytes; may contain fetal meconium, lanugo, or vernix caseosa |
| Lochia serosa | 4 to 10 days | Pink or brownish; watery; odorless | Serum, erythrocytes, shreds of degenerating decidua, leukocytes, cervical mucus, numerous bacteria |
| Lochia alba | 11–21 days, may persist to 6 weeks in lactating women | Yellow to white; may have slightly stale odor | Leukocytes, decidual cells, epithelial cells, fat, cervical mucus, cholesterol, bacteria |

4. **Afterpains**

   a. Caused by intermittent uterine contractions following delivery

   b. Occur in all women but are more painful in multiparous and breast-feeding women

5. Cervix

   a. Soft, irregular, and edematous; may appear bruised with multiple small lacerations

   b. Closes to 2 to 3 cm after several days, admits a fingertip after 1 week

   c. Shape permanently changes after the first delivery from the round, dimple-like os of the nullipara to the lateral slit-like os of the multiparous woman

6. Vagina

   a. Smooth walls, edematous with multiple small lacerations

   b. Client should be free from perineal pain within 2 weeks

   c. Low estrogen levels postpartum lead to decreased vaginal lubrication and vasocongestion for 6 to 10 weeks, which can result in painful intercourse

B. **Abdominal wall**

1. Soft and flabby with decreased muscle tone

2. Striae, or stretch marks, that were red during pregnancy will fade to silver or white in Caucasian women; darker-skinned women will have darker striae that remain darker

3. **Diastisis recti,** separation of the rectus muscles of the abdomen, may improve postpartally depending on the woman's physical condition, number of pregnancies, and type and amount of exercise

C. **Cardiovascular**

1. Returns to prepregnant state within 2 weeks

2. The increase in blood volume by 40 percent during pregnancy is eliminated primarily by diuresis

3. The first 48 hours postpartum are the time of greatest risk of complications for clients with heart disease

4. Blood pressure should remain consistent with pregnancy baseline

5. Bradycardia of 50 to 70 beats per minute is common during the first 6 to 10 days; tachycardia is related to increased blood loss, temperature elevation, or difficult, prolonged labor and birth

6. Increased fibrinogen continues for 1 week resulting in increased sedimentation rate and risk for thrombophlebitis

7. Increased white blood cells up to $30,000/mm^3$ does not necessarily mean infection or may mask signs of infection; an increase of >30 percent in 6 hours indicates pathology

8. Decreased hemoglobin is related to the amount of blood loss during delivery; should return to pre-labor value in 2 to 6 weeks depending on degree of decrease

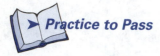

**▶ *Practice to Pass***

A client's white blood cell count is 21,000/mm³ on the first day postpartum. What should you do?

9. Hematocrit increases by 3rd to 5th day postpartum related to diuresis; a drop indicates abnormal blood loss

**D. Urinary**

1. Increased bladder capacity and decreased bladder tone lead to decreased sensation and increased risk of urinary retention and infection

2. Postpartal diuresis of 2,000 to 3,000 mL increases the output in the first 12 to 24 hours after delivery and accounts for a 5-pound weight loss

3. Increased glomerular filtration rate assists in diuresis

4. A full bladder displaces the uterus, increasing the risk of uterine atony and postpartal hemorrhage

5. Fluids are also lost through diaphoresis with increased perspiration most commonly occurring at night

**E. Gastrointestinal**

1. Hunger and thirst are common following birth

2. Risk for constipation increases because of decreased peristalsis, use of narcotic analgesics, dehydration and decreased mobility during labor, and fear of pain from having a bowel movement

3. Risk for hemorrhoids increases because of pressure from pushing during the second stage of labor

**F. Endocrine**

1. Estrogen and progesterone levels drop rapidly after delivery of the placenta

2. Menstruation usually resumes at 7 to 9 weeks for non-lactating women with 90 percent experiencing a menstrual period by 12 weeks; the first cycle is usually anovulatory

3. Ovulation and menstruation return time is prolonged in lactating women and affected by the length of time the woman breast-feeds and whether formula supplements are used; may vary from 2 to 18 months

4. Lactation

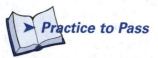

**▶ *Practice to Pass***

A client states she has heard that a woman can't get pregnant again as long as she is breast-feeding. What should you tell her?

   a. Nipple stimulation leads to release of oxytocin from the pituitary gland; this stimulates the release of prolactin from the pituitary gland, which causes production of milk and the **let-down reflex,** release of milk by contractions of the alveoli of the breast

   b. **Colostrum** is the first milk secreted and is rich in protein and immunoglobulins

   c. Primary **engorgement** occurs on the second or third day as the supply of the blood and lymph in the breast is increased and transitional milk is produced

   d. Mature milk is produced after 2 weeks and appears watery and slightly bluish in color, similar to skim milk

## II.  Psychosocial Changes during the Postpartal Period

### A.  Phases of maternal adjustment

1. Taking-in phase

    a. First 3 days postpartum

    b. Preoccupied with own needs

    c. Passive and dependent

    d. Touches and explores infant

    e. Needs to discuss labor and delivery

2. Taking-hold phase

    a. Lasts from the 3rd to 10th day postpartum

    b. Obsessed with body functions

    c. Rapid mood swings

    d. Anticipatory guidance most effective now

3. Letting-go phase

    a. Lasts from 10 days to 6 weeks postpartum

    b. Mothering functions established

    c. Sees infant as a unique person

### B.  *Bonding* (also known as attachment): the process by which parents form an emotional relationship with their infant over time

1. Mother explores the infant first with fingertips, then palms, and finally enfolding the newborn with the whole hands and arms

2. Holds infant in **en face** position, face-to-face position about 20 centimeters apart and on the same plane

3. Uses a soft, high-pitched tone of voice

4. **Engrossment** is the father's absorption, preoccupation, and interest in infant shortly after birth, which can be stimulated by witnessing the birth

### C.  *Postpartum blues:* a maternal adjustment reaction

1. Transient depression usually occurs between the second and third postpartum days and/or within the first 2 weeks postpartum

2. Probably related to changes in hormone levels, fatigue, and psychological stress related to infant dependency

3. Experienced to some degree by a majority of women

4. Characterized by mood swings, anger, tearfulness, feeling let-down, anorexia, and insomnia

5. Usually resolves spontaneously, may need evaluation for postpartum depression if symptoms persist or are severe

### III. Nursing Care of the Postpartal Client

**A. General considerations with postpartal assessment**

1. Evaluate prenatal and intrapartal history for risk factors

2. Provide privacy and encourage client to void prior to assessment

3. Position client in bed with head flat for most accurate findings

4. Proceed in a head-to-toe direction

5. Vital signs are more accurate with woman at rest, will determine the need or priority for other assessments

   **a.** Temperature

      1) Above 100.4°F after first 24 hours may indicate an infection

      2) May be elevated initially after delivery related to dehydration

   **b.** Pulse

      1) Normal range postpartum is 50 to 80 beats per minute

      2) Pulse greater than 100 beats per minute should be reported to the healthcare provider

   **c.** Respirations: normal range is 16 to 24 breaths per minute

   **d.** Blood pressure

      1) Assess for orthostatic hypotension

      2) Monitor more closely if client has a history of preeclampsia

6. Women who experience operative procedures, cesarean delivery, or tubal ligation have postpartal needs similar to those of women who gave birth vaginally and the needs of postoperative clients; monitor breath sounds and have the client cough and take deep breaths

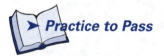

**➤ Practice to Pass**

How should universal precautions be followed during a postpartum assessment?

**B. Postpartum assessment:** the mneumonic BUBBLE-HEB aids the nurse in remembering the components of the assessment

1. Breasts

   **a.** Determine if mother is breast- or bottle-feeding

   **b.** Palpate for engorgement or tenderness

   **c.** Inspect the nipples for redness, cracks, and erectility, if nursing

2. Uterus (see Figure 10-2)

   **a.** Gently place the nondominant hand on the lower uterine segment just above the symphysis pubis; the dominant hand palpates the top of the fundus

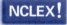

   **b.** Determine the uterine firmness, height of the fundus, and ascertain the position of the fundus in relation to the midline of the abdomen

   **c.** Correlate fundal location with expected descent of 1 centimeter each postpartal day

   **d.** Inspect any abdominal incisions, cesarean delivery, or tubal ligation, for REEDA: redness, edema, ecchymosis, discharge, and approximation of the skin edges

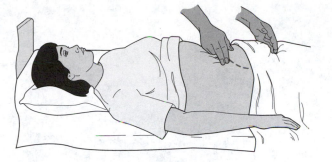

**Figure 10-2**

**Measuring the descent of the fundus.**

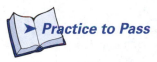

**NCLEX!**

3. **B**ladder

   **a.** The client should void within 6 to 8 hours after delivery

   **b.** Assess frequency, burning, or urgency, which could indicate a urinary tract infection

   **c.** Evaluate the ability to completely empty the bladder

   **d.** Palpate for bladder distention, if unable to void or complete emptying is in question

4. **B**owel

   **a.** Assess for passage of flatus

   **b.** Inspect for signs of distention

   **c.** Auscultate bowel sounds in all four quadrants for postoperative clients

5. Lochia

   **a.** Inspect type, quantity, amount, and odor

   **b.** Correlate findings with expected characteristics of bleeding

   **c.** Cesarean-delivered women may have less lochia

6. **E**pisiotomy or perineal lacerations

   **a.** Inspect the perineum for REEDA

   **b.** Inspect for hemorrhoids

7. **Homan's sign** (see Figure 10-3)

   **a.** Pain in the calf upon dorsiflexion of the foot is recorded as a positive sign and may indicate thrombophlebitis

   **b.** Inspect for pedal edema, redness, or warmth; if abnormal changes are present, assess pedal pulse

8. **E**motional status

   **a.** Assess if the client's emotions are appropriate for the situation

   **b.** Determine the client's phase of postpartal psychological adjustment

   **c.** Assess for signs of postpartum blues

9. **B**onding: describe how the parents interact with the infant

➤ *Practice to Pass*

How should the client be positioned to permit assessment of the perineum?

**Figure 10-3**

Homan's sign.

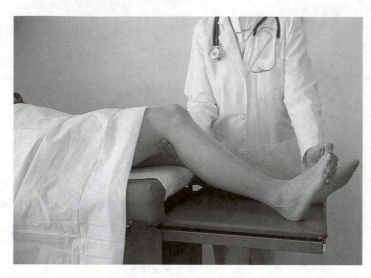

### C. Priority nursing diagnoses

1. Deficient fluid volume

2. Impaired urinary elimination

3. Risk for infection

4. Pain

5. Risk for constipation

6. Interrupted family processes

7. Deficient knowledge

### D. Implementation

1. Prevent hemorrhage

   a. Assess for risk factors

   b. Keep bladder empty

   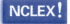

   c. Gently massage fundus, if boggy; teach self-massage of uterus

   d. Administer oxytocic medications, if ordered: oxytocin (Pitocin), methylergonovine maleate (Methergine), ergonovine maleate (Ergotrate)

   e. Monitor for side effects of oxytocics, if administered; hypotension with rapid IV bolus of Pitocin, hypertension with Methergine and Ergotrate

2. Promote comfort

   a. Apply ice to perineum 20 minutes on/10 minutes off for first 24 hours

   b. Encourage sitz bath, warm or cool, tid and prn after first 12 to 24 hours

   c. Teach client perineal care to be used after every elimination

      1) Squirt or pour warm water over the perineum

      2) Blot dry from front to back to prevent tissue trauma and contamination from anal area

3) Apply clean perineal pad from front to back without touching the surface that will be next to client

**d.** Teach client to tighten buttocks, then sit and relax muscles

**e.** Apply topical anesthetics (Dermaplast or Americaine spray) or witch hazel compresses (Tucks)

**f.** Administer analgesics; acetaminophen (Tylenol), non-steroidal anti-inflammatory agents (ibuprofen), narcotics (codeine, hydrocodone, oxycodone)

**g.** Utilize patient-contolled analgesia (PCA pump) or morphine epidural for cesarean deliveries

**h.** Monitor for side effects of morphine epidural, if administered: late-onset respiratory depression (8 to 12 hours), nausea and vomiting (4 to 7 hours), itching (within 3 and up to 10 hours), urinary retention, and somnolence

**3.** Promote bowel elimination

**a.** Encourage early and frequent ambulation

**b.** Encourage increased fluids and fiber

**c.** Administer stool softeners, as ordered; suppositories are contraindicated if the client has a third- or fourth-degree perineal laceration involving the rectum

**d.** Teach client to avoid straining; normal bowel pattern returns in 2 to 3 weeks

**4.** Urinary elimination

**a.** Encourage voiding every 2 to 3 hours even if no urge is felt

**b.** Catheterize, as ordered, for urinary retention; Foley catheter for 12 to 24 hours after cesarean delivery

**5.** Promote successful infant feeding patterns

**a.** Suppression of lactation and successful bottle-feeding

1) Utilize snug bra or breast binder continuously for 5 to 7 days to prevent engorgement

2) Avoid heat and stimulation of the breasts

3) Apply ice packs for 20 minutes qid, if engorgement occurs

4) Encourage demand feedings every 3 to 4 hours, awakening during the day and allowing to sleep at night

**b.** Establishment of lactation and successful breast-feeding

1) Utilize a well-fitting bra for continuous support of the breasts

2) Teach breast care including no use of soap and air drying nipples after feedings

3) Encourage nursing on demand every 2 to 4 hours, awakening during the day and allowing to sleep at night

4) Advise the mother to nurse 10 to 15 minutes on first breast and until the baby lets go of the second; alternate the breast used first and rotate positions

5) Suggest football hold or side-lying position for mothers with cesarean delivery or tubal ligation to avoid discomfort caused by the weight of the baby on the abdominal incision

6) Provide help with positioning, latching on, and breaking suction when done nursing for women nursing multiple births

c. Explore the impact of culture on feeding practices and support family choices as illustrated in Table 10-3

1) Amount of contact and degree of closeness between mother and new-born is often culturally determined

2) Culture may influence how long breast-feeding continues

3) Feeding practices vary across cultures

6. Promote rest and gradual return to activity

a. Organize nursing care to avoid frequent interruptions

b. Plan maternal rest periods when the baby is expected to sleep

c. Teach the woman to resume activity gradually over 4 to 5 weeks; avoid lifting, stair-climbing, and strenuous activity

d. Simple postpartal exercises should be started, per orders; encourage the client to strengthen muscles affected by childbearing; Kegel exercises tighten the perineum by repeatedly attempting to stop the flow of urine and then relaxing; raising the chin to the chest, knee rolls, and buttocks lifts strengthen the abdomen

e. Increased lochia or pain indicates overexertion; modify exercise plan

7. Promote adequate nutritional intake

a. Encourage lactating mothers to add 500 kcal/day to the pre-pregnancy diet; bottle-feeding mothers should return to the pre-pregnancy diet

b. Encourage fluid intake of 2,000 mL/day

c. Continue administration of prenatal vitamins and iron, as ordered; iron is best absorbed in the presence of vitamin C and may increase constipation

8. Promote psychological well-being

a. Plan nursing care based on the client's phase of psychological adjustment and degree of dependence/independence; provide choices whenever possible

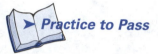

**Practice to Pass**

How would client teaching be modified for a Hmong (southeast Asian) mother who is breastfeeding twins?

| Table 10-3 | Cultural Group | Infant Feeding Practice |
|---|---|---|
| **Cultural Influences on Infant Feeding** | North American and European | Exposing the breast is indecent; weaning is a sign of infant development |
| | Hmong (southeast Asian) | Breast- and bottle-feeding may be combined; expressing or pumping breast milk is unacceptable |
| | Mexican American, Filipino, Navajo, Vietnamese | Colostrum is not offered to the newborn |
| | African-American | Plentiful feeding is emphasized; solids are introduced early |
| | Muslim | Breast-feeding is encouraged to 2 years of age |

   **b.** Encourage and support expression of feelings, positive and negative, without guilt

   **c.** Encourage the client to tell the story of her labor and birth to integrate expectations and fantasies with reality

   **d.** Provide recognition and praise for self- and infant-care activities

9. Promote family well-being

   **a.** Provide an environment that supports family unity and promotes attachment to the newborn

   **b.** Encourage rooming-in, presence of family members

   **c.** Assist parents in preparing siblings with realistic expectations of the newborn, involve siblings in infant care

   **d.** Teach parents that sibling regression is common

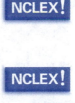

   **e.** Advise the couple to resume sexual activity after the episiotomy has healed and the lochia has stopped, about 3 weeks after delivery; the level of sexual interest and activity may vary, additional water-soluble lubrication may be needed and breast milk may be released with orgasm

   **f.** Counsel couples regarding contraception before discharge, assist the couple to select a method compatible with health needs and individual preferences; a diaphragm or cervical cap will need to be refitted following delivery; oral contraceptives containing estrogen may interfere with lactation

10. Promote maternal safety

   **a.** Give Rho (D) gamma globulin (Rhogam, RhIG, Gamulin) if needed to prevent Rh sensitization and future hemolytic disease of the newborn

     1) Confirm the woman is a candidate: Rh-negative mother not sensitized (negative indirect Coombs' test), Rh-positive newborn not sensitized (negative direct Coombs' test), and no known maternal allergy to globulin preparations

     2) Administer 300 µg IM within 72 hours of delivery

   **b.** Give rubella vaccine to provide activity immunity for mother and avoid fetal malformations if the disease is contracted during a future pregnancy

     1) Confirm the woman is a candidate: titer of < 1:8 (not immune); no known allergy to neomycin

     2) Administer 0.5 mL SC prior to discharge

     3) If mother is a candidate for both Rhogam and rubella vaccine, delay the rubella vaccine at least 6 weeks, and preferably 3 months, to avoid drug interaction and reduced rubella immunity

     4) Teach the client to avoid pregnancy for at least 3 months following vaccination; vaccine contains live virus and can adversely affect the fetus; side effects include burning and stinging at the injection site, warmth and redness, mild symptoms of the disease

   **c.** Teach the client postpartum warning signs to be reported

     1) Bright red bleeding saturating more than 1 pad/hour or passing large clots

2) Temperature greater than 100.4°F

3) Chills

4) Excessive pain

5) Reddened or warm areas of the breast

6) Reddened or gaping episiotomy, foul-smelling lochia

7) Inability to urinate; burning, frequency, or urgency with urination

8) Calf pain, tenderness, redness, or swelling

**E. Evaluation**

1. Assessment findings remain normal

2. Maternal physical and psychological well-being is maintained

3. Client verbalizes/demonstrates techniques of self- and infant-care

4. Parents demonstrate positive signs of attachment with their infant

---

**Case Study**

A client delivered an infant 3 hours ago. The nurse assesses the client and finds the following: fundus firm at 1 centimeter below the umbilicus, small amount of lochia rubra, midline episiotomy well approximated. The client states she is "cramping really bad" when she nurses. She has not ambulated since delivery.

❶ What else would be important to know about this client?

❷ The client states she would like to go to the bathroom. What should the nurse do?

❸ The client is unable to void. What should the nurse do next?

❹ The client's vital signs are: T 100.8°F, P 56, R 16, BP 110/56. How should the nurse interpret these findings, and what interventions are indicated?

❺ What behaviors would the nurse expect to see if this client is bonding positively with her newborn?

*For suggested responses, see page 340.*

---

## Posttest

1   This is the first postoperative day for a client who delivered by cesarean. The client asks the nurse why she has to get up and walk when it hurts her incision so much. The nurse responds that:

(1) Walking decreases the risk of blood clots after surgery.

(2) Walking encourages deep breaths to blow off the anesthetic from surgery.

(3) Early ambulation is important to stimulate milk production.

(4) Walking will decrease the occurrence of afterpains.

**2**  A client delivered by cesarean 2 days ago. While assessing the client's incision, the nurse notes that the skin edges around the incision are red, edematous, and tender to the touch. A scant amount of purulent drainage is noted. What is the most appropriate initial action by the nurse?

(1) Cleanse the wound with betadine.
(2) Notify the physician.
(3) Document this expected response.
(4) Observe the incision closely for the next 24 to 48 hours.

**3**  Which of the following interventions should be omitted when caring for a client with a midline episiotomy with a third-degree laceration?

(1) Increase fiber in diet.
(2) Administer Ducolax suppository.
(3) Increase fluid intake.
(4) Administer an oral stool softener.

**4**  You are caring for a client whose baby was sent to the neonatal intensive care unit because of respiratory distress. The client plans to breast-feed her baby. You understand teaching has been effective when the client states, "I know I need to continue pumping my breasts to:

(1) Prevent engorgement."
(2) Stimulate my milk supply."
(3) Remove the infected milk."
(4) Keep my uterus contracted."

**5**  On the third postpartum day, a client reports that she has voided five times that morning. The nurse should initially:

(1) Collect the next voiding and measure the amount of urine.
(2) Call the physician.
(3) Catheterize the client for residual urine.
(4) Insert a Foley catheter.

**6**  You are assessing a client's fundus and find it firm, 2 centimeters above the umbilicus, and displaced to the right. What is the most appropriate intervention?

(1) Massage the fundus until firm.
(2) Have client void and reassess the fundus.
(3) Notify the physician.
(4) Start a pad count.

**7**  A client's prenatal laboratory findings reveal that she is not immune to rubella. The physician orders rubella vaccine prior to discharge. The nurse knows client teaching has been effective when the client states:

(1) "I'll need another shot in 1 month and again in 6 months."
(2) "This shot may cause a fever and make me vomit."
(3) "I'll need another shot after each baby I have with Rh-positive blood."
(4) "I should not get pregnant for at least 3 months after the vaccine."

**8**  A client's vital signs following delivery are: (Day 1) BP 116/72, T 98.6, P 68; (Day 2) BP 114/80, T 100.6, P 76; (Day 3) BP 114/80, T 101.6, P 80. The nurse should suspect that the client:

(1) Is dehydrated.
(2) May have an infection.
(3) Has normal vital signs.
(4) Is going into shock.

**9**  The nurse is reviewing infection control policies with a nursing student. The nurse knows that the teaching has been effective when the student states, "The best way to prevent postpartum infection starts:

(1) In the recovery room with strict use of sterile technique when palpating the fundus."
(2) On the postpartum unit by teaching the client the principles of perineal care."
(3) In the labor room by limiting the number of sterile vaginal exams."
(4) When the client goes home by avoiding tub baths until the lochia stops."

**10** Which of the following assessments should alert the nurse to hold the scheduled dose of methylergonovine maleate (Methergine) for a postpartal client and call the physician?

(1) Blood pressure 142/86
(2) Apical pulse 56
(3) Blood type O positive
(4) Mother is planning to breast-feed

*See page 233 for Answers and Rationales.*

## Answers and Rationales

### Pretest

**1** **Answer: 3** *Rationale:* The fundus should remain firm after delivery to decrease the risk of postpartum hemorrhage and decrease 1 centimeter below the umbilicus each day. All nursing interventions presented are appropriate, but massaging the fundus until firm is the most important to prevent hemorrhage.
*Cognitive Level:* Application
*Nursing Process:* Implementation; *Test Plan:* PHYS

**2** **Answer: 1** *Rationale:* Afterpains are anticipated in the postpartal client and are effectively treated with analgesics.
*Cognitive Level:* Application
*Nursing Process:* Implementation; *Test Plan:* PHYS

**3** **Answer: 4** *Rationale:* This client should be encouraged to verbalize her disappointment as the first step in resolving her negative feelings.
*Cognitive Level:* Application
*Nursing Process:* Implementation; *Test Plan:* PSYC

**4** **Answer: 3** *Rationale:* Having sexual intercourse before the episiotomy is healed or the lochia has stopped increases the risk of infection. Water-soluble lubricants can be used, if necessary. An IUD is contraindicated during the early postpartum period.
*Cognitive Level:* Application
*Nursing Process:* Planning; *Test Plan:* PSYC

**5** **Answer: 3** *Rationale:* Binding the breasts, either with a snug bra or binder, and applying cold to the breasts will help suppress lactation. Milk supply is stimulated by expressing milk and applying heat to the breasts. Medications to suppress lactation are not recommended.
*Cognitive Level:* Application
*Nursing Process:* Implementation; *Test Plan:* PHYS

**6** **Answer: 1** *Rationale:* Temperature elevation immediately after delivery is often caused by dehydration during labor. Increasing the client's fluid intake will usually decrease the temperature to within normal limits. There is no indication for analgesia or antibiotics at this time. If the fever persists beyond 24 hours or the client has clinical signs of infection, then further investigation and perhaps treatment is warranted.
*Cognitive Level:* Application
*Nursing Process:* Implementation; *Test Plan:* PHYS

**7** **Answer: 1** *Rationale:* Clients are at risk for orthostatic hypotension, especially right after delivery. The nurse should stay with the client the first time she ambulates after delivery to promote safety. Early ambulation prevents circulatory stasis in the lower extremities and should be encouraged. The perineum should be patted (not wiped) dry from front to back to avoid trauma, discomfort, and contamination with bacteria from the anal region.
*Cognitive Level:* Analysis
*Nursing Process:* Implementation; *Test Plan:* SECE

**8** **Answer: 1** *Rationale:* A client with a hemoglobin of 7.2 g/dL would most likely have significant signs and symptoms of anemia, and this could be life-threatening. It would be important to determine if the client had a large estimated blood loss during delivery or if she is currently bleeding excessively. The hematocrit is within normal limits, and mild proteinuria or leukocytosis up to 30,000/mm$^3$ are common in the early postpartum.
*Cognitive Level:* Analysis
*Nursing Process:* Assessment; *Test Plan:* PHYS

**9** **Answer: 4** *Rationale:* An adult client should have a minimum urinary output of 30 cc/hr and this client is below that minimum. In a postpartum client, this is most likely related to urinary retention secondary to perineal edema and trauma from delivery. It is important that postpartal clients are able to empty their bladder without assistance prior to discharge.
*Cognitive Level:* Analysis
*Nursing Process:* Assessment; *Test Plan:* SECE

**10** **Answer: 3** *Rationale:* If a postpartum client is experiencing pain, she will be less likely to ambulate, less receptive to teaching, and more likely to experience constipation because of the fear of pain with a bowel movement. By treating her pain first, interven-

tions for the other nursing diagnoses will be more successful.
*Cognitive Level:* Analysis
*Nursing Process:* Analysis; *Test Plan:* PSYC

## Posttest

1  **Answer: 1** *Rationale:* Clients who have had a cesarean delivery are at risk for complications of surgery, including thrombophlebitis. Early ambulation can significantly decrease the risk of blood clots and other postoperative complications.
*Cognitive Level:* Application
*Nursing Process:* Implementation; *Test Plan:* PHYS

2  **Answer: 2** *Rationale:* This client has signs of an incisional infection. The physician needs to be notified first so that treatment can be started as soon as possible. Betadine has not yet been ordered. Documentation should follow reporting. Continued observation would be an ongoing intervention.
*Cognitive Level:* Analysis
*Nursing Process:* Analysis; *Test Plan:* PHYS

3  **Answer: 2** *Rationale:* A third- or fourth-degree perineal laceration involves the rectal sphincter, therefore, suppositories, enemas, and rectal exams are contraindicated until the rectum heals. Increased fiber and fluids or use of stool softeners are appropriate to promote bowel elimination in all postpartal clients.
*Cognitive Level:* Application
*Nursing Process:* Implementation; *Test Plan:* SECE

4  **Answer: 2** *Rationale:* Breast-milk production is based on supply and demand. The more the breasts are stimulated to produce milk, by nursing the baby or pumping the breasts, the more milk will be produced.
*Cognitive Level:* Analysis
*Nursing Process:* Evaluation; *Test Plan:* HPM

5  **Answer: 1** *Rationale:* Urinary retention can occur because of perineal edema and trauma from delivery. The nursing process begins with assessment. The nurse should accurately assess the client's urinary output first before reporting or determining other interventions that may be indicated.
*Cognitive Level:* Application
*Nursing Process:* Implementation; *Test Plan:* PHYS

6  **Answer: 2** *Rationale:* This client's fundus is already firm, so it is not appropriate to massage the fundus. It is also higher in the abdomen than expected, and it is displaced to the right, which is probably caused by a distended bladder. Having the client void may return the uterus to the expected position; palpating the fundus after voiding will confirm this finding. A pad count would be appropriate if bleeding is increasing; no information given implies that this action is indicated.
*Cognitive Level:* Application
*Nursing Process:* Analysis; *Test Plan:* PHYS

7  **Answer: 4** *Rationale:* The rubella vaccine is a live virus. If a client becomes pregnant within the first 3 months after administration, her fetus is at risk for congenital anomalies related to the virus. Women who are not rubella immune should be vaccinated postpartum, prior to discharge. Teaching should include an effective method of birth control and the importance of avoiding pregnancy for the next 3 months.
*Cognitive Level:* Application
*Nursing Process:* Evaluation; *Test Plan:* SECE

8  **Answer: 2** *Rationale:* The vital signs are not normal. An elevation in body temperature greater than 100.4°F after the first 24 hours postpartum could indicate maternal infection. An elevated temperature within the first 24 hours is usually related to dehydration, although the possibility of infection still exists. Rising pulse and falling blood pressure rather than rising temperature is an indicator of hypovolemic shock.
*Cognitive Level:* Analysis
*Nursing Process:* Analysis; *Test Plan:* PHYS

9  **Answer: 3** *Rationale:* Even when perfect sterile technique is used when doing a vaginal exam, organisms present on the perineum are transported into the vagina and close to the cervix. By limiting the number of vaginal exams, the risk is decreased. Option 1 is incorrect because clean technique, not sterile technique, is used when palpating the fundus. Options 2 and 4 are correct answers, but not the earliest intervention a nurse could perform.
*Cognitive Level:* Application
*Nursing Process:* Evaluation; *Test Plan:* SECE

10  **Answer: 1** *Rationale:* A potential side effect of Methergine is hypertension. If a client's blood pressure is elevated, the nurse should hold the scheduled dose and notify the physician. An apical heart rate of 56 is within normal limits postpartum. Blood type, Rh factor, and chosen feeding method are not related to the use of Methergine.
*Cognitive Level:* Analysis
*Nursing Process:* Implementation; *Test Plan:* PHYS

# References

Alden, K. R. (1999). The newborn: Newborn nutrition and feeding. In Lowdermilk, D. L., Perry, S. E. & Bobak, I. M. (Eds.), *Maternity nursing* (5th ed.). St. Louis: Mosby, pp. 549–577.

Askin, D. (1999). Complications of childbearing: The newborn at risk. In Lowdermilk, D. L., Perry, S. E., & Bobak, I. M. (Eds.), *Maternity nursing* (5th ed.). St. Louis: Mosby, pp. 807–860.

Edwards, L. D. (1999). Postpartum period: Adaptation to parenthood. In Lowdermilk, D. L., Perry, S. E., & Bobak, I. M. (Eds.), *Maternity nursing* (5th ed.). St. Louis: Mosby, pp. 449–488.

Lowdermilk, D. L. & Fishel, A. H. (1999). Complications of childbearing: Postpartum complications. In Lowdermilk, D. L., Perry, S. E., & Bobak, I. M. (Eds.), *Maternity nursing* (5th ed.). St. Louis: Mosby, pp. 742–771.

Morre, M. C. (1999). Pregnancy: Maternal and fetal nutrition. In Lowdermilk, D. L., Perry, S. E., & Bobak, I. M. (Eds.), *Maternity nursing* (5th ed.). St. Louis: Mosby, pp. 258–285.

Olds, S. B., London, M. L., & Ladewig, P. A. (2000). *Maternal-newborn nursing: A family and community-based approach* (6th ed.). Upper Saddle River, NJ: Prentice Hall Health, pp. 705–751, 805–903, 910, 911, 917–919.

Perry, S. E. (1999). Introduction to maternity nursing: Contemporary maternity nursing. In Lowdermilk, D. L., Perry, S. E., & Bobak, I. M. (Eds.), *Maternity nursing* (5th ed.). St. Louis: Mosby, pp. 1–9.

Pillitteri, A. (1999). *Maternal and child health nursing: Care of the childbearing and childrearing family* (3rd ed.). Philadelphia: Lippincott, pp. 594–742.

Piotrowski, K. A. (1999). Childbirth: Nursing care during labor and birth. In Lowdermilk, D. L., Perry, S. E., & Bobak, I. M. (Eds.), *Maternity nursing* (5th ed.). St. Louis: Mosby, pp. 348–406.

Piotrowski, K. A. (1999). Complications of childbearing: Labor and birth at risk. In Lowdermilk, D. L., Perry, S. E., & Bobak, I. M. (Eds.), *Maternity nursing* (5th ed.). St. Louis: Mosby, pp. 694–741.

Sherwin, L. N., Scoloveno, M. A., & Weingarten, C. T. (1999). *Maternity nursing: Care of the childbearing family* (3rd ed.). Stamford, CT: Appleton & Lange, pp. 1019–1062, 1067–1111.

Siegel, R., Gardner, S. L., & Merenstein, G. B. (1998). Families in crisis: Theoretical and practical considerations. In Merenstein, G. B. & Gardner, S. L. (Eds.), *Handbook of neonatal intensive care* (4th ed.). St. Louis: Mosby, pp. 647–672.

Sinclair, B. J. (1999). Reproductive years: Health promotion and prevention. In Lowdermilk, D. L., Perry, S. E., & Bobak, I. M. (Eds.), *Maternity nursing* (5th ed.). St. Louis: Mosby, pp. 41–63.

Stetson, B. (1999). Postpartum period: Assessment and care during the fourth trimester. In Lowdermilk, D. L., Perry, S. E., & Bobak, I. M. (Eds.), *Maternity nursing* (5th ed.). St. Louis: Mosby, pp. 416–448.

Stetson, B. (1999). Postpartum period: Physiological changes. In Lowdermilk, D. L., Perry, S. E., & Bobak, I. M. (Eds.), *Maternity nursing* (5th ed.). St. Louis: Mosby, pp. 407–415.

## CHAPTER 11

# The Complicated Postpartal Experience

A. Jenny Harkey, RNC, MSN, ACCE

## CHAPTER OUTLINE

## OBJECTIVES

- Describe nursing assessments that identify the high-risk postpartal client.

- Discuss nursing interventions for the client with postpartal complications related to hemorrhage.

- Describe the nursing care of a client experiencing a puerperal infection.

- Identify the symptoms and management of thromboembolic disorders.

- List the symptoms exhibited in a client experiencing a postpartal psychiatric disorder.

[ Media Link ]

*Use the CD-ROM enclosed with this text, or log onto the address given to access the free, interactive Companion Website created for this series. The CD-ROM and Companion Website accompanying this book offer additional practice opportunities and information—NCLEX Review, Case Studies, Glossary, In Depth with NCLEX, and more.*

**www.prenhall.com/hogan**

## REVIEW AT A GLANCE

**disseminated intravascular coagulation** *a pathological form of coagulation that is diffuse rather than localized; several clotting factors are consumed to such extent that generalized bleeding may occur*

**early-postpartal hemorrhage** *a loss of blood greater than 500 mL within the first 24 hours following birth*

**endometritis/metritis** *infection of the endometrium*

**hematoma** *a collection of blood resulting from injury to a blood vessel*

**late-postpartal hemorrhage** *a loss of blood greater than 500 mL after the first 24 hours following birth*

**mastitis** *inflammation of the breast connective tissue*

**pelvic cellulitis/parametritis** *inflammation involving the connective tissue of the broad ligament or all pelvic tissue*

**peritonitis** *inflammation of the peritoneum*

**postpartum psychiatric disorders** *according to the DSM-IV, it is one diagnosable syndrome with three subclasses: adjustment reaction with depressed mood; postpartum major mood disorder; and postpartum psychosis*

**puerperal infection** *an infection of the reproductive tract within the 6-week postpartum period*

**subinvolution** *failure of the uterus to return to its normal size after pregnancy*

**thrombophlebitis** *inflammation of a vein wall resulting in a thrombus*

**urinary tract infection/cystitis/ pyelonephritis** *an infection in the urinary tract; cystitis is an infection in the lower urinary tract involving the bladder and urethra; pyelonephritis is an infection in the upper urinary tract including the ureters and kidneys*

**uterine atony** *relaxation of the uterine muscle following birth*

## Pretest

**1** The client is a 36-year-old woman, gravida 6, para 6, who delivered a baby girl at 38 weeks gestation after 8 hours of labor. The baby weighed 7 pounds 14 ounces. The client's vital signs are stable, and her lochia is bright red, heavy, and contains various clots. The largest clot is about half-dollar size. The client is considered to be high risk for uterine atony because of which of the following?

(1) Grand multiparity
(2) Size of the baby
(3) Length of labor
(4) Client's age

**2** A client continues to pass large amounts of clots and bright red lochia despite the nurse's attempt to massage the fundus. Upon reexamination, the nurse finds that the client's uterine fundus remains boggy. The nursing actions and oxytocin (Pitocin) do not seem to be helping to keep the fundus firm. What second medication might the physician request the nurse to administer to manage uterine atony?

(1) Dinoprostone (Cervidil)
(2) Terbutaline sulfate (Brethine)
(3) Magnesium sulfate
(4) Carboprost (Prostin 15-M or Hemabate)

**3** A mother with mastitis is concerned about breastfeeding while she has an active infection. The nurse should explain that:

(1) The infant is protected from infection by immunoglobulins in the breast milk.
(2) The infant is not susceptible to the organisms that cause mastitis.
(3) The organisms that cause mastitis are not passed in the milk.
(4) The organisms will be inactivated by gastric acid.

**4** If the nurse suspects a uterine infection in the postpartum client, the nurse should assess the:

(1) Pulse and blood pressure.
(2) Odor of the lochia.
(3) Episiotomy site.
(4) The abdomen for distention.

**5** A postpartal client develops a temperature during her postpartal course. Which of the following temperatures indicates the presence of postpartal infection?

(1) 99.0°F 12 hours after delivery that decreases after 18 hours
(2) 100. 2°F 24 hours after delivery that decreases the second postpartum day
(3) 100.4°F 24 hours after delivery that remains until the second postpartum day
(4) 100.6°F 48 hours after delivery that continues into the third postpartum day

**6** Which of the following signs of thrombophlebitis must the nurse educate the postpartal client to assess at home after discharge from the hospital?

(1) Muscle soreness in her legs after exercise
(2) Varicose veins in her legs
(3) Local tenderness, heat, and swelling
(4) Bruising

**7** Which of the following instructions should be included in the discharge teaching plan to assist the postpartal client in recognizing early signs of complications?

(1) The passage of clots as large as an orange is expected.
(2) Report any decrease in the amount of brownish-red lochia.
(3) Palpate the fundus daily to make sure it is soft.
(4) Notify your healthcare provider of any increase in the amount of lochia or a return to bright red bleeding.

**8** A client delivered a 9-pound, 10-ounce infant assisted by forceps. When the nurse performs the second 15-minute assessment, the client complains of increasing perineal pain and a lot of pressure. What action should the nurse take?

(1) Put an ice pack on the client's perineum, reassuring the client that this is normal.
(2) Call for assistance.
(3) Assess the fundus for firmness.
(4) Check the perineum for a hematoma.

**9** On the client's third postpartum day, the nurse enters the room and finds the client crying. The client states that she doesn't know why she is crying, and she can't stop. Which of the following is the most appropriate statement for the nurse to make?

(1) "There is no need to cry, you have a healthy baby."
(2) "Are you dissatisfied with your care?"
(3) "Many new mothers have shared with us their same confusion of feelings; would you like to talk about them?"
(4) "This happens to lots of mothers, you'll get over it."

**10** Postpartum depression occurs in 8 to 26 percent of postpartal women. Assessment for factors predisposing a client to postpartum depression should begin prenatally. Which of the following clients would you consider at risk for postpartum depression?

(1) A client who is an unmarried primipara with family support.
(2) A client who has previously had postpartum blues.
(3) A client who is a primipara with documented ambivalence about her pregnancy in the first trimester.
(4) A client who is a primipara with a history of depression and lack of a supportive relationship.

*See pages 258–259 for Answers and Rationales.*

## I. Nursing Care of the High-Risk Postpartal Client

### A. Assessment

1. Degree of homeostasis, amount of intrapartum blood loss, hematocrit, hemoglobin, and CBC results

2. Vital signs: elevated temperature, blood pressure, heart rate; low blood pressure, symptoms of shock

3. Fundus: height, tone, and position

4. Lochia: amount, color, consistency, odor, and presence/size of clots (greater than quarter-size of concern

5. Perineum: edema, ecchymosis, pain, hemorrhoids

6. Bladder: distention and displacement, ability to void

7. Bowel: constipation, distended abdomen, decreased or no bowel sounds (risk of ileus)

8. Breasts: cracked, bleeding, or blistered nipples; engorgement, red streaks, lumps, clogged milk ducts

9. Homan's sign, redness, tenderness, areas of heat in calves, severe abdominal or flank pain

10. Rest, activity tolerance

11. Bonding or attachment behaviors, maternal–infant interaction

**B. Priority nursing diagnoses**

1. Safe, effective care

   a. Risk for injury

   b. Risk for infection

   c. Deficient knowledge

2. Physiologic integrity

   a. Interrupted breast-feeding

   b. Deficient fluid volume

   c. Impaired gas exchange

   d. Fatigue

   e. Pain (perineal)

   f. Imbalanced body temperature

3. Psychosocial integrity

   a. Fear

   b. Disturbed body image

   c. Ineffective coping

   d. Impaired adjustment

4. Health promotion/maintenance

   a. Self-care deficit

   b. Interrupted family processes

   c. Risk for impaired parent–infant attachment

**C. Planning**

1. Develop a nursing care plan that reflects a knowledge of etiology, pathophysiology, and current clinical management for the woman experiencing a postpartal complication

2. The goal of nursing care is that the client will be free from undetected problems and will maintain physiological and psychosocial integrity

**D. Implementation**

1. Teach client normal adaptation

2. Observe for actual or potential problems in the immediate postpartal period (first 2 hours after delivery) and continue into the later postpartal period

3. Administer treatment or medication as ordered

4. Educate client about signs of complications prior to discharge

5. Reinforce importance of keeping appointment for postpartal checkup

6. Provide client with telephone numbers that can be used to ask questions

**E. Evaluation**

1. Abnormal findings are identified early

2. Treatment is effective

3. Client is confident in ability to monitor self and access necessary follow-up care upon discharge from the hospital

## II. Postpartal Hemorrhage

**A. *Early-postpartal hemorrhage***

1. Incidence: approximately one-third of maternal deaths are related to postpartal hemorrhage

2. Definition: a blood loss greater that 500 mL in the first 24 hours after vaginal delivery; may be greater with cesarean delivery

3. Predisposing factors: early postpartal hemorrhage occurs within the first 24 hours of birth; at term, 600 mL/minute of blood perfuses the pregnant uterus; the most common causes of postpartal hemorrhage are uterine atony and lacerations

   **a. Uterine atony**

     1) Description: lack of uterine muscle tone; the normal mechanism for hemostasis after birth of the placenta is contraction of the interlacing uterine muscles to occlude the open areas at the sight of placental attachment; over 75 percent of all postpartal hemorrhages are caused by uterine atony; absence of uterine contraction can cause significant blood loss

     2) Predisposing factors

       a) Conditions that overdistend the uterus

         (1) Delivery of a large infant

         (2) Multiple gestation

         (3) Hydramnios/polyhydramnios

       b) Conditions that affect uterine contractility

         (1) Multiparity

         (2) Precipitous labor

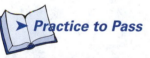

**► *Practice to Pass***

You have received a client on the postpartum unit who delivered a large-for-gestational-age infant via low-outlet forceps. What types of problems would you anticipate this client might experience?

(3) Dysfunctional or prolonged labor

(4) Prolonged third stage of labor

(5) Retained placental fragments

c) Medication use

(1) General anesthesia

(2) Magnesium sulfate (MgSO$_4$)

(3) Oxytocin induction or augmentation of labor

(4) Tocolytics

d) Low platelet count secondary to pregnancy induced hypertension

**b.** Lacerations

1) Description: more common after operative obstetrics, a firm uterus with bright red blood or a steady stream or trickle of unclotted blood

2) Incidence: may make up as much as 20 percent of early postpartal hemorrhage

3) Types/locations

a) Perineal

b) Vaginal

c) Cervical

4) Predisposing factors

a) Primiparous state

b) Epidural anesthesia

c) Precipitous childbirth

d) Macrosomia

e) Forceps or vacuum-assisted birth

f) Mediolateral episiotomy

**c. Hematoma**

1) Description: a collection of blood, often vulvar or vaginal (Figure 11-1), that occurs as a result of injury to a blood vessel during spontaneous delivery; in an assisted vaginal delivery, the most common site is the lateral wall in the area of the ischial spine

2) Incidence: occurs 1 in 300 to 1,500 births

3) Predisposing factors

a) Prolonged pressure of fetal head on vaginal mucosa

b) Operative delivery (forceps or vacuum extraction)

c) Prolonged second stage of labor

d) Precipitous labor

e) Macrosomia

f) Pudendal anesthesia

**Figure 11-1**

**Postpartum vulvar hematoma.**

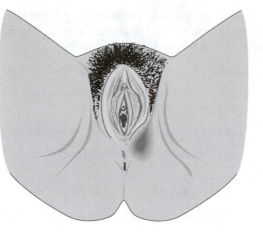

**d. Disseminated intravascular coagulopathy (DIC)**

1) Description: complex disorder of the clotting mechanisms in the blood; consumption of clotting factors that can lead to overwhelming and diffuse hemorrhage; oozing from puncture sites or development of petechiae may be initial clues of coagulopathy

2) Predisposing factors

a) Pregnancy-induced hypertension

b) Amniotic fluid embolism

c) Sepsis

d) Abruptio placentae

e) Prolonged intrauterine fetal demise

f) Excessive blood loss

**e.** Other causes of early postpartal hemorrhage

1) Uterine rupture

2) Uterine inversion

**B. *Late-postpartal hemorrhage***

1. **Subinvolution:** failure of the uterus to return to normal size after pregnancy; late-postpartal hemorrhage occurs most often within 1 to 2 weeks after childbirth because of retention of placental tissue; blood loss at this time may be excessive but usually poses less risk than immediate postpartal hemorrhage; lochia often fails to progress from rubra to serosa to alba normally; lochia rubra that exists longer than 2 weeks is suggestive of subinvolution; subinvolution is most commonly diagnosed at the postpartal exam at 4 to 6 weeks

2. Incidence: 1 in 1,000 births

**C. Nursing assessment**

1. Assess the client's history and labor and delivery record for factors that might predispose the client to postpartal hemorrhage

2. Assess vaginal bleeding after delivery every 10 to 15 minutes for 1 hour, then every 30 minutes for 1 hour until stable; more frequent assessments may be necessary depending upon the client's condition

    a. Bleeding may be slow and continuous or rapid and profuse

    b. Blood may escape from the vagina or pool in the uterus and vagina, becoming evident as clots

    c. Bleeding from a laceration occurs in the presence of a firm uterus

    d. Large and numerous clots may occur

    e. Assist the client to a side-lying position and check the pad underneath frequently; blood may accumulate under the client

    f. Weigh peri-pads to estimate blood loss if careful measurement is deemed necessary

3. Palpate fundus for firmness, assess for height in relation to umbilicus and position

4. Assess for signs of shock

5. Assess bladder for fullness and distention

6. Assess for pelvic pain or backache

D. **Priority nursing diagnoses:** Deficient fluid volume; Risk for injury; Ineffective tissue perfusion: cardiopulmonary; Fear

E. **Planning/goal setting:** client will be free from undetected hemorrhage and shock, will have blood volume restored, and will regain homeostasis

F. **Implementation**

1. Remain with the client

2. Massage boggy uterus gently but firmly, cupping uterus between two hands and avoiding overmassage (see Figure 11-2)

3. Administer uterine stimulants as prescribed by the healthcare provider; see Table 11-1 for commonly prescribed uterine stimulants used to prevent and manage uterine atony and hemorrhage

4. If bleeding is excessive, the healthcare provider may elect to perform a bimanual massage

5. Monitor vital signs, intake and output, level of consciousness, fundal tone and placement, and amount of bleeding during episode of acute hemorrhage; elevate legs 15 to 30 degrees

6. Encourage frequent voiding to prevent bladder distention that contributes to uterine atony; a Foley catheter may need to be inserted or a bed pan may be used during postpartal hemorrhage

7. Replace fluids and administer blood products as ordered

8. Assist with any preoperative preparation as necessary for surgical removal of placental fragments, ligation of a bleeding vessel, or suturing of a laceration

9. Maintain asepsis

10. Assure that surgical consent form is signed, if necessary

11. Support significant other

**Figure 11-2**

**Uterine palpation and massage.**

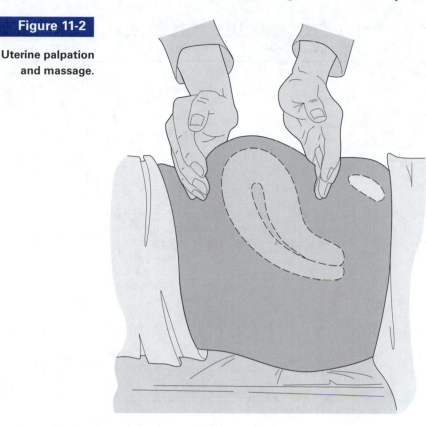

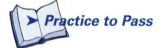

**Practice to Pass**

A postpartal client is going home from the hospital. What symptoms of subinvolution will you include in your discharge teaching?

**G. Evaluation**

1. Client is free from excessive blood loss

2. Lochia is red, moderate in amount, and without clots greater than the size of a quarter

3. Fundus is firm, midline, and at the level of the umbilicus or below

4. Client regains homeostasis

5. Vital signs are normal

6. Intake and output is adequate

7. Client has positive support during postpartum recovery

8. Client's family is informed of client's status and progress

### III. Postpartal (Puerperal) Infections

**A. Reproductive tract infections (Table 11-2)**

1. Incidence: occurs after delivery in about 6 percent of births in the United States

2. Definition: any infection in the reproductive system within 6 weeks of delivery

3. Predisposing factors: anemia, prolonged rupture of membranes, soft tissue trauma or hemorrhage, invasive procedures including the use of internal fetal monitoring, multiple vaginal examinations, retention of placental fragments, chorioamnionitis, preexisting bacterial vaginosis, manual removal of the placenta, lapses in aseptic technique by staff, use of forceps or vacuum-

| Table 11-1 | Uterine Stimulants Used to Prevent and Manage Uterine Atony | | | |
|---|---|---|---|---|
| **Drug** | **Dosing Information** | **Contraindications** | **Expected Effects** | **Side Effects** |
| Oxytocin (Pitocin, Syntocinon) | IV use: 10–40 units in 500–1000 mL crystalloid fluid @ 50 mU/min administration rate. Onset: immediate. Duration: 1 h. **IV bolus administration not recommended.** IM use: 10–20 units. Onset: 3–5 min. Duration: 2–3 h. | | Rhythmic uterine contractions that help to prevent or reverse postpartal hemorrhage caused by uterine atony. | Uterine hyperstimulation, mild transient hypertension, water intoxification rare in postpartum use. |
| Methylergonovine Malaeate (Methergine) | IM use: 0.2 mg q2–4h. Onset: 2–5 min. Duration: 3 h (× 5 dose maximum). PO use: 0.2 mg q6–12h. Onset: 7–15 min. Duration: 3 h (× 1 week). **IV administration not recommended.** | Women with labile or high blood pressure or known sensitivity to drug. | Sustained uterine contractions that help to prevent or reverse postpartal hemorrhage caused by uterine atony; management of postpartal subinvolution. | Hypertension, dizziness, headache, flushing/hot flashes, tinnitus, nausea and vomiting, palpitations, chest pain. Overdose or hypersensitivity is recognized by seizures; tingling and numbness of fingers and toes from vasoconstrictive effect, leading rarely to gangrene; hypertension; weak pulse; chest pain. |
| Ergonovine Maleate (Ergotrate Maleate) | IM use: 0.2 mg q2–4h. Onset 7 min. Duration: 3 h (5 dose maximum). PO use: 0.2 mg q6–12h. Onset: 15 min. Duration: 3 h (× 2–7 days). **IV administration not recommended.** | Women with labile or high blood pressure or known sensitivity to drug. | Sustained uterine contractions that help to prevent or reverse postpartal hemorrhage caused by uterine atony; management of postpartal subinvolution. | Hypertension, dizziness, headache, nausea and vomiting, chest pain. Hypersensitivity is noted by systemic vasoconstrictive effects: seizure, chest pain, and tingling and numbness of fingers and toes that leads rarely to gangrene. |
| Prostaglandin (PGF$_{2a}$, Hemabate, Prostin/15M) | IM use: 0.25 mg repeated up to maximum 5 doses; may be repeated q15–90min. Physician may elect to administer by direct intramyometrial injection. | Women with active cardiovascular, renal, liver disease, or asthma or with known hypersensitivity to drug. | Control of refractory cases of postpartal hemorrhage caused by uterine atony; generally used after failed attempts at control of hemorrhage with oxytoxic agents. | Nausea, vomiting, diarrhea, headache, flushing, bradycardia, bronchospasm, wheezing, cough, chills, fever. |

From Olds, et al. (2000). *Maternal newborn nursing: A family and community-based approach* (6th ed.). Upper Saddle River, NJ: Prentice-Hall, Inc., p. 983.

extraction, and obesity; cesarean delivery is the single most significant risk, with infection occurring in 12 to 51 percent of cases

4. Types of infection

    **a.** Localized lesions of perineum, vulva, and vagina

        1) Local infection may extend through venous circulation resulting in

            a) Infectious thrombophlebitis

            b) Septicemia

| **Table 11-2** | **Type of Infection** | **Assessment Findings** |
|---|---|---|
| **Summary of Specific Reproductive System Infections and Assessment Findings** | Metritis | Fever initially 101–102°F, (38.3–38.9°C); if infection becomes more serious, jagged temperature elevations between 101 and 104°F (38.3 and 40°C). Uterine tenderness on palpation of the fundus or on bimanual examination. Grimacing, guarding, complaints of pain. Prolonged or bothersome afterpains. Subinvolution of uterus. Bacteria revealed on culture of lochia. |
| | Parametrial cellulitis (parametritis) | Prolonged elevation of temperature to 102–104°F (38.9–40°C) with fluctuations. Extension of abdominal pain laterally; possible rebound tenderness. Hypotension, subinvolution, chills. Decreased bowel sounds, nausea, and vomiting. |
| | Peritonitis | Elevation of temperature to as high as 105°F (40.5°C). Severe pain. Paralytic ileus. Abdominal rigidity. Frequent vomiting with dehydration. Weak and thready pulse (possible). Rapid, shallow respirations. Excessive thirst, marked anxiety. |
| | Septic pelvic thrombophlebitis | Elevation of temperature to 105°F (40.5°C); dramatic fluctuations (possible) over short periods. Pain in flank or lower abdomen. |
| | Bacteremia and septic shock | Rapid elevation of temperature to 103–104°F (39.4–40°C). Profuse, foul-smelling lochia. Symptoms of shock. Reduction in urinary output. |

From Sherwen, Scoloveno, Weingarten (2001). *Maternity nursing: Care of the childbearing family* (Media edition). Stamford, CT: Appleton & Lange, p. 900.

2)   Local infection may extend through lymphatic vessels resulting in:

   a)   **Pelvic cellulitis/parametritis:** infection involving connective tissue of the broad ligament or the connective tissue of all the pelvic structures

   b)   **Peritonitis:** infection involving the peritoneal cavity

   b.   **Endometritis/metritis:** localized infection of the lining of the uterus usually beginning at the placental site; endometritis is a common complication after cesarean delivery and is reported to have an incidence ranging from 10 to 50 percent; antibiotic prophylaxis at the time of cord-clamping has been shown to reduce the incidence of postpartum endometritis in both elective and emergent cesarean sections

   c.   Bacterial causative agents

   1)   *Streptococcus hemolyticus:* less common today, virulent onset, and rapid progression

   2)   *Escherichia coli*

   3)   *Staphylococcus aureus*

   4)   *Chlamydia trachomatis*

   5)   β-*hemolytic streptococcus*

   6)   Genital mycoplasmas

   7)   *Clostridia*

   8)   *Klebsiella*

   9)   Anaerobic streptococcus

**5.**   Nursing assessment

   a.   Temperature greater than 100.4°F on any 2 of the first 10 days postpartum excluding the first 24 hours

**NCLEX!**

**NCLEX!**

    **b.** Abnormal lochia

       1) Remains rubra longer

       2) Foul odor

       3) Scant or profuse in amount

    **c.** Tachycardia

    **d.** Delayed involution

       1) Fundal height does not descend as expected

       2) Uterus may feel larger and softer

       3) Client may have pain or tenderness over the uterus

    **e.** Pain, tenderness, or inflammation of perineum

    **f.** Backache

    **g.** Malaise

    **h.** Fatigue

    **i.** Chills

    **j.** Abnormal laboratory results: increased sedimentation rate; leukocytosis—WBC level of 14,000 to 16,000 mm$^3$ is not unusual during the postpartum period; an increase in WBC level of more than 30 percent in a 6-hour period is indicative of infection

**6.** Priority nursing diagnoses: High risk for infection; Pain; Fatigue; Risk for impaired parent–infant attachment; Interrupted family processes; Compromised family coping

**7.** Planning/goal-setting: client will be free from infection, will have infection treated as soon as possible, will participate in prescribed treatment, will develop own maternal role while attaching to newborn, and will have homeostasis restored

**8.** Implementation

    **a.** Administer antibiotics, analgesics, and antipyretics as ordered

    **b.** Promote comfort; frequent linen change

    **c.** Promote adequate nutrition and hydration (3,000 to 4,000 mL/day); monitor and record intake and output

    **d.** Use aseptic technique and good handwashing; provide frequent perineal care and educate client in correct technique

    **e.** Assess vital signs; monitor laboratory results

    **f.** Assess fundus for involution and lochia; encourage semi-Fowler's position to facilitate drainage

    **g.** Promote adequate rest and sleep; allow family and friends to visit per client's wishes

    **h.** Encourage client to care for self first before taking care of baby; allow client to care for and feed infant per client's condition; provide client positive reinforcement

9. Evaluation

   a. Client is comfortable and free of pain

   b. Client obtains adequate nutrition, fluids, and rest

   c. Body temperature decreases and remains normal; infection does not result in more serious complications

   d. Client has support and maintains family contact; client and family state they feel informed of client's condition

   e. Client has minimal delay in bonding with baby; expresses positive feelings toward baby; shows comfort and competence in caring for baby; and has support and assistance in caring for infant when discharged

**B. Wound infections**

1. Description: an infection of the abdominal incision for cesarean delivery or the episiotomy, a perineal incision to faciliate vaginal delivery; the infection rate following cesarean births is 4 to 12 percent, with the highest rate occurring after emergency cesarean because there is more tissue trauma; culture of wound drainage frequently reveals mixed pathogens

2. Predisposing factors

   a. Obesity

   b. Diabetes mellitus

   c. Prolonged postpartal hospitalization

   d. Steroid therapy

   e. Immunosuppression

3. Nursing assessment

   a. REEDA assessment

      1) Redness: erythema around wound

      2) Edema: swelling of tissues

      3) Ecchymosis: skin discoloration

      4) Discharge: purulent drainage from incision site

      5) Approximation of skin edges: gaping of the wound edges

   b. Generalized fever, localized tissue warmth

   c. Tenderness

4. Priority nursing diagnoses: Risk for infection; Deficient knowledge; Pain; Impaired skin integrity

5. Planning/goal-setting: client will be free from infection, will have infection treated as soon as possible, will participate in prescribed treatment, will express increased comfort, and will have homeostasis restored

6. Implementation

   a. Administer antibiotics, analgesics, and antipyretics as ordered

   b. Promote comfort, frequent linen change

    **c.** Promote adequate nutrition and hydration (3,000 to 4,000 mL/day); monitor and record intake and output

    **d.** Use aseptic technique and good handwashing; provide frequent wound or perineal care; educate client in correct technique

    **e.** Assess vital signs; monitor laboratory results

    **f.** Assess incision or episiotomy site every 8 to 12 hours for signs of infection

    **g.** Promote adequate rest and sleep; allow family and friends to visit per client's wishes

    **h.** Encourage client to care for self first before taking care of baby; allow client to care for and feed infant per client's condition; provide client positive reinforcement

  **7.** Evaluation

    **a.** Client is comfortable and free of pain

    **b.** Client obtains adequate nutrition, fluids, and rest

    **c.** Body temperature decreases and remains normal; infection does not result in more serious complications

    **d.** Client has support and maintains family contact; client and family state they feel informed of client's condition

    **e.** Client has minimal delay in bonding with baby; expresses positive feelings toward baby; shows comfort and competence in caring for baby; and has support and assistance in caring for infant when discharged.

**C. Breast infection (mastitis)**

  **1.** Description: **mastitis** is an infection of the breast connective tissue, primarily in women who are lactating; the usual causative organisms are *Staphylococcus aureus, Escherichia coli,* and *Streptococcus* species; *Candida albicans* can also cause mastitis

  **2.** Predisposing factors

    **a.** Traumatized tissue, fissured or cracked nipples

    **b.** Engorgement, milk stasis or poor drainage of milk, missed feedings

    **c.** Lowered maternal defenses caused by fatigue or stress

    **d.** Poor hygiene practices

    **e.** Tight clothing or poor support of pendulous breasts

  **3.** Nursing assessment

    **a.** Breast consistency, nipple condition

    **b.** Warm, reddened, painful area

    **c.** Axillary lymph nodes enlarged or tender

    **d.** Flu-like symptoms

    **e.** Generalized fever

4. Priority nursing diagnoses: Risk for infection; Deficient knowledge; Acute pain; Ineffective breast-feeding; Interrupted breast-feeding

5. Planning/goal-setting: client will be free from infection, have infection treated as soon as possible, participate in prescribed treatment, and successful breast-feeding will be maintained

6. Implementation

   a. Culture and sensitivity of breast milk may be ordered; note that infection usually is not transmitted to breast milk

   b. Administer antibiotics, analgesics, and antipyretics as ordered

   c. Promote comfort: a well-fitting, supportive bra is needed 24 hours a day

   d. Promote adequate nutrition, hydration, rest, and sleep

   e. Remind mother and staff to use good handwashing technique before handling breasts or assisting with breast-feeding; continue breast-feeding as advised by healthcare provider

   f. Assess vital signs as ordered

   g. Educate client regarding breast care, proper latch on, let-down reflex, necessity for frequent breast-feeding, signs of complications, and telephone numbers where client can have questions answered, provide client positive reinforcement

   h. Change position of infant for feeding to relieve pressure on same area of nipple; breast-feed frequently to prevent stasis of milk

7. Evaluation

   a. Client is comfortable and free of pain

   b. Client is adequately hydrated, nourished, and rested

   c. Body temperature decreases and remains normal, infection does not result in breast abscess

   d. Client has support from family in breast-feeding; client and family feel informed of client's condition

   e. Client shows comfort and competence in feeding baby, expresses satisfaction with breast-feeding

**D. Urinary tract infections**

1. Description: **urinary tract infection** occurs in 2 to 4 percent of postpartal women; infection can occur as **cystitis** (lower urinary tract infection) and often appears 2 to 3 days after birth, or as **pyelonephritis** (upper urinary tract infection); post-delivery urinary tract infections are usually caused by *E. coli* bacteria and generally occur soon after vaginal delivery

2. Predisposing factors

   a. Normal postpartal diuresis

   b. Increased bladder capacity

   c. Decreased bladder sensitivity from stretching or trauma

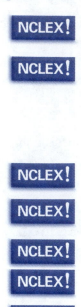

**d.** Possible inhibited neural control of the bladder following the use of general or regional anesthesia

**e.** Contamination from catheterization; as many as 5 percent of women who have one catheterization and 50 percent of those with intermittent catheterization develop bacteriuria

**f.** Obesity

3. Nursing assessment

   **a.** Overdistention of the bladder in the early postpartal period

   **b.** Frequent urination of small amounts, burning, dysuria

   **c.** Hematuria

   **d.** Elevated temperature; low grade temperature occurs with cystitis, higher fever occurs with pyelonephritis

   **e.** Flank pain (pyelonephritis)

   **f.** Costovertebral angle tenderness (pyelonephritis)

   **g.** Chills, nausea, vomiting (pyelonephritis)

4. Priority nursing diagnoses: Risk for infection; Acute pain; Deficient knowledge; Urinary retention; Risk for urinary incontinence; Risk for hyperthermia

5. Planning/goal-setting: client will be free from infection, have infection treated as soon as possible, participate in prescribed treatment and have increased knowledge of measures to prevent urinary tract infections; lower tract infections will not ascend resulting in upper tract infections

6. Implementation

   **a.** Monitor bladder frequently during recovery period to institute preventative measures

   **b.** Culture and sensitivity of urine may be ordered prior to administration of antibiotics

   **c.** Administer antibiotics as ordered; commonly Bactrim or Septra, Macrodantin

   **d.** Promote comfort; administer analgesic, antispasmodic, antippyretic

   **e.** Promote nutrition and hydration; increase oral fluids to 3,000 to 4,000 mL/day

   **f.** Assess vital signs as ordered

   **g.** Promote rest and sleep

7. Evaluation

   **a.** Client is comfortable and free of pain

   **b.** Client is adequately nourished, hydrated, and rested

   **c.** Infection does not result in more serious complications; lower tract infection does not ascend, resulting in upper tract infection

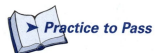

**Practice to Pass**

A lactating client telephones the nursing unit 24 hours after discharge. She is complaining of breast engorgement and a temperature of 99.9°F. What tips would you give her to relieve the engorgement, and what symptoms would you tell her to look for concerning mastitis?

**d.** Body temperature decreases and remains normal

**e.** Client and family feel informed of client's condition

## IV. Thromboembolic Disorders

**A. Description:** thromboembolic disorders may occur antepartally but are usually considered a postpartal complication; when a thrombus occurs in response to inflammation in the vein wall it is called **thrombophlebitis;** in this type of thrombosis, the clot is more firmly attached and is less likely to result in an embolism; thromboembolic disorders are more likely to occur after a cesarean birth

**B. Contributing factors**

1. Increased amounts of blood clotting factors in the postpartal period

2. Postpartal thrombocytosis (increased quantity of circulating platelets and increased adhesiveness)

3. Release of thromboplastin substances from the tissue of the placenta and fetal membranes

4. Increased amounts of fibrinolysis inhibitors

**C. Predisposing factors**

1. Obesity

2. Increased maternal age

3. High parity

4. Anesthesia or surgery resulting in vessel trauma or venous stasis, prolonged bedrest

5. Maternal anemia

6. Hypothermia

7. Heart disease

8. Endometritis

9. Varicosities, injury to the leg

10. History of deep vein thrombosis (DVT)

**D. Types of thromboembolic disorders**

1. Superficial thrombophlebitis (more common in the postpartum)

2. Deep vein thrombosis (DVT)

  **a.** More frequently seen in women with a history of thrombosis

  **b.** Increased incidence in women with obstetric complications such as hydramnios, pregnancy-induced hypertension (PIH), and operative birth

3. Septic pelvic thrombophlebitis

  **a.** A complication that develops in conjunction with infections of the reproductive tract

**NCLEX!**

    **b.** More common in women with a cesarean birth, incidence is 1 in 800 deliveries

    **c.** DVT and septic pelvic thromboemboli predispose clients to pulmonary embolization

**E. Assessment**

  **1.** Superficial thrombophlebitis

    **a.** Symptoms become apparent about the 3rd or 4th postpartal day

    **b.** Tenderness is apparent in a portion of the vein

    **c.** Local heat and redness is present, may have low-grade fever

    **d.** Pulmonary embolism is extremely rare

  **2.** Deep vein thrombosis

    **a.** Frequently occurs in women with a history of thrombosis

    **b.** Characterized by edema of the ankle and leg

    **c.** Initial low grade fever followed by chills and high fever

    **d.** Pain located in lower leg or lower abdomen

    **e.** Homan's sign may or may not be positive, but pain results from calf pressure

    **f.** Peripheral pulses may be decreased

    **g.** May result in pulmonary embolism; signs include dyspnea and chest pain, diagnosis may be verified by V/Q scan, blood gas studies, or x-ray

  **3.** Septic pelvic thrombophlebitis

    **a.** Infection ascends upward along the venous system, and thrombophlebitis develops in the uterine, ovarian, or hypogastric veins

    **b.** Usually unresponsive to antibiotics

    **c.** Characterized by abdominal or flank pain present with guarding

    **d.** Occurs on the 2nd to 3rd postpartal day with fever and tachycardia

    **e.** Intermittent fever and chills may persist

    **f.** Pulmonary embolism may result; signs include dyspnea and chest pain, diagnosis may be verified by V/Q scan, blood gas studies, or x-ray

**F. Priority nursing diagnoses:** Acute pain; Deficient knowledge; Ineffective tissue perfusion; Risk for infection; Impaired physical mobility; Risk for impaired parenting

**G. Planning/goal-setting:** thrombosis will be resolved without further complication and client will participate in prescribed treatment

**H. Implementation**

  **1.** Women with varicosities should be evaluated for the need for support hose during labor and the postpartal period

  **2.** Early ambulation following birth; women who have had a cesarean birth should be encouraged to perform regular leg exercises to promote venous return

3. If the diagnosis of DVT is made, the nurse should monitor the woman for signs of pulmonary embolism

4. The nurse needs to monitor for signs of bleeding related to heparin or Coumadin therapy, and keep protamine sulfate, the antagonist for heparin, available; keep vitamin K available if receiving oral warfarin (Coumadin)

5. Warm, moist soaks are maintained with legs elevated, if ordered

6. Obtain clotting times as ordered in client who is on anticoagulant therapy

7. Maintain bedrest as ordered; if client may get up, educate client to avoid standing or sitting for long periods of time; advise client against crossing legs

8. Review need for client to wear support stockings, if ordered, and to plan for rest periods with legs elevated

9. Promote increased fluid intake

10. Promote comfort

    a. Administer non-aspirin analgesic for pain

    b. Elevate extremities on pillow to decrease venous aching

    c. Promote adequate rest and sleep

11. Serial measurements of both of the extremities should be made daily to compare for any increase in swelling

12. Report to the physician any heavy vaginal bleeding, generalized petechiae, bleeding from the mucous membranes, hematuria, or oozing from venipuncture sites

**I. Evaluation**

1. Client is comfortable, free of pain, and adequately rested

2. Thromboembolic disorder does not result in more serious complications

3. Client and family state they feel informed of client's condition

4. Client has minimal delay in interaction with baby, support and assistance in caring for infant when discharged

5. Client feels comfortable with self-administration of heparin or oral medication upon discharge

**V. Postpartal Psychiatric Disorders**

**A. Description**

1. Many types of psychiatric problems may occur in the postpartum

2. The *Diagnostic and Statistical Manual of Mental Disorders, 4th edition* (DSM-IV) classifies postpartum onset mood disorders and proposes that postpartal psychiatric disorders be considered one diagnostic syndrome with three subclasses; a fourth area, postpartum onset of panic disorder, has also been described

    a. Adjustment reaction with depressed mood is also known as postpartum, maternal, or baby blues

       1) Occurs in as many as 50 to 80 percent of mothers and is characterized by mild depression interspersed with happier feelings

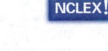

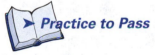

**➤ Practice to Pass**

A newly delivered postpartal client complains of pain in her thighs and lower legs. How would you assess this client for a potential thromboembolic complication?

2) The blues typically occur within a few days after the baby's birth and are self-limiting, lasting from 1 to 10 days, more severe in primiparas

3) Seems to be related to the rapid alteration in estrogen, progesterone, and prolactin levels after birth

4) New mothers feel overwhelmed, unable to cope, fatigued, anxious, irritable, and oversensitive; episodic tearfulness occurs without any reason

b. Postpartum major mood disorder, also known as postpartum depression

1) Develops in about 8 to 26 percent of all postpartal women

2) May occur anytime in the first postpartum year, most often occurs around the fourth week

3) Symptoms: sadness, frequent crying, insomnia, appetite change, difficulty concentrating and making decisions, feelings of worthlessness, obsessive thoughts of inadequacy as a person/parent, lack of interest in usual activities, lack of concern about personal appearance; irritability and hostility toward the new baby may be seen

4) Risk factors: primiparity, ambivalence about maintaining the pregnancy throughout the pregnancy, history of postpartum depression or bipolar illness, lack of social support, lack of a stable relationship with parents or partner, body image and eating disorders, and lack of a supportive relationship with parents, especially the client's father, as a child

5) Treatment: medication, primarily the selective serotonin reuptake inhibitors such as sertaline (Zoloft), paroxetine (Paxil) and fluoxetine (Prozac), individual or group psychotherapy, and practical assistance with child care and other demands of daily life; in lactating women, very small amounts of these drugs were found in breast milk and in their infants' serum samples

c. Postpartum psychosis

1) Has an incidence rate of 1 to 2 per 1,000

2) Evident within the first 3 months postpartum

3) Symptoms: agitation, hyperactivity, insomnia, mood lability, confusion, irrationality, difficulty remembering or concentrating, poor judgment, delusions, and hallucinations

4) Risk factors: previous postpartum psychosis, history of bipolar disorder, prenatal stressors such as lack of support, obsessive personality, and a family history of mood disorder

5) 10 to 25 percent reoccurrence rate in subsequent pregnancies

6) Treatment: hospitalization, antipsychotic medications, sedatives, electroconvulsive therapy, removal of the infant, social support, and psychotherapy

d. Postpartum onset panic disorder: characterized by frightening panic attacks that includes acute onset of anxiety, fear, rapid breathing, palpitation, and a sense of doom

**B. Assessment**

1. History of previous psychological problems

2. Adequacy of coping skills

3. Degree of self-esteem

4. Presence of mood swings, emotional distress, restlessness, irritability, guilt, extreme anxiety about the baby, anorexia, inability to complete activities of daily living, or trouble concentrating or expressing self

**C. Priority nursing diagnoses:** Risk for impaired parenting; Ineffective coping; Risk for impaired parent–child attachment; Risk for compromised family coping

**D. Planning/goal-setting:** client and family will recognize common postpartum psychological changes; client will be free from psychological maladaptation; client and family will recognize signs of psychological impairment and will contact appropriate resources identified at time of discharge; and client will function adequately as a parent

**E. Implementation**

1. Observe client with baby, by herself, and with family and friends

2. Recognize early signs of problems

3. Seek client referral to psychiatrist for evaluation of psychological status

4. Support positive parenting behaviors

5. Discuss client's plans for her baby and herself

6. Refer client to social services, if indicated

**F. Evaluation**

1. Client uses appropriate coping strategies to care for self and baby

2. Client has realistic expectations for self and baby

3. Client perceives that she is receiving the support she needs

4. Client has support for depressive episodes

5. Client and family share feelings and concerns openly

6. Appropriate bonding is observed and baby is safe

7. Home is a safe environment

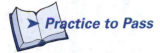

**Practice to Pass**

You are assessing a client's interaction with her newborn infant. What types of behavior would you see if the client was suffering from a postpartal psychiatric disorder?

**Case Study**

The client is a 16-year-old gravida 1, para 1 who delivered her infant by cesarean at 37 weeks gestation following prolonged rupture of membranes and failure to progress during labor.

❶ What factors increase the client's risk for a postpartal infection?

❷ What ongoing nursing assessments are necessary to identify an infection?

❸ What signs and symptoms are used to diagnose an infection?

❹ What is the first step in treating an infection?

❺ What nursing diagnoses are pertinent to a client with a postpartal infection?

*For suggested responses, see pages 340–341.*

## Posttest

**1** Which of the following items of clothing worn by a postpartal client could possibly promote a problem for the woman?

(1) Pantyhose
(2) Short athletic socks
(3) Knee-highs
(4) Colored tights

**2** Which of the following nursing interventions is appropriate to help a lactating client prevent mastitis?

(1) Apply Vitamin E cream to soften the nipples.
(2) Wear a tight, supportive bra.
(3) When the client's nipples are sore, offer the infant a bottle.
(4) Encourage the client to breast-feed her infant frequently.

**3** Upon assessment of a postpartal client, the home visit nurse observes symptoms of infection. Which of the following symptoms indicates infection?

(1) Pinkish lochia
(2) Bradycardia
(3) Abdominal tenderness
(4) Oral temperature of 99.2°F

**4** Which of the following nursing interventions, if prescribed, would have the most direct effect on reducing postpartal hemorrhage?

(1) Continuous fundal massage to decrease bleeding and facilitate uterine contraction
(2) Trendelenburg position to facilitate cardiac function
(3) Bladder catheterization to maintain uterine contraction
(4) Administration of a tocolytic drug

**5** What factor in a client's history places the client at greatest risk for postpartal endometritis?

(1) Cesarean delivery after 24 hours labor and failure to progress
(2) External fetal monitoring during labor
(3) Ruptured membranes for 4 hours prior to delivery
(4) Spontaneous vaginal delivery after 8 hours labor

**6** After the delivery of a large-for-gestational-age infant, a client is noted to have bright red blood continuously trickling from the vagina. Her fundus is firm and located in the midline. What is the most likely cause of this bleeding?

(1) Lacerations
(2) Hematoma
(3) Uterine atony
(4) Retained fragments of conception

**7** A client is in the immediate postpartal period after delivery of a 9 pound, 14 ounce baby. The client is a gravida 6, para 5. The nurse has been checking the client every 15 minutes for the last 45 minutes. The client has been stable with a firm fundus and moderate amount of lochia. As the nurse begins her final 15-minute assessment, she notices some new blood stains on the top sheet and discovers the client lying in a pool of blood that covers the protective bed pad. The fundus is located above the umbilicus and is boggy. What would the nurse's first action be?

(1) Take the client's blood pressure.
(2) Put the client on a bedpan in case she needs to empty her bladder.
(3) Start an IV.
(4) Massage the uterus.

**8** A woman who delivered 3 weeks ago calls the postpartum unit with breast-feeding questions. She wants to know if it is all right to continue to breast-feed while she has the flu. She states that she feels achy all over, has been having chills, and her temperature is 103°F. What other question is important for the nurse to ask?

(1) "Have you been sleeping well?"
(2) "What does your lochia look like now?"
(3) "Do you have any reddened areas or tenderness on your breasts, or unusual breast discharge?"
(4) "Do you have any swelling in your legs or visual disturbances?"

**9** It is most important for the nurse to have which drug readily available when the client is being treated with heparin therapy for thrombophlebitis?

(1) Calcium gluconate
(2) Aquamephyton
(3) Protamine sulfate
(4) Ferrous sulfate

**10** Which client is exhibiting symptoms of a postpartum psychosis?

(1) A client delivered an infant 6 months ago. A policeman who found her walking down the street in her bathrobe has brought her to the Emergency Department. She was holding a knife and a baby blanket and screaming, "My baby is a demon, and I have to destroy her."
(2) A client delivered an infant 3 days ago. The nurse walked into her room and found her crying. The client stated, "I am so confused. I am happy that I had my baby, but I am so unsure of what to do!"
(3) A client's husband called the postpartum unit and stated his wife has not gotten out of bed for the last 2 days, doesn't want to eat, and is not interested in the things that she used to be interested in. He is having to take care of the baby by himself.
(4) A client delivered a baby 6 weeks ago. At her 6-week check-up, she complained of episodes of anxiety, fear, rapid breathing, palpitations, and a sense of doom.

*See pages 259–260 for Answers and Rationales.*

# Answers and Rationales

## Pretest

**1  Answer: 1  *Rationale:*** Women that are parity of 6 or above (grandmultiparity) are at the greatest risk of uterine atony because of repeated distention of uterine musculature during pregnancy. Labor leads to muscle stretching, diminished tone, and muscle relaxation. The client's age is not a factor in uterine atony, the length of labor is not considered to be prolonged or precipitous, and the size of the baby is considered appropriate for gestational age and is not considered to be macrosomic.
***Cognitive Level:*** Analysis
***Nursing Process:*** Analysis; ***Test Plan:*** PHYS

**2  Answer: 4  *Rationale:*** Cervidil is used to ripen the cervix before labor; terbutaline sulfate is a tocolytic, and could cause further muscle relaxation; magnesium sulfate is used to decrease contractions or prevent seizures; and Hemabate is a prostaglandin, used to manage uterine atony. Oxytocin remains the first-line drug, the prostaglandins now are more commonly used as the second-line drug, and carboprost (Prostin 15-M or Hemabate) is the most commonly used uterotonin. As many as 68 percent of clients respond to a single carboprost injection, with 86 percent responding by the second dose.
***Cognitive Level:*** Application
***Nursing Process:*** Planning; ***Test Plan:*** PHYS

**3  Answer: 3  *Rationale:*** The organisms are localized in breast tissue and are not excreted in the breast milk.
***Cognitive Level:*** Application
***Nursing Process:*** Implementation; ***Test Plan:*** PHYS

**4  Answer: 2  *Rationale:*** An abnormal odor of the lochia indicates infection in the uterus. The vital signs may be affected by an infection, but that is not definitive enough to suspect a uterine infection. A distended abdomen usually indicates a problem with gas, perhaps a paralytic ileus. Inspection of the episiotomy site would not provide information regarding a uterine infection.
***Cognitive Level:*** Application
***Nursing Process:*** Assessment; ***Test Plan:*** HPM

**5  Answer: 4  *Rationale:*** A temperature elevation greater than 100.4°F on two postpartum days not including the first 24 hours meets the criteria for infection. This criteria has existed since early in the 20th

century, and remains the most common standard in the United States. It is not abnormal for a postpartal client to run a low-grade fever in the first 24 hours. This can be caused by the body's reaction to labor, dehydration, or a reaction to epidural anesthesia. Postpartum nurses should assess other signs and symptoms of infection in addition to fever and WBCs when evaluating the possibility of infection in mothers who had epidural analgesia.
***Cognitive Level:*** Analysis
***Nursing Process:*** Assessment; ***Test Plan:*** PHYS

**6  Answer: 3  *Rationale:*** These are classic signs of thrombophlebitis that appear at the site of inflammation; the others listed are not.
***Cognitive Level:*** Application
***Nursing Process:*** Implementation; ***Test Plan:*** HPM

**7  Answer: 4  *Rationale:*** An increase in lochia or a return to bright red bleeding after the lochia has changed to pink indicates a complication. The other statements are false.
***Cognitive Level:*** Application
***Nursing Process:*** Planning; ***Test Plan:*** HPM

**8  Answer: 4  *Rationale:*** Bleeding into the connective tissue beneath the vulvar skin may cause the formation of vulvar hematomas. Hematomas develop as a result of injury to tissues with spontaneous as well as operative deliveries (use of forceps). One of the first signs of a hematoma may be complaint of pressure, pain, or an inability to void. An ice pack to the perineum can be used to reduce swelling, but a hematoma is abnormal and should be reported to the physician. The fundus should be assessed, but the client's complaints warrant perineal or vaginal assessment.
***Cognitive Level:*** Application
***Nursing Process:*** Assessment; ***Test Plan:*** PHYS

**9  Answer: 3  *Rationale:*** Creating an environment where a client and her family can discuss emotional concerns is essential. Sharing time with the new mother to discuss thoughts and feelings is important to clients. Responding with patronizing answers (options 1 and 4) does nothing to assist the mother to talk about her thoughts and feelings and may increase her sense of isolation and feelings of inadequacy and despair.
***Cognitive Level:*** Application
***Nursing Process:*** Implementation; ***Test Plan:*** PSYC

**10**  **Answer: 4**  *Rationale:* Risk factors for postpartum depression include primiparity, ambivalence about maintaining the pregnancy throughout the pregnancy, history of previous depression or bipolar illness, lack of a stable support system, lack of a stable relationship with parents or partner, poor body image, and lack of a supportive relationship with parents, especially her father as a child. Ambivalence regarding pregnancy is a normal response in the first and into the second trimester, but should be resolved by the third trimester. Postpartum blues occurs in approximately 50 to 80 percent of postpartum women; the blues does not particularly indicate that a woman will develop postpartum depression.
*Cognitive Level:* Analysis
*Nursing Process:* Assessment; *Test Plan:* PSYC

## Posttest

**1**  **Answer: 3**  *Rationale:* The postpartal woman is prone to develop superficial thrombophlebitis due to increased amounts of clotting factors in the blood during the postpartal period as well as an increased amount of platelets and increased adhesiveness. Any restrictive clothing on the legs should be avoided.
*Cognitive Level:* Analysis
*Nursing Process:* Implementation; *Test Plan:* HPM

**2**  **Answer: 4**  *Rationale:* Preventing stasis of the milk and emptying the breast frequently will help prevent mastitis. The other options are false.
*Cognitive Level:* Application
*Nursing Process:* Implementation; *Test Plan:* HPM

**3**  **Answer: 3**  *Rationale:* The signs of a postpartal infection would include a temperature of greater than 100.4°F on two successive days after the first 24 postpartal hours, tachycardia, foul-smelling lochia, and pain and tenderness of the abdomen. The pinkish lochia is normal, and the temperature might indicate a cold or that breast milk is coming in.
*Cognitive Level:* Analysis
*Nursing Process:* Assessment; *Test Plan:* HPM

**4**  **Answer: 3**  *Rationale:* A full bladder may cause uterine atony and contribute to bleeding. If a client has hemorrhage, a Foley catheter may also be needed to allow accurate measurement of urine output, which is an indicator for kidney function. Overly aggressive stimulation of the fundus may cause decreased uterine tone; this is detrimental because overstimulation of the uterine muscle fibers can contribute to uterine atony. Avoid the Trendelenburg

position because it has been reported to interfere with cardiac and respiratory function by increasing pressure on chemoreceptors and decreasing the area for lung expansion. A tocolytic agent relaxes the uterus; in this case, an oxytocic drug to contract the uterus would be indicated.
*Cognitive Level:* Analysis
*Nursing Process:* Implementation; *Test Plan:* HPM

**5**  **Answer: 1**  *Rationale:* Factors contributing to postpartal endometritis include the introduction of pathogens with invasive procedures, prolonged labor, and prolonged rupture of membranes. The risk of endometritis is greatest after a cesarean delivery, especially after a long labor and prolonged rupture of membranes. Options 2, 3, and 4 are neither invasive, nor do they increase the client's risk for infection.
*Cognitive Level:* Comprehension
*Nursing Process:* Analysis; *Test Plan:* HPM

**6**  **Answer: 1**  *Rationale:* Suspect lacerations if the client is bleeding and the fundus is firm. If the cause were uterine atony, the fundus would not be firm. When there are fragments of the placenta or the membranes, the uterus will not contract effectively.
*Cognitive Level:* Analysis
*Nursing Process:* Analysis; *Test Plan:* PHYS

**7**  **Answer: 4**  *Rationale:* Of the options given the only one that immediately affects the bleeding is uterine massage. It might be important to start an IV with oxytocin at a rapid rate, and to allow the client to empty her bladder; however, the first action is to massage the uterus to stop or slow down the blood flow.
*Cognitive Level:* Analysis
*Nursing Process:* Implementation; *Test Plan:* PHYS

**8**  **Answer: 3**  *Rationale:* Mastitis most frequently occurs at 2 to 4 weeks after delivery with initial flu-like symptoms plus breast tenderness and redness. The client may be describing symptoms of a breast infection. Sleep, lochia, and edema with visual disturbances are not associated with breast problems.
*Cognitive Level:* Analysis
*Nursing Process:* Assessment; *Test Plan:* PHYS

**9**  **Answer: 3**  *Rationale:* Protamine sulfate is the drug used to combat bleeding problems related to heparin overdose. Option 1 raises serum calcium levels. Option 2 is the antidote for warfarin. Option 4 is an iron supplement.
*Cognitive Level:* Application
*Nursing Process:* Implementation; *Test Plan:* SECE

**10 Answer: 1** *Rationale:* The client in option 1 is exhibiting a loss of reality; she is delusional and threatening her baby, indicative of psychosis. The client in option 2 is exhibiting what is commonly called postpartum blues; it is temporary and goes away. The client in option 3 is exhibiting major depression. The client in option 4 is having postpartum anxiety attacks.
*Cognitive Level:* Analysis
*Nursing Process:* Assessment; *Test Plan:* PSYC

## References

Beck, C. T. (1998). A checklist to identify women at risk for developing postpartum depression. *Journal of Obstetric, Gynecologic, and Neonatal Nursing 27*(1): 39–46.

Beck, C. T. (1998). Postpartum onset of panic disorder. *Image: Journal of Nursing Scholarship 30*(2): 131–135.

Beck, C. T. (1999). Postpartum depression: Stopping the thief that steals motherhood. *AWHONN Lifelines 3*(4): 41–44.

Bell, K. K. & Rawlings, N. L. (1998). Promoting breast-feeding by managing common lactation problems. *The Nurse Practitioner 23*(6): 102–123.

Brown, C., Stettler, W., Twickler, D., & Cunningham, F. (1999). Puerperal septic pelvic thrombophlebitis: Incidence and response to heparin therapy. *American Journal of Obstetrics and Gynecology 181*(1): 143–148.

Brumfield, C. Hauth, J., & Andrews, W. (2000). Puerperal infection after cesarean delivery: Evaluation of a standardized protocol. *American Journal of Obstetrics and Gynecology 182*(5): 1147–1151.

Christoforidis, N., Dawlatly, B., Gouk, E., & Murray, B. (1999). Massive secondary postpartum haemorrhage three weeks after caesarean section. *Journal of Obstetrics & Gynaecology 19*(2): 197–199.

Ernest, J. M. & Mead, P. B. (1998). Postpartum endometritis. *Contemporary OB/GYN 43*(1): 33–38.

Fehder, W. & Gennaro, S. (1998). Immune alterations associated with epidural analgesia for labor and delivery. *American Journal of Maternal Child Nursing (MCN) 23*(6): 292–299.

Lamberg, L. (1999). Safety of antidepressant use in pregnant and nursing women. *Journal of the American Medical Association (JAMA) 282*(3): 222–223.

Mattson, S. & Smith, J. (2000). *Core curriculum for maternal newborn nursing* (2nd ed.). Philadelphia: W. B. Saunders, pp. 638–639.

Montgomery, A. M. (2000). Breastfeeding and postpartum maternal care. *Primary Care 27*(1): 237–250.

Morey, S. S. (1998). ACOG releases report on risk factors, causes and management of postpartum hemorrhage. *American Family Physician 58*(4): 1002–1004.

Morin, K. H. (1998). Perinatal outcomes of obese women: A review of the literature. *Journal of Obstetric, Gynecologic, and Neonatal Nursing 27*(4): 431–440.

Morrison, E. H. (1998). Common peripartum emergencies. *American Family Physician 58*(97): 1593–1605.

Olds, S., London, M., & Ladewig, P. (2000). *Maternal newborn nursing: A family and community-based approach* (6th ed.). Upper Saddle River, NJ: Prentice-Hall, Inc., pp. 907, 982, 988–989, 996–1008.

Olson, H. & Nunnelee, J. (1998). Incidence of thrombosis in pregnancy and postpartum: A retrospective review in a large private hospital. *Journal of Vascular Nursing 16*(4): 84–86.

Payton, R. G. & Brucker, M. C. (1999). Drugs and uterine motility. *Journal of Obstetric, Gynecologic, and Neonatal Nursing 28*(6): 628–638.

Sherwen, L., Scoloveno, M., & Weingarten, C. (2001). *Maternity nursing: Care of the childbearing family—media edition.* Stamford, CT: Appleton & Lange, pp. 878, 890–901, 906–909.

Vogel, A., Hutchison, L., & Mitchells, E. (1999). Mastitis in the first year postpartum. *Birth 26*(4): 218–225.

Winkler, M. & Rath, W. (1999). A risk-benefit assessment of oxytocics in obstetric practice. *Drug Safety 20*(4): 323–345.

## CHAPTER 12

# Normal Newborn Experience

Anita Kyle, MS, CNS-MCH, RNC

## CHAPTER OUTLINE

*Nursing Care of the Normal
    Newborn*

*Physiologic Changes
    Newborn Nutrition*

## OBJECTIVES

▪ Identify nursing assessments to be performed on the newborn on admission to the nursery.

▪ Describe the changes required in each body system for successful transition from intrauterine to extrauterine life.

▪ Identify client teaching for the new mother related to infant nutrition.

[ *Media Link* ]

*Use the CD-ROM enclosed with this text, or log onto the address given to access the free, interactive Companion Website created for this series. The CD-ROM and Companion Website accompanying this book offer additional practice opportunities and information—NCLEX Review, Case Studies, Glossary, In Depth with NCLEX, and more.*

**www.prenhall.com/hogan**

## REVIEW AT A GLANCE

**acrocyanosis** *peripheral cyanosis; blue color of hands and feet*

**Babinski reflex** *a neurological reflex where newborn toes will hyperextend and fan apart from dorsiflexion of big toe when foot is stroked upward from heel and across ball of foot*

**Barlow's maneuver** *when the infant's thigh is adducted and gently pressed downward and dislocation is felt as femoral head slips out of acetabulum*

**caput succedaneum** *swelling of tissue over the presenting part of the fetal head caused by pressure during labor; crosses suture lines*

**cephalhematoma** *blood from ruptured vessels between the skull bone and the external covering, the periosteum; does not cross the suture line*

**ductus arteriosus** *in fetal circulation, an anatomic shunt between the pulmonary artery and arch of the aorta*

**ductus venosus** *in fetal circulation, shunts arterial blood into inferior vena cava*

**Epstein's pearls** *small white specks on the gum lines of newborns*

**Erb-Duchenne paralysis (Erb's palsy)** *paralysis of arm and chest wall from a*

birth injury to the brachial plexus or 5th to 6th cervical nerves

**foramen ovale** *in fetal circulation, a shunt that connects the right and left atria*

**grasp reflex** *elicited by placing an object in the newborn's hand, resulting in a firm hold of the object*

**lanugo** *fine, downy hair found on all body parts of fetus (except palms of hands and soles of feet), from 20 weeks gestation to birth; begins to decrease at 36 to 40 weeks*

**latch-on** *proper position of the infant on the nipple/aerola to allow the transfer of milk, tongue down with lactiferous sinuses covered*

**meconium** *dark green or black material present in the large intestine of a full-term infant; the first stool passed*

**milia** *tiny, white pustules on the face and chin resulting from unopened sebaceous glands*

**Mongolian spots** *dark, flat pigmented areas of lower back and buttocks in some infants of African-American, Hispanic, or Asian heritage*

**Moro reflex** *elicited by startling the newborn; flexion of thighs and knees and*

fingers that fan, then clench as arms are thrown out, then brought together

**Ortolani's maneuver** *a manual procedure performed to rule out the possibility of congential hip dysplasia*

**pilonidal dimple** *dimple located on skin surface at base of spine not connected to the spine*

**plantar grasp** *pressure applied with the finger against the ball of the infant's foot causes the toes to flex*

**rooting reflex** *an infant's tendency to turn head and open lips to suck when one side of the mouth is touched*

**sucking reflex** *elicited by inserting a finger or nipple in newborn's mouth*

**tonic neck reflex** *elicited when infant's head is turned to one side, the arm and leg of that side extend while the extremities on the opposite side flex; fencing position*

**trunk incurvature** *stroking the spine causes the pelvis to turn to that side (Galant reflex)*

**vernix caseosa** *a protective cheese-like whitish substance present on the fetal skin; decreases with increased gestational age*

## Pretest

**1** A newborn's head circumference is 34 cm and chest circumference is 32 cm. Which nursing action would be appropriate?

(1) Refer the newborn for evaluation for psychomotor retardation.
(2) Prepare the mother for the probability that the physician will want to transilluminate the cranial vault.
(3) Measure the occipitofrontal circumference daily.
(4) Record the findings and take no further action.

**2** The nurse tests the newborn's Babinski reflex by:

(1) Touching the corner of the newborn's mouth or cheek.
(2) Changing the newborn's equilibrium.
(3) Placing a finger in the palm of the newborn's hand.
(4) Stroking the lateral aspect of the sole from the heel upward and across the ball of the foot.

**3** A new mother questions the nurse about the "lump" on her baby's head and says the physician told her it was a "collection of blood between a skull bone and its covering (periosteum)." The nurse explains that this is called:

(1) Caput succedaneum.
(2) Molding.
(3) Cephalhematoma.
(4) Subdural hematoma.

**4** Risk management, a standard for nursing care, requires the nurse to evaluate all assessment findings. To uphold that standard, the nurse evaluates a newborn for which of the following normal heart rates within 3 minutes of birth?

(1) 100–130 beats per minute
(2) 110–180 beats per minute
(3) 120–160 beats per minute
(4) 130–170 beats per minute

**5** Which of the following criteria of gestational age must be assessed within 2 hours of birth for the results to be valid?

(1) Breast tissue
(2) Posture
(3) Soles of feet creases
(4) Scarf sign

**6** A newborn is admitted to the nursery 15 minutes after birth. He is moderately cyanotic, has a mottled trunk, active movement of the extremities, and is wrapped in a cotton blanket. The primary assessment by the nurse would be to check:

(1) The umbilical stump for bleeding.
(2) The baby's temperature.
(3) For visible abnormalities.
(4) For a patent airway.

**7** The nurse observes that a client, who is one day postpartum and breast-feeding her first child, appears frightened. The client says, "The baby has been breathing funny, fast and slow, off and on." To reassure the client, a nursing response would be:

(1) "That's normal when the baby breast-feeds."
(2) "There's nothing to worry about. I'm going to take the baby back to the nursery now."
(3) "I'll watch the baby for a while to see if there is something wrong."
(4) "Don't be frightened. It's a normal breathing pattern. I'll sit here while you finish feeding him."

**8** Which behavior observed by the nurse indicates good bottle-feeding technique? The mother:

(1) Keeps the nipple full of formula throughout the feeding.
(2) Props the bottle on a rolled towel.
(3) Points the bottle at the infant's tongue.
(4) Enlarges the nipple hole to allow for a steady stream of formula to flow.

**9** A breast-feeding mother is beginning to experience nipple discomfort while breast-feeding. The nurse's first priority in the plan of care would be to:

(1) Have the mother pump until the nipples heal and give breast milk from the bottle.
(2) Remove the baby from the breast and reposition.
(3) Give the mother a nipple shield to wear.
(4) Have the mother breast-feed only from the nipple that is not injured.

**10** A mother asks, "Is it true that breast milk will prevent my baby from catching colds and other infections?" The nurse should make which of the following replies based on current research findings?

(1) "Your baby will have increased resistance to illness caused by bacteria and viruses, but she may still contract infections."
(2) "You shouldn't have to worry about your baby's exposure to contagious diseases until she stops breast-feeding."
(3) "Breast milk offers no greater protection to your baby than formula feedings."
(4) "Breast milk will give your baby protection from all illnesses to which you are immune."

*See pages 277–278 for Answers and Rationales.*

## I. Nursing Care of the Normal Newborn

### A. Physical assessment

1. Vital signs

   a. Heart rate is 120–160 beats/min, irregular, especially when crying, and perhaps a functional murmur; may be as high as 170 when crying, or below 120 when resting; count the apical pulse for one full minute

   b. Respirations are 30–60 breaths/min with short periods of apnea, irregular; cry is vigorous and loud; may be slightly elevated during crying, but over 60/min (tachypnea) 2 hours after delivery or less than 30/min (bradypnea) may indicate a problem; count for one full minute

   c. Temperature is 36.5–37°C (97.7–98.6°F) axillary; stabilizes about 8 to 10 hours after birth; poor thermo-stability is related to heat loss via *convection* (loss to cooler air currents), *radiation* (indirect heat transfer from body to cooler surfaces), *evaporation* (from wet skin) and *conduction* (direct heat loss to cooler objects)

   d. Blood pressure is 80/46; varies with changes in newborn's activity and blood volume; more accurate when newborn is resting

2. Pain assessment: intermittent crying not lasting more than 60 seconds, not high-pitched, quiets easily, and no tears noted

3. Priority nursing diagnosis: Ineffective thermoregulation; Ineffective breathing pattern; Decreased cardiac output

4. Planning and implementation

   a. Maintain newborn on radiant warmer or in isolette with servocontrol to maintain skin temperature 36.5 to 37°C (97.5 to 98.6°F)

   b. Allow infant to assume a flexed position to decrease surface area of skin exposed to environment, thereby reducing heat loss

   c. Monitor axillary and skin probe temperature per institution's protocol

   d. Monitor respirations for tachypnea and skin color changes for mottling

5. Evaluation: at 2 hours of age the newborn maintains an axillary temperature of 97.7–98.6°F, a heart rate of 120–160/min, respirations 30–60/min with no signs of distress, skin color pink, and remains in flexed position

### B. General assessment (performed in cephalocaudal or head to toe/tail manner)

1. Head

   a. ¼ of body size, molding of fontanels and suture spaces, round, and moves easily from left to right and up to down

   b. Frontal occipital circumference (FOC), measured around the forehead and occipital area, is 32 to 37 cm. (12.5 to 14.5 in.) or 2 cm greater than chest circumference

   c. Symmetric exception may be caused by birth trauma, i.e., **caput succedaneum** (swelling of soft tissue under the scalp), or **cephalhematoma** (collection of blood beneath the cranial bone and the periosteum)

    **d.** Anterior and posterior fontanels should be open, the posterior closing sooner (8 to 12 weeks) than the anterior (18 months)

**3.** Hair: silky smooth, grows toward face, high above eyebrow, variations in texture depend on ethnic background

**4.** Face: symmetric movement

**5.** Eyes

    **a.** Clear blue/slate-gray or brown in color

    **b.** Pupils equal and reactive to light, blink reflex present, sclera is bluish white

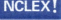

    **c.** May have subconjunctival hemmorrhage (small broken tiny capillaries on sclera, will disappear in few weeks)

    **d.** Edametous eyelids

    **e.** Lacrimal structures (tearing) functions at about 2 months

**6.** Nose: patent nares bilaterally, no discharge, may have flat bridge, sneezing done to clear nostrils

**7.** Mouth

    **a.** Symmetrical when cries, hard palate intact, uvula midline, reflexes present

    **b.** **Rooting reflex** (infant turns to side stimulated and opens mouth to suck), **sucking reflex** (when object placed in mouth or touches lips)

    **c.** May have **Epstein pearls** (small white specks, inclusion cysts, on gum ridges), tongue not protruding

**8.** Ears: well-formed notch of ear on straight line with outer canthus of eye

**9.** Neck: short, freely movable, has **tonic neck reflex** or fencer position (when head is turned to one side, extremities on same side extend and extremities on opposite side flex

**10.** Chest

    **a.** Clavicles straight and intact, barrel-shaped chest with bilateral expansion with inspirations

    **b.** Breath sounds clear

    **c.** Heart rate ausculated at border of left sternum extending left to mid-clavicle; regular rate and rhythm

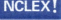

    **d.** Point of maximum impulse (PMI) lateral to midclavicular line at 3rd to 4th intercostal space.

**11.** Breasts: nipples symmetric, may have whitish discharge or supernumerary (extra, small) nipples on chest surface

**12.** Abdomen

    **a.** Soft, dome-shaped, round, some laxness of muscles, moves with respirations

    **b.** Bowel sounds when relaxed

      **c.** Umbilical cord is white, gelatinous with two arteries and one vein, clamped with no foul odor

      **d.** Femoral pulses palpable and equal, no bulges or nodes along bilateral inguinal areas

**13.** Genitalia

      **a.** Male: pendulous scrotum with rugae, testes descended into scrotum, penis with urinary meatus at tip of glans on ventral surface of penile shaft

      **b.** Female: labia minora may have **vernix caseosa** (white cheesy protective covering that decreases as gestational age increases) and smegma in creases, labia majora normally covers the minora and clitoris, discharge (blood-tinged mucus or pseudomenstruation) may be present because of maternal hormones

**14.** Extremities and trunk

      **a.** Trunk: short, flexed synchronized movement

      **b.** **Trunk incurvature reflex (Galant reflex):** newborn lies prone and when side is stroked causes pelvis to turn to stimulated side

      **c.** Hips: stable with no clicks or snaps upon movement

      **d.** To rule out hip dislocation, **Barlow's maneuver** adducts legs over hips and a snap is felt as femur leaves the acetabulum and with **Ortolani's maneuver,** the hip joint is abducted and lifted, and a click is felt as femur enters the acetabulum

      **e.** Arms: equal in length with symmetrical movement; **grasp reflex** present, newborn grasps when object is placed in hand; non-movement may indicate **Erb-Duchenne paralysis** or **Erb's palsy,** newborn unable to move upper arms, or asymmetric Moro response may be caused by damage to 5th and 6th cervical roots of the brachial plexus; five digits on each hand with normal palmar creases, nails present

      **f.** Legs: equal length, bowed, well-flexed, symmetric skin folds, peripheral pulses present

      **g.** Feet: creases on soles, may have "positional" clubfoot caused by intrauterine position but should be able to turn toward midline; **plantar grasp**—pressure on soles of feet elicits curling of toes; **Babinski reflex**—stroking sole upward and across the ball of the foot elicits fanning and extension of toes, disappears at 12 months

      **h.** Back: spine straight and flexible, may have small **pilonidal dimple,** a small dimple at the base of the spine but without connection to spinal cord

      **i.** Anus: patent, well-placed, may have meconium stool

**15.** Skin

      **a.** Color consistent with ethnic background, pink-tinged

      **b.** **Acrocyanosis:** bluish discoloration of the hands and feet may be present

      **c.** May have mottling: lacy pattern of dilated blood vessels under skin caused by fluctuation of general circulation

**d.** May have **milia**—obstructed secretions of sebaceous glands

**e.** May have **Mongolian spots**—bluish pigmented areas on dorsal area of buttocks of Asian, African-American, or Hispanic descent

**f.** May have **lanugo**—downy, fine hair of fetus between 20 weeks and birth, noticeably found on shoulders, forehead and cheeks

**C. Gestational age assessment using the Ballard tool**

1. An assessment that evaluates six neuromuscular and six physical characteristics performed during the first few hours of birth

2. A score of 1 to 5 is assigned to each characteristic and the total score correlates to a gestational age, i.e., a term newborn given a score of 3 for each characteristic scores an 18 for the neuromuscular assessment and 18 for the physical characteristics; the total of 36 points correlates to 38+ weeks' gestation

3. The rating is then marked on the graph along with the newborn's birth weight, length, and head circumference in order to classify the newborn based on maturity and intrauterine growth

4. An overall rating below the tenth percentile indicates the infant is *small for gestational age* (*SGA*); between the 10th and the 90th percentile indicates the infant is *appropriate for gestational age* (*AGA*); above the 90th percentile indicates that the infant is *large for gestational age* (*LGA*)

5. Determining ratings for each of the subscores

   **a.** The nurse should wear gloves when assessing the newborn after birth prior to the first bath

   **b.** The nurse first evaluates observable characteristics without disturbing the newborn then proceeds to characteristics that require more handling of the baby

   **c.** Maternal conditions such as pregnancy-induced hypertension (PIH), diabetes, and maternal analgesia and anesthesia in the intrapartal period may affect some gestational age components

   **d.** Neuromuscular maturity: during the first 24 hours, the newborn's nervous system is unstable; reflexes and assessments dependent on his/her brain centers may be unreliable and need to be repeated in 24 hours

      1) Posture: well-flexed with elbow, hip, and knee joints at 90-degree angle

      2) Square window sign (wrist): elicited by flexing the newborn's hand toward the ventral forearm until resistance is felt and measuring the angle

      3) Arm recoil: in the supine position, elbows are flexed and held for 5 seconds, then extended at the newborn's side and released; upon release, the term newborn will form an angle of less than 90 degrees and recoil back to a flexed position

      4) Popliteal angle: in the supine position, the thigh is flexed on the abdomen and chest with one hand; with the index finger of the other hand behind the ankle, try to extend the lower leg until resistance is felt

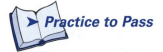

**Practice to Pass**

An anxious new mother asks you, "What's wrong with my baby? What are those white spots on her nose and chin?" What is your response?

5) Scarf sign: in the supine position, draw an arm across the chest toward the opposite shoulder until resistance is felt; note the location of the elbow in relation to the midline of the chest

6) Heel-to-ear extension: in the supine position, gently draw the foot toward the ear on the same side until resistance is felt; the knee may bend; hold the buttocks down to avoid rolling the newborn and note the proximity of the foot to ear and degree of knee extension

e. Physical maturity: not influenced by labor and birth and do not change significantly within the first 24 hours after birth

1) Skin: opaque texture, few distinct larger veins, dry, some peeling

2) Lanugo: minimal, decreases as gestational age increases

3) Plantar surface: a reliable indicator of gestational age in the first 12 hours of life; beginning at the top of the foot, creases should cover at least ⅔ of the entire foot surface

4) Breast: using the forefinger and middle finger, gently measure the breast tissue between them in millimeters; at term gestation, the measurement should be between 5 to 10 mm; the nipple should be raised above the skin level

5) Eye/Ear: eyes are open and clear; ears—when top and bottom of pinna are folded over each other, the pinna will spring back quickly when released; the upper ⅔ of the pinna incurves

6) Male genitalia: testes descended, scrotum pendulous and covered with rugae

7) Female genitalia: labia majora increases as gestation increases and nearly covers the clitoris at 36 to 40 weeks; at 40 weeks, the majora cover the labia minora and clitoris

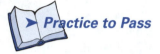

**▶ Practice to Pass**

Many factors can influence the term newborn's gestational age score. What factors might affect the posture, sole creases, and amount of breast bud tissue?

## II. Physiologic Changes

A. **Cardiovascular:** expansion of the lungs with the first breath increases pulmonary blood flow and decreases pulmonary vascular resistance

1. Increased aortic pressure and decreased venous pressure: clamping of the umbilical cord increases vascular resistance, and aortic blood pressure increases

2. Increased systemic pressure and decreased pulmonary artery pressure caused by the loss of the placenta; lung expansion increases pulmonary blood flow and dilates pulmonary vessels; pulmonary vascular beds open and perfuse other body systems

3. The **foramen ovale** (an opening that previously connected the right and left atria), functionally closes in about 1 to 2 hours, and anatomically closes in a few weeks to 1 year, increasing the left atrial pressure; some shunting may occur early in transition and with crying

4. The **ductus arteriosus** (in fetal circulation, an anatomic shunt between the pulmonary artery and arch of the aorta) closes, reversing the blood flow, so now blood flows from the aorta to the pulmonary artery because of the increased left arterial pressure

5. The **ductus venosus** closes (in fetal circulation, shunts arterial blood into inferior vena cava) thought to be related to severance of the cord, results in redistribution of blood and cardiac output; closure forces perfusion of the liver

B. **Respiratory:** initial respirations are triggered by physical, sensory, and chemical factors

1. Physical: the effort required to expand the lungs and fill the collapsed alveoli, changes in pressure gradient

2. Sensory: temperature, noise, light, sound

3. Chemical: changes in blood (decreased $O_2$ level, increased $CO_2$ level, decreased pH) as a result of the transitory asphyxia during delivery

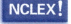

4. The newborn is an obligatory nose-breather, and any obstruction will cause respiratory distress; the newborn's ability to maintain respiratory function is influenced by his or her large heart that reduces lung space and weak intercostal muscles, and horizontal ribs and high diaphragm, which restrict the space available for lung expansion

5. Priority nursing diagnoses: Impaired gas exchange; Ineffective breathing pattern

6. Planning and implementation

   a. Monitor newborn's respirations for any signs of respiratory distress (increased rate, audible grunting, nasal flaring, retractions) per institutional protocol; normal limits are 30 to 60/min

   b. Monitor color of skin, oral area, and extremities for any signs of hypoxia

   c. Keep newborn on warmer for closer observation

   d. Keep infant NPO if respirations are above 60/min

   e. Maintain oral area free from mucus or emesis

7. Evaluation: newborn's respirations are within normal limits, color is pink, temperature stable with no signs of respiratory distress

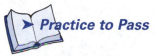

**What position do most newborns usually assume during transition? Why?**

C. **Neurologic:** the newborn's brain is ¼ the size of an adult's and myelination of nerve fibers is incomplete

1. Newborn exhibits uncoordinated movements, labile temperature regulation, poor control over musculature, easy startling, and tremors of the extremities

2. Newborn reflexes are important indicators of normal development; these include **Moro reflex** (elicited by startling the newborn; flexion of thighs and knees and fingers that fan, then clench as arms are thrown out, then brought together) and previously discussed Babinski grasp, plantar grasp, sucking, and tonic neck reflexes

3. Periods of reactivity: pattern of behavior during first several hours after birth

   a. First period of reactivity: 30 to 60 minutes after birth; awake and alert; may display nursing and attachment behaviors with random diffuse movements

**b.** Period of inactivity to sleep phase: activity diminishes, heart and respiratory rates decrease, and newborn enters sleep phase lasting from a few minutes to 2 to 4 hours; will be difficult to awaken

**c.** Second period of reactivity: awakes from deep sleep, lasting 4 to 6 hours; close observation is required for changes in heart rate, respiration, and color

**D. Musculoskeletal:** newborn should have full range of motion—when the extremities are fully extended, they should return to a flexed position; any variations should be further investigated

**E. Gastrointestinal changes**

1. Digestive enzymes are active at birth and can support extrauterine life by 36 to 38 weeks gestation

2. Necessary muscular and reflex developments for transporting food are present at birth

3. Digestion of protein and carbohydrates is easily accomplished, but fat digestion and absorption are poor due to absence of pancreatic enzymes

4. Little saliva is manufactured until 3 months

5. An immature lower esophageal sphincter often leads to regurgitation or spitting up

6. **Meconium,** stool that contains bile, epithelial cells, and amniotic cells, is excreted within 24 hours in 90 percent of normal newborns

7. Wide variations occur among newborns regarding interest in food

**F. Genitourinary changes**

1. Functioning nephrons are complete by 34 to 36 weeks gestation

2. Glomerular filtration rate (reabsorption and filtration) is low, therefore, newborn may tend to reabsorb sodium and excrete large amounts of water

3. Decreased ability to excrete drugs and excessive fluid loss can lead to acidosis and fluid imbalance; uric acid crystals may cause a reddish stain in the diaper

**G. Hepatic**

1. If the mother's iron intake has been adequate, iron stores from mother are sufficient to carry the newborn through the fifth month of extrauterine life; iron supplements may be given after this age

2. Liver controls the amount of circulating unconjugated bilirubin, a pigment derived from the hemoglobin that is released with the breakdown of red blood cells

3. Unconjugated bilirubun can leave the vascular system and permeate other extravascular tissues (e.g., skin, sclera, oral mucous membranes), resulting in a yellow coloring termed jaundice or icterus

4. Because unconjugated bilirubin binds to albumin (protein) and is eliminated in the stools, early and increased feeding may be encouraged to promote increased excretion of stool

5. Priority nursing diagnoses: Risk for deficient fluid volume; Risk for injury; Risk for impaired skin integrity; Diarrhea; Imbalanced nutrition: less than body requirements

6. Planning and implementation

   a. Record intake (oral and parental) and output (weigh diapers) every 2 to 4 hours

   b. Monitor for adequate hydration; skin turgor, specific gravity with each voiding, noting quality and characteristics of urine

   c. Phototherapy; maintain "bili-mask" over eyes, check eyes for pressure from mask

   d. Monitor diaper area for skin breakdown and rash

7. Evaluation: newborn is breast-feeding every 2 to 3 hours with balanced intake and output, skin is elastic, oral mucous membranes are moist, urine is clear straw-colored and passes bili-stools × 6 in 24 hours; bili-mask positioned over eyes; diaper area is clean with no signs of skin breakdown

**H. Integumentary**

1. The more mature the newborn, the more mature the skin and more likely the newborn will be protected from heat loss and infection

2. Skin color depends on activity level, temperature, hematocrit levels, and race

3. Plethora is a ruddy (red) appearance and usually indicates a hematocrit greater than 65 percent and should be evaluated

4. A polycythemic infant should be monitored closely for signs and symptoms of cyanosis, respiratory distress, hypoglycemia, and jaundice

5. When the infant cries, skin becomes bright red because of immature capillary system; acrocyanosis is common

**I. Immune system**

1. Of the three major types of immunoglobulins (IgG, IgA, and IgM), only IgG crosses the placenta; therefore, infants receive passive immunity from the mother in the form of IgG near the end of gestation or passive acquired immunity

2. Infants eventually produce antibodies (active acquired immunity) beginning at about 3 months, but IgA is missing from the respiratory, urinary, and gastrointestinal tract until approximately 4 to 6 months of age, unless the newborn is breast-fed or until the infant produces the antibodies him- or herself

3. Infants who are breast-fed are provided antibodies from the breast milk for as long as the mother chooses to breast-feed and are provided protection from many infectious diseases, including influenza, mumps, and chickenpox

**III. Newborn Nutrition**

A. **Nutrition guidelines:** a well, healthy newborn needs 90 to 120 kcal/24 hr of nutrition and 140 to 160 mL/kg/24 hr of fluid intake; weight gain is 4 to 8 ounces/week; weight doubles by 6 months of age, and triples by the age of 1 year

**B. Priority nursing diagnosis:** Deficient knowledge; Ineffective breast-feeding; Imbalanced nutrition: less than body requirements; Imbalanced nutrition more than body requirements

**C. Planning and implementation:** teaching guidelines for formula/bottle feeding

1. Formula meets the energy and nutrient requirements of newborn/infants, but does not have the immunologic properties and digestibility of human milk

2. Standard formulas are available in three types

   a. Concentrated liquid: diluted with water at a 1:1 ratio

   b. Powder: mixed with water, usually 1 scoop to 2 ounces of water

   c. Ready-to-feed: can be poured directly into a bottle; must be refrigerated once opened and discarded after 24 hours

   d. The American Academy of Pediatrics (AAP) recommends that infants be given formula or breast-milk until 12 months of age

   e. Soy formulas are available for infants who cannot tolerate cow's milk protein and lactose

3. Preparation of formula

   a. Aseptic sterilization: supplies are sterilized separately from the formula by boiling water for 20 minutes

   b. Terminal sterilization: formula is poured into unsterilized bottles that are sterilized together for 25 minutes

   c. With sanitary conditions, bottles and formula are not routinely sterilized, but all equipment is cleaned thoroughly, including the top of the can of formula

   d. Formula may be warmed to room temperature in a container of warm water; bottles should never be warmed in a microwave; hot spots may develop and burn infant's mouth/throat; heating also changes the nutritional composition of the formula

4. Feeding techniques

   a. Hold infant close with head elevated

   b. Keep bottle tipped so that nipple remains full of formula

   c. Never prop bottle or put the infant to bed with a bottle in his or her mouth; propping can cause aspiration and middle ear infections

   d. Discard any formula left in bottle because of the risk of bacterial growth

**D. Planning and implementation:** teaching guidelines for breast-feeding

1. Influences on supply and demand (infant need)

   a. Maternal supply is related to the frequency of the feedings until about 3 to 4 weeks when the milk supply is well-established; thereafter, the critical factor for supply to meet demand is breast emptying

   b. Infants self-regulate their intake and control breast milk production by the degree to which they "empty" the breast; the lactating breast is never "emptied" completely, but the infant chooses how much to take

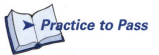

**Practice to Pass**

A new mother asks, "How long should I continue to feed my newborn formula? It's so expensive. When can I give him cow's milk?" How should the nurse respond?

NCLEX!

NCLEX!

2. The suckling sequence and proper **latch-on** (see Figure 12-1)

   a. The nipple and areola are drawn into the mouth enough for the lips to cover 1 to 1½ inches of the areola

   b. The jaw should move up and down in a rhythmic motion during milk transfer; the ears may wiggle; cheeks should be full and rounded, not sucked in

   c. Upper and lower lips should be flanged

   d. Tongue should be troughed—cup-shaped, beginning at the bottom of the mouth and extending over the lower alveolar ridge; in this way, the tongue draws the nipple in and presses it against the hard palate forming a teat; the tongue then humps up from back to front of the areola in a "rolling-like" movement for the milk transfer

3. Frequency of feedings: increasing the frequency will not increase the supply unless transfer of milk is successfully occurring; audible swallowing is the best indicator of milk transfer, more frequent as more milk is transferred

   a. Schedules should not be imposed on breast-feeding newborns as they have a stomach capacity of about 30 mL, and breast milk is more easily digested than artificial milk (formula)

   b. Breast-feeding infants should be fed when hunger cues are displayed; rooting, sucking on fists, clenched fists; these cues may be exhibited from 90 minutes to 3 hours after the last feeding; crying is the last sign of hunger

   c. Night feedings will be necessary during the first 6 to 8 weeks; the fat content of breast-milk is high in the evening, which may help the infant to consume more calories and therefore feel more satiated; infants who consume more calories during the day may be able to have longer stretches of sleep at night

4. Duration of feedings

   a. Research does not document the common myth that limiting time at the breast will minimize or prevent sore nipples; sore nipples are almost always caused by incorrect positioning at the breast or poor latch-on

**Figure 12-1**

**Latch-on position**.

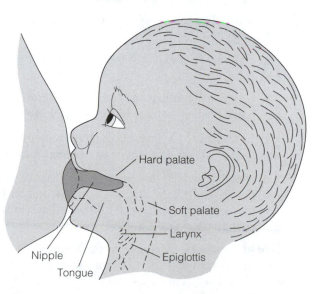

Hard palate

Soft palate

Larynx

Epiglottis

Nipple

Tongue

**b.** Mothers should watch the baby, not the clock; what the infant is doing at the breast is a better indicator of milk transfer than the time spent there

**c.** Newborns/infants with different sucking styles take different amounts of time to complete a feeding, anywhere from 10 to 30 minutes; foremilk is the milk that is produced and stored between feedings, looks like skimmed milk—bluish in tint and usually has less fat content than hindmilk, which is produced during and released at the end of a feeding and looks much richer with a yellowish tint

**d.** Signs of satiation are slowing of audible swallowing, pauses between sucking bursts, infant takes him- or herself off breast, hunger cues disappear, relaxed, drowsy, sleeping

5. Positioning for feeding; good positioning is paramount for proper latch-on and effective suckling

**a.** Body position for mother starts with good posture; straight back, pillows under arms (and under infant), feet touching floor or a footstool beneath her feet

**b.** Hand position: in the early weeks, the breast should be supported with the hand; use caution that the fingers do not cover the lactiferous sinuses or the areola that the infant needs to take into his or her mouth; later on, the infant will be able to support the breast after the initial latch-on

**c.** Cradle hold: infant is in chest-to-chest position, facing breast close enough to touch with nose and chin, with shoulder resting slightly lower on mother's forearm and hand supporting the infant's buttocks; opposite hand is used to support the breast

**d.** Side-lying position: infant is lying alongside the mother with a rolled-up blanket behind infant and a pillow behind mother to help maintain position; this position is suggested for night-time feedings and mothers who had cesarean deliveries

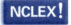

**e.** Football or clutch position: infant is positioned in mother's arm with his or her head, back, and shoulders in palm of hand; infant is tucked up under mother's arm, lining up the infant's lips with the nipple

6. Breast-feeding support is necessary for the beginning or continuing of breast-feeding

**a.** Encourage use of breast-feeding support groups or telephone hotlines at hospitals

**b.** Lactation consultants are trained and certified to provide assistance to breast-feeding mothers who experience problems

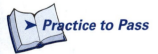

**c.** La Leche League is an international breast-feeding support and information group, with local groups often meeting in neighborhoods

**d.** Hospitals and birthing centers that subscribe to the World Health Organization's (WHO) Baby Friendly Hospital promote the "ten steps to successful breast-feeding" and stop the distribution of breast milk substitutes (Box 12-1)

**Practice to Pass**

A new breast-feeding mother says she isn't sure that her newborn is "getting any milk." How do you respond?

**E. Evaluation:** infant is gaining ½ to 1 ounce per day, doubles weight by 6 months of age and triples weight by 1 year of age; infant has 8 to 10 wet or soiled diapers per day and is alert and responsive

| **Box 12-1** | **Every facility providing maternity services and care for newborn infants should:** |
|---|---|
| **Ten Steps to Successful Breastfeeding** | 1. Have a written breast-feeding policy routinely communicated to all healthcare staff. |
| | 2. Train all healthcare staff in the skills necessary to implement this policy. |
| | 3. Inform all pregnant women about the benefits and management of breast-feeding. |
| | 4. Help mothers initiate breast-feeding within a half-hour of birth. |
| | 5. Show mothers how to breast-feed and how to maintain lactation even if they are separated from their infants. |
| | 6. Give newborn infants no food or drink other than breast-milk unless it is medically indicated. |
| | 7. Practice rooming-in—allow mothers and infants to stay together—24 hours a day. |
| | 8. Encourage breast-feeding on demand. |
| | 9. Give no artificial teats or pacifiers (also called dummies or soothers) to breast-feeding infants. |
| | 10. Foster the establishment of breast-feeding support groups and refer mothers to them on discharge from the hospital or clinic. |

**Case Study**

The client delivered her first child by cesarean delivery. She had an uneventful recovery. Her clinical status is within normal limits, and her vital signs are stable but her blood pressure is somewhat elevated 1 hour after delivery. She emphatically tells you that she does not want to feed the baby, even though before delivery she stated, "I really want to breast-feed immediately after delivery." Now, she wants you to feed her newborn in the nursery. You want to comply with the client's wishes but you are concerned about the conflicting statements made by the mother prior to and after delivery and the benefits of early breast-feeding.

❶ What does your assessment data reveal about the mother?

❷ What is your first nursing action based on your assessment data?

❸ When do you take the newborn to his mother?

❹ How much instruction do you give the mother when you take the newborn to her?

❺ What are the priorities for helping the newborn and his mother have a positive experience?

*For suggested responses, see page 341.*

# Posttest

1  At 2 days of age, a murmur is heard over the right and left auricles of the newborn's heart. This may represent a patent:

(1) Umbilical vein.
(2) Foramen ovale.
(3) Ductus arteriosus.
(4) Ductus venosus.

**2** From the following, select a nursing goal for a newborn in transition.

(1) To facilitate development of a close parent-infant relationship
(2) To assist parents in developing healthy attitudes about childrearing practices
(3) To identify actual or potential problems that may require immediate or emergency attention
(4) To provide the parents of the newborn with information about well-baby programs

**3** To meet the standard of care for risk management, the nurse assessing a newborn must be aware that asymmetric Moro reflex responses are often associated with:

(1) Injury to the cerebrum or cerebellum.
(2) Injury to cranial nerve VII.
(3) Injury to the brachial plexus, clavicle, or humerus.
(4) Poor muscle tone secondary to a genetic aberration such as Down syndrome.

**4** Most newborns void in the first 24 hours after birth. Which of the following may cause a reddish stain, sometimes called "red brick dust" on the diaper?

(1) Uric acid crystals in the urine
(2) Mucus and urate in the urine
(3) Bilirubin in the urine
(4) Excess iron in the urine

**5** A nurse providing care to a newborn would use knowledge of which of the following concepts underlying adaptation of the newborn's immune system?

(1) Iron stores from the mother are sufficient to carry the newborn through the fifth month of extrauterine life.
(2) Unconjugated bilirubin can leave the vascular system and permeate the other extravascular tissues.
(3) The newborn is unable to limit invading organisms at their point of entry.
(4) Most newborns void in the first 24 hours after birth and 5 to 20 times thereafter.

**6** The nurse who is trying to prevent heat loss in the newborn would realize that which of the following physical characteristics serves to decrease a newborn's loss of heat?

(1) Flexed position
(2) Blood vessel dilation
(3) Limited subcutaneous fat
(4) Larger body surface relative to that of an adult

**7** A client is bottle-feeding her newborn. The nurse should teach her that when her baby regurgitates small amounts of formula, she should:

(1) Take a rectal temperature.
(2) Recognize this as a normal occurrence.
(3) Discontinue feedings for 6 to 8 hours.
(4) Report this immediately to the pediatrician.

**8** A mother recently gave birth to her second child. She began breast-feeding in the birthing room. An appropriate nursing intervention would be to suggest that the mother, for now:

(1) Bottle-feed the baby between breast-feeding sessions.
(2) Routinely use plastic-lined nipple shields.
(3) Impose time limits for breast-feeding sessions.
(4) Offer both breasts at each feeding.

**9** Which of the following is an acceptable guideline for the use and storage of canned formula?

(1) The nutrients in canned formula may be enhanced with whole milk.
(2) Tap water in cities is clean and need not be sterilized for preparing infant formula.
(3) Refrigerating unused portions of the infant's formula after feeding is a good practice.
(4) Formula in an opened can should be used or discarded in 24 hours.

**10** The nurse is assisting a new mother in breast-feeding. The mother asks how she will know if her infant is getting anything from her breasts. The nurse's response is based on the knowledge that the best indicator that the infant is getting breast milk is:

*See pages 278–279 for Answers and Rationales.*

(1) Very loud burping.
(2) Finishing the feeding in 3 to 5 minutes.
(3) Audible swallowing.
(4) Sleeping 4 hours between feedings.

# Answers and Rationales

**Pretest**

**1** **Answer: 4** *Rationale:* This finding is normal. No further action is required.
*Cognitive Level:* Analysis
*Nursing Process:* Implementation; *Test Plan:* HPM

**2** **Answer: 4** *Rationale:* A Babinski reflex is elicited by stroking the lateral aspect of the sole of the heel upward and across the ball of the foot. A positive test (in newborns) of fanning the toes and dorsiflexing the big toe is an indicator of fetal well-being. Touching the corner of the mouth or cheeks (option 1) elicits the rooting reflex. Changing the newborn's equilibrium (option 2) elicits the Moro reflex. Placing a finger in the palm of the newborn's hand (option 3) elicits the palmar grasp reflex.
*Cognitive Level:* Application
*Nursing Process:* Implementation; *Test Plan:* HPM

**3** **Answer: 3** *Rationale:* Cephalhematoma is a collection of blood between a skull bone and its covering (periosteum). Caput succedaneum is swelling of the tissue over the presenting part of the fetal head caused by pressure during labor. Molding refers to the overlapping of cranial bones or shaping of the fetal head to accommodate and conform to the bony and soft parts of the mother's birth canal during labor. Subdural hematoma refers to bleeding between the dural and arachnoid membranes of the brain.
*Cognitive Level:* Analysis
*Nursing Process:* Implementation; *Test Plan:* HPM

**4** **Answer: 3** *Rationale:* The normal range is 120–160 beats/min. The rate varies with activity, increasing to 160 while crying and decreasing to 120 while in deep sleep. Bradycardia, rates below 120 (included in options 1 and 2), and tachycardia, rates above 160 (included in options 2 and 4), are not normal and require further evaluation and intervention.
*Cognitive Level:* Analysis
*Nursing Process:* Evaluation; *Test Plan:* HPM

**5** **Answer: 3** *Rationale:* After 12 hours, the edema of tissues present in most newborns begin to resolve and creases appear; these creases do not have the same predictive value as those assessed before resolution of newborn edema (option 3). All of the criteria in options 1, 2, and 4 remain predictive beyond the first 12 hours after birth.
*Cognitive Level:* Analysis
*Nursing Process:* Assessment; *Test Plan:* HPM

**6** **Answer: 2** *Rationale:* These symptoms reflect cold stress and require the temperature to be taken immediately (option 2). These symptoms are not associated with bleeding from the umbilical stump (option 1), congenital abnormalities (option 3), or respiratory distress (option 4).
*Cognitive Level:* Application
*Nursing Process:* Assessment; *Test Plan:* HPM

**7** **Answer: 4** *Rationale:* Periodic breathing with no color or heart rate changes is normal in the newborn adapting to extrauterine life. Option 4 provides verbal reassurance and also physical reassurance by the presence of the nurse. Option 2 doesn't reassure the mother and option 3 confirms the mother's fears. Option 1 provides information but doesn't address the mother's subjective sense of fear.
*Cognitive Level:* Analysis
*Nursing Process:* Implementation; *Test Plan:* PSYC

**8** **Answer: 1** *Rationale:* Keeping the nipple full of formula prevents the infant from sucking air. Options 2 and 4 can cause aspiration of formula and option 3 could cause the infant to gag and vomit.
*Cognitive Level:* Analysis
*Nursing Process:* Evaluation; *Test Plan:* PHYS

**9** **Answer: 2** *Rationale:* Discomfort while breastfeeding is almost always caused by improper latch-on. Removing the infant from the breast and repositioning with proper position can reduce the discomfort. Having the mother pump and give the breast milk

from a bottle can interfere with the breast-feeding process and may cause nipple confusion. Giving the mother a nipple shield to wear and having the mother breast-feed from the uninjured nipple will not solve the poor latch-on, and feeding from one breast will cause engorgement in the other breast.
*Cognitive Level:* Application
*Nursing Process:* Planning; *Test Plan:* HPM

**10** **Answer: 1** *Rationale:* Breast milk will not protect the baby from *all* illnesses (options 2 and 4). Lacto-ferrin (a whey protein in human milk) inhibits the growth of iron-dependent bacteria in the GI tract together with secretory IgA (another whey protein in human milk), which protects against respiratory and GI bacteria, viral organisms, and allergies. Breast milk does have other enzymes and proteins that protect the infant from illness.
*Cognitive Level:* Application
*Nursing Process:* Implementation; *Test Plan:* HPM

## Posttest

**1** **Answer: 2** *Rationale:* The foramen ovale is an opening between the right and left atria that should close shortly after birth so the newborn will not have a murmur or mixed blood traveling through the vascular system. Options 1, 3, and 4 are incorrect as they do not connect the right and left atria.
*Cognitive Level:* Analysis
*Nursing Process:* Assessment; *Test Plan:* PHYS

**2** **Answer: 3** *Rationale:* One of the nursing goals of newborn care during the first few hours after birth is to identify actual and potential problems that might require immediate attention. Options 1, 2, and 4 are all considered to be continuing care goals. All of these should be carried out after the initial goals are met.
*Cognitive Level:* Application
*Nursing Process:* Planning; *Test Plan:* HPM

**3** **Answer: 3** *Rationale:* An asymmetric Moro reflex response is often associated with injury to the brachial plexus, clavicle, or humerus, preventing abductive and adductive movements of the upper extremities. Injury to the cerebrum or cerebellum (option 1) could result in symmetric loss of the reflex. Cranial nerve VII (option 2) is the facial nerve; even if it is paralyzed, there is no effect on the Moro response. Down syndrome (option 4) is not responsible for an asymmetric Moro response.
*Cognitive Level:* Comprehension
*Nursing Process:* Analysis; *Test Plan:* HPM

**4** **Answer: 1** *Rationale:* Uric acid crystals in the urine may produce the reddish "brick dust" stain on the diaper. Mucus and urate do not produce a stain. Bilirubin and iron are from hepatic adaptation.
*Cognitive Level:* Analysis
*Nursing Process:* Assessment; *Test Plan:* PHYS

**5** **Answer: 3** *Rationale:* The newborn cannot limit the invading organism at the port of entry. Options 1, 2, and 4 are true adaptations in other body systems.
*Cognitive Level:* Analysis
*Nursing Process:* Implementation; *Test Plan:* SECE

**6** **Answer: 1** *Rationale:* The flexed position of the term infant decreases the surface area exposed to the environment, thereby, reducing heat loss (option 1). Blood vessels are closer to the skin than in an adult and constrict when exposed to cooler temperatures (option 2). Limited subcutaneous fat will increase a newborn's heat loss (option 3). Larger body surface than an adult increases the newborn's heat loss (option 4).
*Cognitive Level:* Analysis
*Nursing Process:* Assessment; *Test Plan:* HPM

**7** **Answer: 2** *Rationale:* Small amounts of regurgitation of formula is common, often caused by "over-feeding" or an immature cardiac sphincter (option 2). Regurgitation of formula is not necessarily a sign of infection, or a reason to take a temperature (option 1), or discontinue a feeding (option 3). Vomiting, forceful, or persistent expulsion of formula should be further investigated (option 4).
*Cognitive Level:* Application
*Nursing Process:* Planning; *Test Plan:* HPM

**8** **Answer: 4** *Rationale:* Mothers are encouraged to offer both breasts to the infant in the beginning for simultaneous stimulation, but it is not imperative nor harmful if the infant doesn't feed off of one breast at a session. Giving supplemental feedings can upset the natural supply and demand and can shorten the breast-feeding experience (option 1). Prolonged exposure to plastic liners or wet nursing pads may result in skin breakdown (option 2). Time limits should not be imposed on breast-feeding infants as they each have different styles of suckling (option 3).
*Cognitive Level:* Application
*Nursing Process:* Implementation; *Test Plan:* HPM

**9** **Answer: 4** *Rationale:* Opened cans of formula must be used within a 24-hour period (option 4). There are no nutrients in whole milk that can enhance formula, and the Academy of Pediatrics strongly recommends that infants only take mother's milk or formula for the first 12 months of life to decrease the chance of allergies (option 1). Tap water is not always safe (option 2). Any formula not taken by the infant should be disposed of as bacteria from the infant's mouth can enter the bottle and contaminate the remaining formula (option 3).

*Cognitive Level:* Application
*Nursing Process:* Planning; *Test Plan:* SECE

**10  Answer: 3** *Rationale:* Audible swallowing during a feeding produces sounds heard as a soft "ka" or "ah." Burping is related to how much air the infant swallows during feedings (option 1). Newborns usually spend 15 to 20 minutes at the breast in the first few weeks. Some older infants may be able to finish a feeding in 3 to 5 minutes (option 2). Because breastmilk is more digestible than formula, and a newborn's stomach is small, feeding is usually needed more frequently than every 4 hours. Frequent feedings are important in the early days to establish lactation (option 4).

*Cognitive Level:* Analysis
*Nursing Process:* Implementation; *Test Plan:* HPM

# References

American Academy of Pediatrics, Work Group on Breastfeeding (1997). Breastfeeding and the use of human milk. *Pediatrics 100*(6): 1035–1039.

Biancuzzo, M. (1999). *Breastfeeding the newborn.* St. Louis: Mosby, pp. 47–53, 73, 85–120, 254.

Bobak, I. M. (1998). *Nurses notes: Maternal-newborn core content at a glance.* Philadelphia: Lippincott-Raven, pp. 167–172.

Lawrence, R. & Lawrence, R. (1999). *Breastfeeding: A guide for the medical profession.* St. Louis: Mosby, pp. 261–285.

Lowdermilk, D. L., Perry, S. E., & Bobak, I. M. (1999). *Maternity nursing* (5th ed.). St. Louis: Mosby, pp. 489–490, 514–521.

McKinney, E. S., Ashwill, J. W., Murray, S. S., James, S. R. Gorrie, T. M., & Droske, S. C. (2000). *Maternal child nursing.* Philadelphia: W. B. Saunders, pp. 568–596.

Nichol, F. & Humerick, S. (2000). *Childbirth education* (2nd ed.). Philadelphia: W. B. Saunders, pp. 134–135.

Olds, S. B., London, M. L., & Ladewig, B. W., (2000). *Maternal newborn nursing* (6th ed.). Upper Saddle River, NJ: Prentice-Hall, Inc., pp. 681, 685–723, 732–771, 799–800, 890–894.

Riordan, J. & Auerbach, K. (1999). *Breastfeeding and human lactation* (2nd ed.). Boston: Jones & Bartlett, pp. 137–140, 301–303.

## CHAPTER 13

# The Complicated Newborn Experience

Deborah Bartnick RN, MSN

## CHAPTER OUTLINE

## OBJECTIVES

▮ Describe nursing assessments that identify the high-risk newborn.

▮ Discuss nursing interventions for the newborn with problems related to maturity or size.

▮ Identify the components of nursing care for the newborn experiencing birth trauma.

▮ Relate the consequences of maternal infections to the care of the newborn.

▮ Identify nursing actions to prevent cold stress in the newborn.

▮ Differentiate between physiologic and pathologic jaundice.

▮ Identify nursing responsibilities in the care of newborns receiving phototherapy.

▮ Discuss nursing care of the newborn experiencing respiratory distress.

▮ Describe the components of care for the infant of a diabetic mother.

▮ Relate the consequences of maternal substance abuse to the care of the newborn.

[ Media Link ]

**Use the CD-ROM enclosed with this text, or log onto the address given to access the free, interactive Companion Website created for this series. The CD-ROM and Companion Website accompanying this book offer additional practice opportunities and information—NCLEX Review, Case Studies, Glossary, In Depth with NCLEX, and more.**

www.prenhall.com/hogan

## REVIEW AT A GLANCE

**bronchopulmonary dysplasia (BPD)** *chronic pulmonary disease occurring in infants who required mechanical ventilation and high levels of oxygen in the first weeks of life*

**continuous positive airway pressure (CPAP)** *pressurized air delivered to lungs to keep them expanded during exhalation*

**exchange transfusion** *replacement of 70 to 80% of circulating blood by withdrawing the recipient's blood and injecting donor's blood in equal amounts*

**extracorporeal membrane oxygenation (ECMO)** *prolonged heart-lung bypass to allow lungs to heal*

**intrauterine growth restriction (IUGR)** *fetal undergrowth from any cause*

**intraventricular hemorrhage (IVH)** *bleeding into ventricle in brain, causing increased intracranial pressure*

**kernicterus** *damage to nervous system caused by very high levels of bilirubin in blood*

**meconium aspiration syndrome (MAS)** *respiratory disease of term, postterm, and SGA neonates caused by inhalation of meconium into lungs*

**necrotizing enterocolitis (NEC)** *acute gastrointestinal disorder in the sick neonate*

**neutral thermal environment** *An environment that provides for minimal heat loss or expenditure*

**oxygen hood** *method of delivering oxygen through a plastic hood placed over the infant's head*

**phototherapy** *treatment of infants with hyperbilirubinemia by exposing them to bright lights called bililights*

**retinopathy of prematurity (ROP)** *formation of fibrotic tissue behind lens of eye causing blindness; occurs in preterm infants who experience high blood oxygen levels*

**respiratory distress syndrome (RDS)** *respiratory disease that affects premature babies; caused by lack of surfactant*

**transient tachypnea of the newborn (TTN)** *Respiratory distress in a term infant related to delayed absorption of fluid in lungs from delivery*

**umbilical artery line (UAL)** *catheter threaded through umbilical artery; used to monitor blood pressure, give IV fluids and obtain blood samples*

**umbilical venous line (UVL)** *catheter threaded through umbilical vein; used to obtain blood samples and give IV fluids and medications*

## *Pretest*

**1** The nurse is admitting a neonate 2 hours after delivery. Which assessment data should the nurse be concerned about?

(1) Hands and feet blue
(2) Nasal flaring
(3) Minimal response to verbal stimulation
(4) Apical heart rate 156

**2** Of the following nursing diagnoses for a high-risk newborn, which requires the most immediate intervention by the nurse?

(1) Acute pain related to frequent heelsticks
(2) Imbalanced nutrition: less than body requirements related to limited oral intake
(3) Ineffective airway clearance related to pulmonary secretions
(4) Deficient knowledge related to infant care needs

**3** On admission to the nursery it is noted that the mother's membranes were ruptured for 48 hours before delivery and her temperature is 102°F. What information from this newborn's assessment should the nurse evaluate further?

(1) Axillary temperature 97.2°F
(2) Irregular respiratory rate
(3) Jitteriness
(4) Excessive bruising of presenting part

**4** Nursing care of the baby experiencing neonatal abstinence syndrome should include which of the following?

(1) Place stuffed animals and mobiles in the crib to provide visual stimulation.
(2) Position the baby's crib in a quiet corner of the nursery.
(3) Avoid the use of pacifiers.
(4) Spend extra time holding and rocking the baby.

**5** A mother was diagnosed with gonorrhea immediately after delivery. When providing nursing care for her baby, an important goal is to:

(1) Prevent the development of ophthalmia neonatorum.
(2) Lubricate the eyes.
(3) Prevent the development of thrush.
(4) Teach the danger of breast-feeding with gonorrhea.

**6** A full-term newborn weighed 10 pounds 5 ounces at birth. A priority nursing diagnosis for this baby is:

(1) Ineffective thermoregulation related to lack of subcutaneous fat.
(2) Risk for injury related to macrosomia.
(3) Impaired gas exchange related to lack of surfactant.
(4) Deficient knowledge related to newborn care.

**7** The nurse finds the mother of a 28-week gestation infant crying in her room. The mother states, "I just know my baby is going to die." What is the most therapeutic response by the nurse?

(1) "Don't worry, everything will be fine."
(2) "Why do you think that?"
(3) "You seem very worried about what will happen to your baby."
(4) "My baby was born at 27 weeks and he is fine now."

**8** A nurse is admitting an infant of a diabetic mother (IDM). At 1 hour of age, the nurse notices that the newborn is very jittery. Which action by the nurse is most appropriate?

(1) Begin oxygen by nasal cannula.
(2) Assess the newborn's blood glucose.
(3) Place the newborn under a radiant warmer.
(4) Initiate use of a cardiac/apnea monitor.

**9** A newborn's temperature is 97.4°F. The priority nursing intervention is to:

(1) Notify the physician/nurse practitioner immediately.
(2) Take the newborn to the nursery and observe for 2 hours.
(3) Reassess the temperature in 4 hours.
(4) Wrap the newborn in two warm blankets and place a cap on the head.

**10** A nurse is assessing a neonate born 12 hours ago and notes a yellow tint to the sclera. What else would be important for the nurse to assess?

(1) Blood glucose
(2) Blood type and Rh factor of mother and newborn
(3) Blood pressure
(4) Length of time membranes ruptured prior to delivery

*See page 310 for Answers and Rationales.*

## I. Nursing Care of the High-Risk Newborn

### A. Assessments that identify high-risk newborns

1. Certain prenatal and intrapartal risk factors will increase the risk of a neonate experiencing complications after delivery

   a. Maternal preexisting diabetes or development of gestational diabetes during the pregnancy; a primary concern in infants of diabetic mothers (IDM) is hypoglycemia after delivery

   b. Mother received narcotic analgesics/anesthetics during labor, especially systemically and immediately before delivery; narcotics cross the placenta and can cause respiratory depression in the neonate after delivery

   c. Fetal asphyxia causes the fetus to pass meconium into the amniotic fluid, which could be aspirated during delivery; common causes of fetal asphyxia include placental insufficiency, prolapsed cord, placental abruption, and placenta previa

> **d.** Difficult or prolonged labor, which increases the risk of birth trauma
>
> **e.** Multiple gestation pregnancy
>
> **f.** Preterm or postterm delivery
>
> **g.** Life-threatening congenital anomalies
>
> **h.** Maternal or neonatal infection
>
> **i.** Small for gestational age (SGA) or large for gestational age (LGA)

2. Apgar scores: an Apgar score of less than 6 at 1 minute or 7 at 5 minutes indicates the neonate is not making a satisfactory transition to extrauterine life and requires careful monitoring

3. Changes in physical assessment are often vague, so a thorough assessment is essential (see Box 13-1)

4. Gestational age

   **a.** Gestational age less than 37 weeks gestation based on due date

   **b.** Do a quick assessment if due date unknown; follow up with a thorough gestational age assessment as soon as possible

   1) Eyelids fused until 26 weeks gestation

   2) Creases cover a third of the soles of the feet at 36 weeks gestation

   3) Breast buds are absent until 37 weeks gestation

   4) Ear cartilage has little recoil until 30 weeks gestation

   5) Vernix covers body by 31 to 33 weeks gestation

   6) Lanugo covers shoulders by 33 to 36 weeks gestation

**B. General planning and implementation for all high-risk newborns**

1. Constantly monitor infant for subtle changes in condition and intervene promptly when necessary

   **a.** Decrease risk of nosocomial infections; each neonate should have his or her own supplies; handwashing is the most important method of preventing infection

---

| **Box 13-1** |  |
|---|---|
| **Critical Neonatal Assessment Indicators** | **The appearance of any of these signs in a neonate could indicate the presence of a serious complication:**<br><br>• Respiratory: bradypnea or tachypnea, respiratory distress, weak or absent respiratory effort<br>• Cardiovascular: bradycardia or tachycardia, murmur<br>• Neuromuscular: lethargy, temperature instability, tremors, unusual behaviors such as lip-smacking<br>• Gastrointestinal: poor feeding tolerance, poor suck/swallow reflex<br>• Skin color: cyanosis (acrocyanosis is normal for the first 24 to 48 hours after delivery), jaundice (especially within the first 24 hours)<br>• Obvious major anomalies |

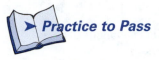

**b.** Conserve infant's energy and decrease physiologic stress by organizing care and minimizing interruptions; monitor each neonate for signs of stress

**c.** Provide appropriate stimulation for infant growth and development; high-risk neonates have the same developmental needs as the healthy neonate

**2.** Common procedures/tests/equipment

**a.** Pulse oximeter

1) Estimates arterial oxygen saturation through a sensor placed on the skin

a) Sensor should be placed on palm of hand, sole of foot, or wrapped around finger

b) Assess skin integrity at sensor site every 4 hours and rotate site every 12 hours

2) Pulse oximeter reading of 88 to 92 percent reflects safe clinical range

**b.** Arterial blood gas (ABG)

1) Direct measurement of amount of oxygen, carbon dioxide, and select electrolytes in a sample of arterial blood by arterial puncture or from umbilical artery line (UAL)

2) Compare oximeter reading at time blood sample obtained to correlate values

3) Apply pressure to puncture site for 3 to 5 minutes if obtained by arterial puncture

**c.** Blood glucose monitoring (Dextrostick, Accucheck)

1) Warm the foot prior to obtaining blood sample to increase circulation

2) Lance the heel to obtain the blood sample; this test is performed at the bedside; the heel is the preferred site (see Figure 13-1)

### Figure 13-1

**Newborn heel sticks.**

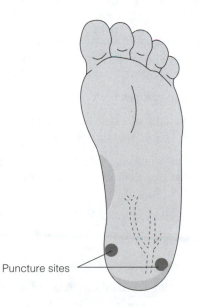

Puncture sites

**d.** Umbilical lines

1) An **umbilical arterial line (UAL)** is inserted into an umbilical artery and is used primarily to obtain arterial blood gasses

2) An **umbilical venous line (UVL)** is inserted into the umbilical vein and can be used for IV fluids, medications and to obtain blood for lab tests

3) All babies with umbilical lines should be closely assessed for blue discoloration or blanching on the lower extremities or buttocks, which could indicate an emboli or vasospasm and may necessitate the removal of the line

4) Assess closely for line placement, bleeding from the umbilicus or disconnected tubing; position the infant in a side-lying or prone position for close monitoring

**e.** Oxygen administration

1) Oxygen can be administered by **oxygen hood** (hood placed over infant's head), nasal cannula, **continuous positive airway pressure (CPAP)** (pressurized air), or endotracheal tube (ET)

2) Oxygen should be warmed and humidified prior to administration to decrease insensible fluid loss and heat loss

3) Monitor the amount of oxygen being administered and oxygen saturation and/or ABGs; it is important to administer the minimum amount of oxygen to meet the infant's oxygen needs to prevent complications

**f.** Gavage tubes

1) Used to decompress the stomach or to administer formula, breast-milk, or oral medications

2) It is preferred to insert the tube orally instead of nasally because infants are obligate nose-breathers

3) A 5 Fr. or 8 Fr. tube is commonly used; measure the tube from the earlobe to the nose and then to the tip of the xyphoid process; insert the tube and secure placement

4) Check placement of the tube prior to administering any feeding or medication; feedings should be administered over 3 to 5 minutes to avoid dumping syndrome; offer a pacifier during the feeding

**3.** Parenting the high-risk newborn

**a.** Parents are initially in a state of shock and disbelief and may grieve the loss of the "perfect baby" that they fantasized about during pregnancy

**b.** Priority nursing diagnoses for parents of high-risk infants: Compromised family coping; Deficient knowledge; Anticipatory grieving; Powerlessness; Social isolation

**c.** Planning and intervention

1) Assess bonding

2) Explain equipment and infant's condition

3) Present positive, realistic attitude and establish trust

4) Encourage parents to touch infant and perform care-taking activities as infant's condition allows

5) Encourage parents to verbalize feelings

6) Teach parents care of infant in preparation for discharge

7) Give Polaroid pictures of infant to parents prior to transfer to the Neonatal Intensive Care Unit (NICU)

**d.** Evaluation: parent(s) demonstrate effective coping with newborn's situation

## II. Problems Related to Maturity

### A. Prematurity

**1.** Description: infant born before completion of 37th week of pregnancy

**a.** Prognosis and severity of complications related to level of maturity: the earlier the infant is born, the greater the chance of complications

**b.** Major complications are related to **respiratory distress syndrome** (disorder caused by lack of surfactant), difficulty regulating body temperature, infection, and hemorrhage

**c.** Generally ready for discharge near their due date

**2.** Etiology

**a.** Incidence of preterm births in United States is 8 percent

**b.** Earliest age of viability is 23 to 24 weeks gestation

**c.** Maternal risk factors: age, smoking, poor nutrition, placental problems (placenta previa, placental abruption, preeclampsia/eclampsia), previous preterm delivery, incompetent cervix

**d.** Fetal risk factors: multiple gestation pregnancy, infection

**e.** Other risk factors: low socioeconomic status, environmental exposure to harmful substance

**3.** Assessment and pathophysiology

**a.** Respiratory

1) Insufficient surfactant allows alveoli to collapse with each expiration

2) Inadequate number and maturity of alveoli makes adequate alveolar gas exchange difficult

3) Skeletal muscles weak so may not be able to reposition head and body to maintain patent airway

4) Signs of respiratory distress typically develop within 1 to 2 hours after delivery (see Box 13-2)

5) Respiratory failure is most common cause of death in preterm infants within the first 72 hours of life

**b.** Temperature regulation

1) Lack of subcutaneous fat to insulate body

2) Large body surface area in proportion to body weight, so more likely to lose heat faster

| Box 13-2 |
|---|

**Signs of Neonatal Respiratory Distress**

- Tachypnea
- Intercostal and/or subcostal retractions
- Nasal flaring
- Expiratory grunting
- Seesaw respiratory movements
- Diminished breath sounds
- $PaO_2$ less than 50 mm Hg
- $PCO_2$ above 60 mm Hg
- Increasing exhaustion
- Cyanosis (late finding)

     3) Small muscle mass

     4) Absent sweat or shiver mechanisms

     5) Increased insensible fluid loss

     6) Increased risk of hypothermia

  **c.** Low resistance to infection

     1) Lack of immunoglobulins from the mother (these usually cross the placenta in the third trimester)

     2) Difficulty localizing infection and poor WBC response

     3) Increased risk of infection

  **d.** Immature liver

     1) Increased risk of hyperbilirubinemia caused by difficulty in eliminating bilirubin released by normal breakdown of red blood cells

     2) Immature production of clotting factors resulting in increased risk of bleeding disorders

     3) Increased risk of hypoglycemia related to inadequate glucose stores

  **e.** Hematopoetic: bruises easily related to fragile capillaries and prolonged prothrombin time

  **f.** Hepatic

     1) Increased risk of hyperbilirubinemia related to immature liver

     2) Decreased liver glycogen stores so infant is prone to hypoglycemia

     3) Prolonged drug metabolism related to immature liver

  **g.** Gastrointestinal

     1) Weak suck/swallow reflex until 33 to 34 weeks gestation and poor gag/cough reflexes increase risk of aspiration

     2) Increased risk of **necrotizing enterocolitis (NEC),** a neonatal disorder related to immature GI system and hypoxia

     **h.** Renal

       1) Unable to concentrate urine effectively increasing the risk of dehydration

       2) Prolonged drug excretion time related to immature kidneys

     **i.** Neuromuscular

       1) Immature control of vital functions

       2) Increased risk of **intraventricular hemorrhage (IVH),** which is bleeding into the ventricles of the brain

       3) Increased risk of apnea

       4) Poor muscle tone

       5) Weak or absent reflexes

       6) Weak, feeble cry

**4.** Priority nursing diagnoses: Impaired gas exchange; Ineffective thermoregulation; Imbalanced nutrition: less than body requirements

**5.** Planning and implementation

     **a.** Respiratory

       1) Maintain respirations at 30 to 60/min, assess every 1 to 2 h and prn

       2) Assess oxygenation and administer $O_2$ as ordered

         a) Auscultate breath sounds

         b) Monitor for signs of respiratory distress

         c) Suction prn

         d) Monitor oxygen saturation and/or blood gasses

     **b.** Thermoregulation

       1) Maintain **neutral thermal environment** (temperature that prevents heat loss) and prevent cold stress

         a) Place infant under radiant warmer or in double-wall isolette

         b) Warm equipment and linen before contact with infant

         c) Generally, infant can be weaned to an open bassinet when his or her temperature is stable and the infant is gaining weight

       2) Assess infant's temperature q 2 to 3 hours and prn

     **c.** Monitor for signs of sepsis

     **d.** Feeding

       1) Feed according to abilities

       2) Assess tolerance of feedings

         a) Monitor suck/swallow reflex to assess the risk of aspiration; if poor, gavage feed as indicated

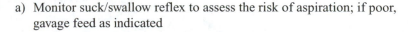

b) Use "preemie" nipple if bottle feeding; burp frequently

c) Assess for abdominal distention and emesis, which could indicate the neonate is not tolerating the feedings

3) Monitor I & O, daily weight; assess for dehydration

e. Monitor for hypoglycemia

f. Monitor for hyperbilirubinemia

g. Organize care to minimize stress

h. Skin care with special attention to cleanliness and careful positioning to prevent skin breakdown

i. Assess apical heart rate for 1 min q 1 to 2 h

j. Monitor potential bleeding sites (umbilicus, injection sites)

k. Monitor overall growth and development; check daily weight, measure length and occipital frontal circumference (OFC) weekly

l. Monitor closely for medication side effects caused by decreased ability to metabolize and excrete medications

6. Evaluation: infant will not develop complications related to preterm birth

7. Potential complications related to prematurity

a. Respiratory distress syndrome (RDS)

1) Also known as hyaline membrane disease

2) Primarily associated with prematurity

3) Usually appears during first 24 to 48 hours after birth and peaks around 72 hours

4) Other predisposing factors include: fetal hypoxia and postnatal hypothermia

5) Factors protecting neonate against RDS

a) Chronic fetal stress, such as maternal hypertension and preeclampsia

b) Prenatal administration of betamethasone to mother, which accelerates fetal lung maturity

c) Administration of artificial surfactant (Exosurf, Survanta) in the infant's airway after delivery, which helps keep the alveoli from collapsing and causing atelectasis

6) At risk for **bronchopulmonary dysplasia (BPD),** a chronic pulmonary disease requiring mechanical ventilation and high oxygen levels in the first weeks of life

b. **Retinopathy of Prematurity (ROP)**

1) Etiology: prolonged exposure to high concentrations of oxygen causes hemorrhage within the retina and leads to retinal detachment and loss of vision

2) Preventable with cautious administration of oxygen; it is critical to administer the minimum amount of oxygen to maintain a $PaO_2$ of 50 to 70 mm Hg

3) All premature infants who received oxygen should be screened prior to discharge by an ophthalmologist

**c.** Intraventricular hemorrhage (IVH)

1) Etiology: rupture of thin, fragile capillaries within the ventricles of the brain leading to increased intracranial pressure

2) Prematurity and hypoxia are primary risk factors

3) Assessment: neurological changes such as hypotonia and lethargy, bulging fontanels, increasing OFC, bradycardia, apnea

**d.** Necrotizing enterocolitis (NEC)

1) Etiology: intestinal ischemia related to shunting of blood to brain and heart in response to fetal or neonatal distress

2) Assessment: abdominal distention, poor feeding, vomiting, blood in stool

3) Treatment involves NPO, IV fluids and antibiotics until intestines healed

**e.** Apnea and bradycardia

1) Preterm neonates are at risk for apnea related to immature regulation of vital functions; if the apnea is prolonged, eventually bradycardia occurs

2) Infants almost always go into respiratory arrest first, followed by cardiac arrest; by supporting respiratory function, the heart rate should return to normal range

3) If apnea occurs, first stimulate respirations with gentle tactile stimulation; if this is unsuccessful, reposition the neonate and finally support respirations with an ambu bag if necessary

**B. Postmaturity**

**1.** Definition and etiology

**a.** Born after completion of 42 weeks of pregnancy

**b.** Problems caused by progressively less efficient actions of placenta

**c.** At risk for birth injury related to dystocia

**d.** Placental insufficiency may occur with an aging placenta that can no longer meet the needs of the fetus; increases the risk of fetal asphyxia, which can result in the passage of meconium in utero and increased risk of **meconium aspiration syndrome (MAS),** inhalation of meconium into the lungs

**2.** Assessment

**a.** Absence of vernix and minimal lanugo

**b.** Dry, cracked skin related to metabolism of fat to meet energy needs in utero

      **c.** Hypoglycemia related to metabolism of glycogen to meet energy needs in utero

      **d.** Minimal subcutaneous fat

      **e.** Skin and cord yellow/green caused by meconium staining

      **f.** Long fingernails and often has scratches on face and trunk

  **3.** Priority nursing diagnoses: Risk for injury; Hypothermia; Imbalanced nutrition: less than body requirements

  **4.** Interventions

      **a.** Assess for presence of meconium at delivery

      **b.** Assess for presence of birth injuries

      **c.** Assess for signs of hypoglycemia

  **5.** Evaluation: neonate will make a successful transition to extrauterine life

## III. Problems Related to Size

### A. Small for gestational age (SGA)

  **1.** Definition: birth weight below 10th percentile

  **2.** Etiology: placental insufficiency, infections, smoking, hypertension, malnutrition

  **3.** Assessment

      **a.** Skin: loose and dry, little fat or muscle mass

      **b.** Little scalp hair

      **c.** Hypoglycemia

      **d.** Weak cry

  **4.** Priority nursing diagnoses: Hypothermia; Risk for injury; Imbalanced nutrition: less than body requirements

  **5.** Interventions

      **a.** Assess for the presence of meconium during labor and delivery; thoroughly suction airway immediately after delivery if present

      **b.** Assess temperature and provide neutral thermal environment

      **c.** Assess for signs of hypoglycemia

      **d.** Weigh daily and assess changes in weight

  **6.** Evaluation: infant maintains stable temperature and blood glucose level and gains weight

### B. Large for gestational age (LGA)

  **1.** Definition: birthweight above 90th percentile

  **2.** Etiology

      **a.** Primary cause: infant of diabetic mother (IDM)

      **b.** If preterm, at risk for respiratory distress syndrome

      **c.** If postterm, at risk for meconium aspiration

3. Increased risk of:

   a. Hyperbilirubinemia related to increased bilirubin released from damaged red blood cells secondary to traumatic delivery

   b. Birth injury: fractured clavicle, Erb-Duchenne paralysis secondary to shoulder dystocia

4. Assessment

   a. Macrosomia (large body size and high birthweight)

   b. Signs of birth trauma related to cephalopelvic disproportion (CPD)

   c. Hypoglycemia, especially with an IDM

5. Priority nursing diagnosis: Risk for injury

6. Interventions

   a. Assess for signs of birth injury

   b. Assess for signs of hypoglycemia

7. Evaluation: infant will transition to extrauterine life without birth trauma or injury

## IV. Problems Related to Birth Trauma

### A. Facial paralysis

1. Etiology: temporary facial paralysis caused by pressure on the facial nerve during delivery

2. Assessment: face on affected side is unresponsive when neonate cries, eye remains open, forehead will not wrinkle

3. Self-resolves within hours or days of delivery, permanent paralysis is rare

4. Assess and support ability to feed orally

### B. Erb-Duchenne paralysis

1. Definition: brachial paralysis of upper portion of the arm

2. Etiology

   a. Most common type of paralysis associated with difficult delivery

   b. Incidence: 0.5 to 1.9 per 1,000 live births

   c. Paralysis is related to stretching or pulling the head away from shoulder during difficult delivery

3. Assessment

   a. Flaccid arm with elbow extended and hand rotated inward

   b. Moro reflex absent on affected side

   c. Grasp reflex intact

4. Interventions

   a. Intermittent immobilization

   b. Brace, splint, or pin sleeve to mattress

**c.** Reposition q 2 to 3 hours

**d.** Delay range-of-motion until 10th day to prevent further damage

### C. Fractures

1. Etiology

    **a.** Clavicle is the bone most frequently fractured during delivery

    **b.** Other bones fractured during delivery are skull, humerus and femur

    **c.** Cephalopelvic disproportion (CPD) is often a predisposing factor

2. Assessment (fractured clavicle): limited range-of-motion, crepitus over the affected bone and absence of Moro reflex on affected side

3. Priority nursing diagnoses: Risk for injury; Acute pain

4. Interventions (fractured clavicle)

    **a.** Instruct parents to handle affected arm gently

    **b.** Usually self-resolves

5. Evaluation: infant will not show signs of permanent damage related to birth trauma

### D. Asphyxia

1. Definition: inadequate tissue perfusion which fails to meet the metabolic needs of the tissues

2. Etiology

    **a.** Nonreassuring fetal heart rate pattern during labor (late or variable decelerations, loss of variability, bradycardia), difficult delivery, prematurity, passage of meconium in utero

    **b.** Initial goal is to identify neonates at risk so resuscitation can begin immediately if necessary

3. Assessment

    **a.** Fetal scalp pH during labor; 7.20 or less considered ominous sign of fetal asphyxia

    **b.** Apgar score of 4 to 7 indicates need for stimulation; score less than 4 indicates need for resuscitation; resuscitative efforts should begin immediately if needed

    **c.** Passage of meconium prior to or during delivery

4. Priority nursing diagnoses: Ineffective breathing pattern; Decreased cardiac output

5. Interventions

    **a.** At delivery, hold neonate in a head-down position and thoroughly suction the mouth and nares

    **b.** Place neonate under pre-warmed radiant warmer

    **c.** Stimulate respiratory effort by rubbing the back and feet

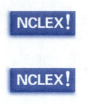

**d.** If respirations inadequate, place neonate in "sniffing" position; inflate neonate's lungs with positive pressure using bag and mask with 100 percent oxygen at rate of 40 to 60 breaths/min

**e.** Once breathing is established, check the heart rate; if heart rate is less than 60, or 60 to 80 and not increasing, begin cardiac compressions; the lower third of the sternum should be compressed with two fingertips or both thumbs at rate of 90 beats/min; a 3:1 ratio of compressions to assisted ventilation is used (see Figure 13-2)

**f.** Resuscitative medications, primarily epinephrine, should be administered after 30 seconds of assisted ventilation and compressions if the neonate's heart rate is not above 80 beats/min

**g.** Administer naloxone (Narcan) if mother received narcotics near time of delivery

**6.** Evaluation: the newborn's metabolic and physiologic processes are stabilized, and recovery proceeds without complications

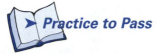

**➤ *Practice to Pass***

How should interventions differ during resuscitation if meconium is present in the amniotic fluid?

## V. General Care of the Neonate Experiencing Respiratory Distress

### A. Common causes of respiratory distress in neonates

**1.** Respiratory distress syndrome (RDS); typically preterm infants

**2.** Meconium aspiration syndrome (MAS); typically term and postterm infants

**3.** **Transient tachypnea of the newborn (TTN)** from delayed absorption of fluid in lungs from delivery; typically term and postterm infants

### B. Assessment (see Box 13-2)

### C. Interventions

**1.** Maintain neutral thermal environment due to increased oxygen demand if neonate is hypothermic

**2.** Administer warmed, humidified oxygen as ordered, generally attempting to keep the oxygen saturation greater than 88 to 90 percent and the $PaO_2$ between 50 and 70 mm Hg

**Figure 13-2**

**External cardiac massage.**

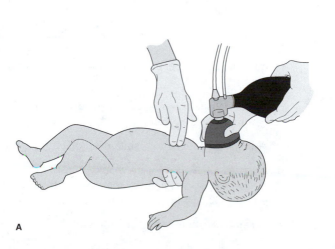
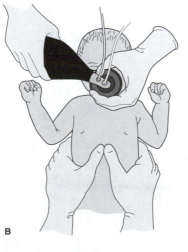

A   B

3. Withhold oral feedings if respiratory rate greater than 60 breaths/min because of increased risk of aspiration; notify healthcare provider

4. Position neonate side lying or supine with neck slightly extended ("sniffing position"); arms at sides

5. Suction prn to maintain a patent airway

6. Monitor oxygen saturation and/or arterial blood gasses (ABGs) as ordered

**D. Meconium aspiration syndrome (MAS)**

1. Definition: aspiration of meconium into the tracheobronchial tree during the first few breaths after delivery in a term neonate

2. Etiology

   a. Prenatal asphyxia causes increased fetal intestinal peristalsis, relaxation of the anal sphincter and passage of meconium into the amniotic fluid; this fluid may be aspirated into the lungs during the first few breaths after delivery

   b. Meconium-stained fluid occurs in 8 to 29 percent of all pregnancies

   c. Meconium in the lungs produces a ball-valve action (air is allowed in but cannot be exhaled) and is irritating to the airway; as the lungs become hyperinflated, pulmonary perfusion decreases leading to increased hypoxia

   d. Can lead to persistent pulmonary hypertension of the newborn (PPHN)

3. Assessment

   a. May demonstrate signs of fetal distress during labor and delivery

   b. Apgar score less than 6 at 1 and 5 minutes

   c. Immediate signs of respiratory distress at delivery (cyanosis, tachypnea, retractions)

   d. Overdistended, barrel-shaped chest

   e. Diminished breath sounds

   f. Yellow staining of skin, nails, and umbilical cord

4. Priority nursing diagnosis: Ineffective gas exchange

5. Interventions

   a. Suction baby's oropharnyx then nasopharnyx after the neonate's head is born and the shoulders and chest are still in the birth canal to remove as much meconium as possible before the baby's first breath

   b. If the meconium is thick in the amniotic fluid, place neonate under radiant warmer, visualize the glottis, and suction any meconium from the trachea before stimulating respirations

   c. Administer oxygen to maintain adequate $PO_2$ and oxygen saturation

   d. Anticipate the need for mechanical ventilation, high-frequency ventilation or **extracorporeal membrane oxygenation (ECMO),** which is used for prolonged heart-lung bypass to allow lungs to heal

   e. Perform chest physiotherapy routinely

**6.** Evaluation

   **a.** The risk of MAS is promptly identified and early intervention is initiated

   **b.** The neonate is free of respiratory distress and acid-base imbalance

**E. Transient tachypnea of the newborn (TTN)**

  **1.** Etiology

    **a.** Failure to clear the airway of excess lung fluid at delivery

    **b.** Primarily occurs in term infants, especially if delivered by cesarean because they have not experienced the mechanical squeeze that occurs during a vaginal delivery

  **2.** Assessment

    **a.** Expiratory grunting, nasal flaring, mild cyanosis

    **b.** Tachypnea by 6 hours of age, respiratory rate may get as high as 100 to 140 breaths/min

  **3.** Priority nursing diagnosis: Ineffective gas exchange

  **4.** Interventions

    **a.** Administer oxygen as needed to maintain $PO_2$ and oxygen saturation within normal limits

    **b.** Usually self resolves within 72 hours

  **5.** Evaluation: the neonate is free of respiratory distress and acid–base imbalance

## VI. Congenital Infections

**A. TORCH**

  **1.** Toxoplasmosis

    **a.** Etiology

      1) Caused by the protozoan *Toxoplasma gondii*

      2) Contracted by eating raw or undercooked meat or contact with feces of infected cats; maternal-fetal transmission during pregnancy

      3) Often results in spontaneous abortion if contracted during first trimester

      4) Severe neonatal disorders associated with congenital infection include convulsions, coma, microcephaly and hydrocephalus

    **b.** Interventions: to prevent maternal-fetal transmission, women should:

      1) Use good handwashing

      2) Avoid eating raw meat

      3) Avoid exposure to cat litter during pregnancy

      4) Have toxoplasma titer checked prenatally if cats live in the household

  **2.** Other infections, usually Hepatitis B (HBV)

    **a.** Transmitted from mother to neonate in about 90 percent of cases

    **b.** Transmitted transplacentally and by contact with blood and body fluids

c. Associated with a 32 percent increased risk of preterm labor

d. Infected neonates may be symptom free or have acute hepatitis, with a 75 percent mortality rate

e. Infants of mothers with positive HbsAg should receive hepatitis B immune globulin (HBIG) 0.5 mL IM within first 12 hours of life. They should also receive the hepatitis B vaccine, with the first dose within the first 12 hours of life, the second dose at 1 month and the third dose at 6 months

f. Center for Disease Control (CDC) recommends all women be screened prenatally for HbsAg to determine newborns at risk

3. Rubella

a. Etiology

1) Also called German measles

2) Up to 20 percent of women of childbearing age are not rubella immune; a rubella titer of 1:8 or greater indicates immunity

3) Eighty to ninety percent of fetuses exposed during the first trimester will be affected either by spontaneous abortion or congenital anomalies

b. Assessment: clinical signs of congenital infections are congenital heart disease, **intrauterine growth restriction (IUGR)** or fetal undergrowth, and hearing loss

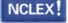

c. Interventions: infants born with congenital rubella syndrome are infectious and should be isolated

4. Cytomegalovirus (CMV)

a. Respiratory or sexual transmission; neonate can contract during delivery through an infected birth canal

b. Most common cause of congenital viral infection, occurring in 1 percent of all newborns. Most (90 to 95 percent) of these infants are asymptomatic at birth; remaining 5 to 10 percent may experience hemolytic anemia and jaundice, hydrocephaly or microcephaly, pneumonitis, deafness, and fetal or neonatal death

c. Disease is usually progressive through infancy and childhood

5. Herpes (HSV)

a. Etiology: herpes simplex virus type 1 or type 2

b. Maternal symptoms include vesicles on genitalia that are usually painful; fetal symptoms include fever or hypothermia, jaundice, seizures, poor feeding; 50 percent develop vesicular skin lesions

c. There is no known cure

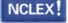

d. Virus can be lethal to fetus and is transmitted during birth; cesarean delivery is indicated if the mother has active lesions at the time of delivery

B. **Sexually transmitted infections**

1. Syphilis

a. Etiology

1) Caused by treponema palladium, a spirochete

2) Organism crosses the placenta after 16 weeks gestation and infects fetus; Langhans' layer in the chorion prevents fetal infection early in pregnancy until this layer begins to atrophy between 16 and 18 weeks gestation

3) There is no increase risk of anomalies, but spirochete may cause inflammatory and destructive changes in the liver, spleen, kidneys, and bone marrow

4) If syphilis is untreated during pregnancy, 25 percent of pregnancies will end in stillbirth and 40 to 50 percent of neonates born to these women will have symptomatic congenital syphilis

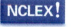

b. Assessment: clients with syphilis have a positive serologic test (VDRL)

2. Gonorrhea

a. Causative organism is *Neisseria gonorrhea*

b. Incidence in pregnant women is 2 to 7 percent

c. Neonate can be exposed to organism during birth; this can result in sepsis or ophthalmia neonatorum, which can cause permanent blindness

e. Penicillin is the treatment of choice

f. Eye prophylaxis with erythromycin (Ilotycin) ointment within 4 hours after birth can decrease the risk of ophthalmia neonatorum

3. Chlamydia

a. Most common sexually transmitted disease

b. Caused by *Chlamydia trachomatis*

c. Can be transmitted to neonate during delivery and cause neonatal conjunctivitis and pneumonia

d. Eye prophylaxis with erythromycin ointment shortly after birth can prevent neonatal conjunctivitis; silver nitrate has been used prophylactically in the past but is not effective against *Chlamydia trachomatis*

4. Candidiasis

a. Etiology

1) Neonatal oral yeast infection is commonly called thrush

2) Caused by yeast normally found in the vagina, most commonly *Candida albicans*

3) Excessive yeast growth occurs more commonly in sick newborns and those receiving antibiotics or steroids

4) Neonate may contract thrush during birth process or from contaminated hands or feeding equipment

b. Assessment

1) Thrush presents as white patches on oral mucosa, gums, and tongue, which cannot be manually removed and may bleed when touched

2) Occasional difficulty in swallowing

c. Priority nursing diagnoses: Acute pain; Imbalanced nutrition: less than body requirements

d. Interventions

1) Anti-fungal medications are applied to the affected area to treat the infection; feed sterile water prior to administration to rinse out milk

2) Nystatin (Mycostatin) is applied to the newborn's mouth with a medicine dropper or swabbed over mucosa, gums, and tongue after a feeding

3) Gentian violet may also be swabbed over the mucosa, gums, and tongue, being careful to guard against staining the skin, clothes, and equipment

e. Evaluation

1) The neonate's mouth is intact, lesions are healed, with no evidence of infection

2) The neonate eats orally and maintains weight or regains weight lost, if any

5. HIV/AIDS

a. Etiology

1) During childbearing, transmission can occur across the placenta or through breast-milk or contaminated blood

2) Maternal to newborn transmission rates are 20 to 30 percent; transmission rate decreases by 2/3 when mothers are given zidovudine (ZDV) prenatally and intrapartally as well as administered to the newborn after delivery

3) It may take up to 15 months for infants to form own antibodies against HIV

4) For infants, the average survival time between testing positive for HIV infection and death is 9 months; with a 70 to 80 percent mortality rate by 2 years of age

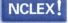

5) HIV testing should be done at birth and 1 to 2 months of age

b. Assessment

1) Typically asymptomatic at birth

2) By 1 year of age most manifest some symptoms similar to those in adults

3) Failure to thrive with developmental delays

4) Hepatomegaly and/or splenomegaly

5) Lymphoid interstitial pneumonitis

6) Recurrent infections, persistent thrush

7) Chronic diarrhea

c. Priority nursing diagnoses: Imbalanced nutrition: less than body requirements; Risk for impaired skin integrity; Risk for infection; Impaired physical mobility

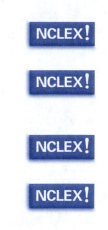

    **d.** Interventions

        1) Universal precautions; specific isolation not required

        2) Promote comfort

        3) Keep well nourished; encourage bottle-feeding as the AIDS virus has been found in breast-milk

        4) Thorough cord care to prevent infection, prevent exposure to infections

        5) The infant should receive all vaccines except oral poliovirus

        6) Skin and mouth care

        7) Administer zidovudine (ZDV) as ordered

    **e.** Evaluation: potential opportunistic infections are identified early and treated promptly

**C. Sepsis**

  **1.** Definition: generalized infection that has spread rapidly through the bloodstream

  **2.** Pathophysiology: immature immune system, inability to localize infection, and lack of IgM immunoglobulin, which is necessary to protect against bacteria and does not cross the placenta

  **3.** When sepsis is suspected, cultures will be obtained and antibiotics started immediately; after 72 hours of treatment, antibiotics may be discontinued if final culture reports are negative and symptoms have subsided; antibiotics will generally be continued for 10 to 14 days if final culture reports are positive

  **4.** Etiology

    **a.** Prolonged rupture of membranes

    **b.** Long, difficult labor

    **c.** Resuscitation and other invasive procedures

    **d.** Maternal infection

    **e.** Beta-hemolytic streptococcal vaginosis is the most common cause of neonatal sepsis and meningitis; cervical culture should be obtained prior to delivery; if positive, antibiotics given during intrapartum period decrease the risk of transmission

    **f.** Aspiration of amniotic fluid, formula, or mucus

    **g.** Nosocomial: caused by infected healthcare workers or equipment

  **5.** Assessment

    **a.** Symptoms often vague initially

    **b.** Temperature instability, especially hypothermia

    **c.** Feeding intolerance as evidenced by decreased intake, abdominal distention, vomiting, poor sucking

    **d.** Subtle behavior changes, "the infant just doesn't look right," lethargy, seizure activity, pallor

       **e.** Progressive respiratory distress

       **f.** Hyperbilirubinemia

       **g.** Tachycardia initially, followed by periods of apnea and bradycardia

  **6.** Priority nursing diagnoses: Risk for infection; Deficient fluid volume

  **7.** Interventions

       **a.** Obtain cultures (blood, urine, cerebral spinal fluid) before antibiotics are initiated

       **b.** Administer antibiotics as ordered

       **c.** Observe for changes in vital signs and physical assessment

  **8.** Evaluation

       **a.** The newborn will remain free from sepsis

       **b.** The newborn's early signs of sepsis will be recognized, and appropriate therapy will be initiated

       **c.** If therapy is necessary, the newborn will not suffer negative consequences

## VII. Cold Stress

  **A. Pathophysiology:** neonates produce body heat by non-shivering thermogenesis; this process requires increased oxygen and glucose consumption to burn brown fat; subcutaneous fat acts as an insulator and helps conserve body heat; a flexed position decreases exposed surface area and conserves body heat

  **B. Etiology**

    **1.** At risk for hypothermia because of large surface-area-to-mass ratio

    **2.** Large amount of heat is lost from head

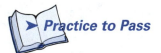

    **3.** All newborns are at risk for hypothermia, especially preterm and small-for-gestational-age infants

  **C. Interventions**

    **1.** Maintain neutral thermal environment

      **a.** Reduce or eliminate heat lost through drafts and contact with cold objects

      **b.** Postpone initial bath until temperature has stabilized

      **c.** Dry infant immediately after delivery and when bathing

    **2.** Place newborn under servo-controlled warmer or on mother's abdomen immediately after delivery

    **3.** Assess body temperature; keep axillary temperature 97.6° to 99.2°F

    **4.** If axillary temperature is less than 97.6° F:

      **a.** Put hat on infant's head

      **b.** Wrap newborn with warm blankets

      **c.** Assess oxygenation status and assess for hypoglycemia

      **d.** Rewarm infant slowly to prevent hypotension and apnea

    **5.** Chronic hypothermia could be an early sign of sepsis

*Practice to Pass*

You are caring for an infant in an isolette and you notice that the isolette temperature has been steadily increasing over the past 12 hours. This means that the isolette has to stay warmer to keep the infant's temperature stable; for what problems should the nurse assess closely?

## VIII. Hyperbilirubinemia

### A. Etiology

1. Bilirubin is formed by the breakdown of hemoglobin from red blood cells; there are two types of bilirubin: direct (conjugated), which is water-soluble and easier for the body to eliminate, and indirect (unconjugated), which is fat-soluble so it can more easily cross the blood-brain barrier but is harder for the body to eliminate

2. Before birth, unconjugated bilirubin is eliminated by the placenta; after delivery, the bilirubin is converted from an unconjugated to a conjugated form in the liver and is excreted via the bile ducts into the intestines; it can be reabsorbed from the intestines if peristalsis slows

3. **Kernicterus** is a potential complication of hyperbilirubinemia; bilirubin is deposited in the basal ganglia of the brain and causes permanent impaired neurological function; bilirubin level, gestational age, condition, and poor fluid-caloric balance increase the risk of kernicterus at low serum-bilirubin levels

### B. Physiologic jaundice

1. A normal newborn has two times as much bilirubin as an adult related to a higher concentration of circulating red blood cells, an impaired ability of the liver to conjugate bilirubin related to immaturity and transition from fetal to neonatal circulation, and a shorter lifespan of the fetal red blood cell

2. Factors that increase risk of physiologic jaundice

   a. Resolution of enclosed hemorrhage (cephalhematoma, large amount of bruising from difficult delivery)

   b. Infection

   c. Dehydration

   d. Sepsis

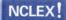

3. Physiologic jaundice usually begins after the first 24 hours of life

### C. Pathologic jaundice

1. Usually related to hemolytic disease of the newborn

   a. Rh incompatibility

      1) If the mother is Rh-negative and the fetus is Rh-positive, the fetus's Rh-positive red blood cells enter the maternal bloodstream through breaks in the maternal–fetal circulation late in pregnancy and after separation of the placenta at delivery, causing maternal antibody formation; in a subsequent pregnancy with another Rh-positive fetus, the maternal antibodies will cross the placenta, enter the fetal bloodstream and attack the red blood cells causing hemolysis and fetal anemia; Rhogam is given to the mother to prevent the development of these antibodies, but it cannot reverse the reaction once it occurs

      2) Erythroblastosis fetalis is the most severe hemolytic reaction; it causes severe anemia, cardiac decompensation, edema, ascites, hypoxia, and may result in fetal death

**b.** ABO incompatibility

    1) If mother has type O blood and is carrying a fetus with blood type A, B, or AB, the fetus's red blood cells enter the maternal bloodstream through breaks in the maternal–fetal circulation late in pregnancy and after separation of the placenta at delivery, causing maternal antibody formation; in a subsequent pregnancy with another fetus with that blood type, the maternal antibodies will cross the placenta, enter the fetal bloodstream and attack the red blood cells causing hemolysis and anemia; this reaction tends to be less severe than with Rh incompatibility

 **c.** Jaundice begins within the first 24 hours of life

**D. Assessment**

    **1.** Determine mother's blood type and Rh factor; if mother is Rh-negative or type-O blood, determine infant's blood type and Rh factor

    **2.** Evaluate results of Coombs' tests

       **a.** Indirect Coombs' determines the presence of maternal antibodies (sensitization) in maternal blood; a positive test indicates the presence of antibodies

       **b.** Direct Coombs' determines the presence of maternal Rh antibodies in fetal blood; cord blood is generally used; a positive test indicates the presence of antibodies

    **3.** Golden amniotic fluid indicates severe hemolytic disease

    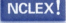 **4.** Assess for jaundice by gently pressing on the sternum or forehead; in dark-skinned infants, assess the sclera, palms of the hands, and soles of the feet

    **5.** Evaluate the results of bilirubin levels

       **a.** Bilirubin can be assessed noninvasively with a bilimeter

       **b.** Total serum bilirubin levels greater than 13 to 15 mg/dL indicates hyperbilirubinemia

    **6.** Enlarged liver and spleen

    **7.** Anemia

    **8.** Concentrated, dark urine

**E. Priority nursing diagnoses:** Deficient fluid volume (red blood cell); Risk for injury (brain damage); Disturbed thought processes (mental retardation)

**F. Interventions**

    **1.** Early and frequent feedings to stimulate peristalsis

    **2. Phototherapy** (exposure of infant to bright light)

       **a.** Cover closed infant's eyes when under phototherapy light; remove eye covers every 2 hours when under light to assess for conjunctivitis and when not under phototherapy to promote bonding

       **b.** Infant should be undressed to maximize the amount of circulating blood exposed to the phototherapy light; genitalia can be covered to prevent soiling

       **c.** Change infant's position every 2 hours and assess for skin breakdown

     **d.** Assess for loose green stools as bilirubin is excreted through the intestines

     **e.** Increase fluid intake to prevent dehydration

     **f.** Assess temperature every 2 hours and monitor for hypo- or hyperthermia

     **g.** Monitor bilirubin levels

  **3. Exchange transfusion**

     **a.** Used to quickly decrease high bilirubin level by exchanging the infant's circulating blood volume with donor blood; also removes anti-Rh antibodies and fetal cells coated with antibodies from infant's blood and corrects anemia

     **b.** Only use Rh-negative blood to decrease risk of a transfusion reaction

     **c.** Warm blood to room temperature to prevent cardiac arrest

     **d.** Give calcium gluconate, as ordered, after each 100 mL

     **e.** Assess vital signs before procedure, every 15 minutes during procedure and post-procedure

     **f.** Record time, amount of blood withdrawn, time and amount injected, medications given

     **g.** Assess for dyspnea, listlessness, bleeding, cyanosis, bradycardia or arrythmias, hypoglycemia

**G. Evaluation**

  **1.** Infant's bilirubin levels decrease to within normal range

  **2.** Infant does not demonstrate any long-term effects of hyperbilirubinemia

## IX. Hypoglycemia

**A. Etiology**

  **1.** Definition: blood glucose less than 30 to 35 mg/dL in a term newborn

  **2.** Glucose levels are assessed with a heel-stick

  **3.** Newborns at risk: infants of diabetic mothers (IDM), small for gestational age, premature, and infants experiencing cold stress, hypothermia, or delayed feedings

  **4.** Poor prognosis if hypoglycemia is not treated

  **5.** Blood glucose usually stabilizes within 48 to 72 hours

**B. Assessment**

  **1.** Tremors, jitteriness

  **2.** Lethargy

  **3.** Decreased muscle tone

  **4.** Apnea

  **5.** Anorexia

**C. Priority nursing diagnosis:** Imbalanced nutrition: less than body requirements

**D. Interventions**

1. Check blood glucose on all infants at risk by 1 hour of age (30 minutes if IDM), and any symptomatic newborn as ordered

2. Treat hypoglycemia by breast-feeding immediately or feeding D5W or D10W, either orally or intravenously; do not attempt to feed a lethargic infant orally because of an increased risk of aspiration

3. If treated for hypoglycemia, reassess blood glucose level before next feeding

## X. Infant of a Diabetic Mother (IDM)

**A. Etiology**

1. Hormones secreted during pregnancy (HPL) increase maternal resistance to insulin, increasing insulin requirements; in diabetic clients, the pancreas can not secrete the additional insulin needed during pregnancy and blood glucose levels increase

2. Maternal insulin cannot cross the placenta but glucose can; fetal glucose levels rise; the fetus's pancreas responds by secreting more insulin, which metabolizes the additional glucose and acts as a growth hormone; increased insulin needs decrease surfactant production

**B. Assessment**

1. Large for gestational age; birth trauma more likely

2. Maternal dystocia related to cephalopelvic disproportion (CPD)

3. Enlarged internal organs: cardiomegaly, hepatomegaly, splenomegaly

4. Hypoglycemia

5. Hypocalcemia

6. Hyperbilirubinemia

7. Respiratory distress syndrome (RDS)

8. False positive L/S ratio

9. Increased risk for congenital anomalies, particularly cardiac and spinal defects

**C. Priority nursing diagnoses:** Risk for injury; Imbalanced nutrition: less than body requirements; Impaired gas exchange

**D. Interventions**

1. Assess for birth trauma

2. Assess blood glucose at 30 minutes and 1, 2, 4, 6, 9, 12, and 24 hours after birth

3. Treat hypoglycemia per orders

**E. Evaluation**

1. The newborn experiences minimal or no episodes of hypoglycemia, hypocalcemia, or hyperbilirubinemia

2. The newborn exhibits adequate respiratory function and gas exchange

**Practice to Pass**

How could chronic diabetes cause a baby to be small for gestational age (SGA)?

## XI. Substance Abuse

### A. Fetal alcohol syndrome (FAS)

1. Etiology

   a. Alcohol crosses the placenta and interferes with protein synthesis

   b. Increased risk of congenital anomalies, mental deficiency, intrauterine growth restriction (IUGR)

2. Assessment

   a. Small for gestational age

   b. Facial features: epicanthal folds, maxillary hypoplasia, long and thin upper lip

   c. Irritable, hyperactive

   d. High-pitched cry

3. Interventions

   a. Reduce environmental stimuli

   b. Swaddle to increase feeling of security

   c. Administer sedatives as ordered to decrease side effects of withdrawal

   d. Maintain nutrition and hydration

4. Priority nursing diagnosis: Risk for injury

5. Evaluation: the newborn maintains adequate respirations, gains weight, demonstrates normal newborn reflexes, and shows no evidence of CNS hyper-irritability

### B. Neonatal abstinence syndrome (NAS)

1. Etiology

   a. Repeated intrauterine absorption of drugs from maternal bloodstream causes fetal drug dependency

   b. Increased risk of spontaneous abortion, preterm labor, stillbirth

   c. Degree of drug withdrawal depends on type and duration of addiction and maternal drug levels at delivery

2. Assessment

   a. Hyperactivity, jitteriness

   b. Absence of "step" reflex and "head-righting" reflex

   c. Shrill, persistent crying

   d. Frequent yawning and sneezing; nasal stuffiness

   e. Respiratory distress

   f. Sweating

   g. Feeding difficulties (regurgitation, vomiting, and diarrhea), increased need for non-nutritive sucking

   h. Developmental delays

3. Priority nursing diagnoses: Risk for injury; Impaired gas exchange; Imbalanced nutrition: less than body requirements

4. Interventions

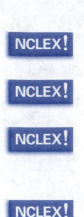

**a.** Position infant on side to facilitate drainage of mucus

**b.** Suction prn to maintain patent airway

**c.** Decrease environmental stimuli, swaddle for comfort

**d.** Intake and output, daily weight

**e.** Obtain meconium and/or urine for drug screening as ordered

**f.** Administer medications as ordered

   1) Paregoric elixir is used to wean the infant

   2) Chlorpromazine (Thorazine) and diazepam (Valium) are used to decrease hyperirritability; valium predisposes to hyperbilirubinemia and is contraindicated in jaundiced newborns

   3) Methadone

   4) Phenobarbital is used to decrease hyperirritability and hyperbilirubinemia

**g.** Pacifier for non-nutritive sucking

5. Evaluation: the newborn maintains adequate respirations, gains weight, demonstrates normal newborn reflexes, and shows no evidence of CNS hyperirritability

---

**Case Study**

**A 29-week-gestation newborn is 6 hours of age. You are the nurse assigned to care for him in the neonatal intensive care unit.**

❶ What additional information do you need before planning care for this newborn?

❷ What are the priorities for the newborn's care at this time?

❸ The parents are concerned because they have heard oxygen can cause blindness in preterm infants. How would you respond?

❹ Discuss how you can meet the newborn's psychosocial and developmental needs.

❺ The mother asks if she can still breast-feed. How should you respond?

*For suggested responses, see page 341.*

## Posttest

1. The parents of a 28-week-gestation neonate ask the nurse, "Why does he have to be fed through a tube in his mouth?" The nurse's best response is that:

(1) It allows an accurate assessment of intake.
(2) The baby's sucking, swallowing, and breathing are not coordinated yet.
(3) The baby's stomach cannot digest formula.
(4) It helps prevent thrush.

**2** Which nursing diagnosis should be the highest priority when caring for a preterm newborn?

(1) Ineffective thermoregulation related to lack of subcutaneous fat
(2) Anticipatory grieving related to loss of "perfect delivery."
(3) Imbalanced nutrition related to immature digestive system
(4) Risk for injury related to thin epidermis

**3** A nurse is caring for a 12-hour-old newborn. The nurse notes a yellow tint to the baby's skin and sclera. What lab test should the nurse anticipate being ordered?

(1) Blood glucose
(2) Direct Coombs'
(3) Blood culture
(4) Arterial blood gas (ABG)

**4** A newborn is admitted with a diagnosis of transient tachypnea of the newborn (TTN). When planning nursing care for this baby, a goal should be to:

(1) Promote adequate quantity of surfactant.
(2) Promote absorption of fetal lung fluid.
(3) Assist in removal of meconium from airway.
(4) Stimulate respirations.

**5** The nurse is assigned to a baby receiving phototherapy. Which assessment warrants further investigation?

(1) Loose, green stools
(2) Yellow tint to skin
(3) Temperature 97.2°F
(4) Fine, red rash on trunk

**6** A mother is crying at her baby's bedside. The most therapeutic response by the nurse is:

(1) "Don't worry. Everything will be fine."
(2) "Why are you upset?"
(3) "Would you like me to call the hospital chaplain?"
(4) "This must be hard for you."

**7** A baby's mother is HIV-positive. Which of the following interventions is most important when planning care for this newborn?

(1) Encourage the mother to breast-feed.
(2) Administer zidovudine (ZDV) after delivery.
(3) Cuddle the baby as much as possible.
(4) Place the baby's crib in a quiet corner of the nursery.

**8** The nurse is preparing to initiate bottle-feeding in a preterm infant. In which of the following situations should the nurse withhold the feeding and notify the healthcare provider?

(1) Apical heart rate 120
(2) Axillary temperature 97.2°F
(3) Yellow tint to skin and sclera
(4) Respiratory rate 72

**9** A newborn's mother has a history of prenatal narcotic abuse. Which of the following nursing interventions would be most appropriate for this infant?

(1) Hold and rock infant as much as possible.
(2) Offer infant a pacifier.
(3) Place mobile on crib.
(4) Encourage family members to stroke and talk to the infant.

**10** The nurse is caring for a preterm infant who is at risk for an intraventricular hemorrhage (IVH). Which daily assessment is most critical for this infant?

(1) Blood pressure
(2) Occipital frontal circumference (OFC)
(3) Intake and output
(4) Moro reflex

*See pages 310–311 for Answers and Rationales.*

# Answers and Rationales

## Pretest

**1** **Answer: 2** *Rationale:* Nasal flaring could be a sign of respiratory distress and requires immediate intervention. The other assessment data are normal findings for a neonate at 2 hours of age.
*Cognitive Level:* Analysis
*Nursing Process:* Analysis; *Test Plan:* PHYS

**2** **Answer: 3** *Rationale:* Maintaining a patent airway is the highest priority when providing care for a newborn. A newborn's condition will deteriorate rapidly without a patent airway.
*Cognitive Level:* Analysis
*Nursing Process:* Analysis; *Test Plan:* SECE

**3** **Answer: 1** *Rationale:* This newborn is at risk for sepsis caused by prolonged rupture of membranes and maternal fever. A primary sign of sepsis in the newborn is temperature instability, particularly hypothermia. An irregular respiratory pattern is normal. Jitteriness may be a sign of hypoglycemia. Excessive bruising is often related to a difficult delivery with an increased risk of hyperbilirubinemia.
*Cognitive Level:* Analysis
*Nursing Process:* Analysis; *Test Plan:* PHYS

**4** **Answer: 2** *Rationale:* Neonatal abstinence syndrome, or drug withdrawal, causes hyperstimulation of the neonate's nervous system. Nursing interventions should focus on decreasing environmental and sensory stimulation during the withdrawal period.
*Cognitive Level:* Application
*Nursing Process:* Implementation; *Test Plan:* PHYS

**5** **Answer: 1** *Rationale:* A newborn can become infected with gonorrhea as it passes through the birth canal. Gonorrhea can cause permanent blindness in the newborn, called ophthalmia neonatorum. All babies' eyes are treated with an antibiotic prophylactically after birth.
*Cognitive Level:* Application
*Nursing Process:* Planning; *Test Plan:* HPM

**6** **Answer: 2** *Rationale:* Newborns experiencing macrosomia are more likely to experience birth injuries during delivery. Nursing care after delivery should focus on assessing for signs of birth injuries and intervening if appropriate.
*Cognitive Level:* Application
*Nursing Process:* Analysis; *Test Plan:* SECE

**7** **Answer: 3** *Rationale:* Reflecting on what the client said offers the client an opportunity to share her feelings. Avoid giving false reassurance or asking clients "why" they feel the way they do.
*Cognitive Level:* Application
*Nursing Process:* Implementation; *Test Plan:* PSYC

**8** **Answer: 2** *Rationale:* Infants of diabetic mothers are at risk for hypoglycemia after delivery. A primary sign of hypoglycemia is jitteriness. The newborn is not showing any signs of hypoxia so oxygen would not be appropriate. Putting the newborn under a warmer or on a monitor would not harm the infant, but they are not the priority interventions at this time.
*Cognitive Level:* Analysis
*Nursing Process:* Implementation; *Test Plan:* PHYS

**9** **Answer: 4** *Rationale:* This newborn has a low temperature and the nurse must intervene quickly to prevent complications related to hypothermia. Wrapping the baby in warm blankets and covering the head will help prevent heat loss through conduction, convection and radiation and is the most important initial intervention. Babies can lose a large amount of heat from their head, so keeping it covered will help stabilize the temperature.
*Cognitive Level:* Application
*Nursing Process:* Implementation; *Test Plan:* PHYS

**10** **Answer: 2** *Rationale:* This newborn has signs of jaundice, which include a yellow tint to the sclera and skin. Jaundice is considered pathologic if it occurs within the first 24 hours of life, when it is most often caused by Rh- or ABO-incompatibility. It would be important to assess both the mother's and newborn's blood type and Rh-factor to determine if this could be causing the jaundice. A bilirubin level should also be obtained.
*Cognitive Level:* Analysis
*Nursing Process:* Assessment; *Test Plan:* PHYS

## Posttest

**1** **Answer: 2** *Rationale:* Neonates generally aren't able to effectively coordinate sucking, swallowing, and breathing until 34 to 36 weeks gestation. If fed orally before that time, they are at greater risk of aspiration. Typically they will be fed through a gavage tube until they are able to drink from a bottle- or breast-feed. Intake can be accurately assessed with oral and gavage feedings. The stomach of a preterm infant can digest small amounts of formula or breast-milk. Thrush is an oral yeast infection commonly

caused during passage through the birth canal, and gavage feedings will not prevent it from occurring.
*Cognitive Level:* Application
*Nursing Process:* Implementation; *Test Plan:* SECE

**2 Answer: 1** *Rationale:* Newborns compensate for hypothermia by metabolizing brown fat. This process requires glucose and oxygen. Preterm newborns are at risk for hypoglycemia and respiratory distress, so hypoglycemia can further increase their needs for oxygen and glucose and cause serious complications. The other diagnoses are appropriate but not the highest priority.
*Cognitive Level:* Analysis
*Nursing Process:* Analysis; *Test Plan:* SECE

**3 Answer: 2** *Rationale:* Jaundice in an infant less than 24 hours of age is often caused by Rh or ABO incompatibility. A direct Coombs' test determines the presence of maternal antibodies in the baby's blood. The other lab tests are not related to hyperbilirubinemia.
*Cognitive Level:* Application
*Nursing Process:* Planning; *Test Plan:* PHYS

**4 Answer: 2** *Rationale:* Transient tachypnea of the newborn (TTN) is caused by delayed absorption of fetal lung fluid. Nursing care is focused on supporting oxygenation needs to allow the newborn's body to reabsorb the fluid. TTN causes tachypnea so stimulating respirations is not appropriate. Inadequate surfactant is related to prematurity and respiratory distress syndrome. Meconium in the airway results in meconium aspiration syndrome and is usually associated with fetal asphyxia.
*Cognitive Level:* Application
*Nursing Process:* Planning; *Test Plan:* PHYS

**5 Answer: 3** *Rationale:* Infants should be unclothed while receiving phototherapy to increase the circulating blood volume exposed to the phototherapy light. However, this increases the risk of temperature instability, and infant temperatures should be monitored carefully. Any temperature below 97.6°F is considered hypothermia and requires immediate attention. Loose green stools and a yellow tint to the skin are expected findings with hyperbilirubinemia. A fine, raised red rash may appear on the infant's skin as a side effect of the phototherapy and does not require intervention.
*Cognitive Level:* Analysis
*Nursing Process:* Analysis; *Test Plan:* PHYS

**6 Answer: 4** *Rationale:* Reflection allows the client to verbalize their feelings. The nurse should not give the client false hope. Clients often do not know why they feel the way they do, and it is not helpful to ask them to determine this. Some clients may find comfort in a religious leader, but care should be taken not to stereotype the client's religious beliefs.
*Cognitive Level:* Application
*Nursing Process:* Implementation; *Test Plan:* PSYC

**7 Answer: 2** *Rationale:* Administering zidovudine (ZDV, formally AZT) to the mother prenatally and intrapartally, as well as to the infant immediately after delivery decreases the prenatal risk of transmission of HIV by 60 to 70 percent. Breast-feeding is contraindicated in an HIV-positive mother because the virus can be passed through breast-milk. Cuddling the infant is important, but not the highest priority in this situation. Decreasing environmental stimulation is not indicated.
*Cognitive Level:* Application
*Nursing Process:* Implementation; *Test Plan:* SECE

**8 Answer: 4** *Rationale:* Any sustained respiratory rate greater than 60 breaths/minute increases the risk of aspiration in the infant. Oral feedings should be withheld on infants experiencing tachypnea to decrease the risk of aspiration. An apical heart rate of 120 is a normal finding. Although an infant temperature of 97.2°F is considered hypothermia, it would not be a contraindication to oral feedings. Jaundice may be considered abnormal, but it alone would not be an indication to withhold an oral feeding.
*Cognitive Level:* Analysis
*Nursing Process:* Assessment; *Test Plan:* SECE

**9 Answer: 2** *Rationale:* Infants experiencing neonatal abstinence syndrome (NAS) often have an increased need for non-nutritive sucking, and offering a pacifier would help meet this need. The other three answers are incorrect because they all involve increasing the environmental stimulation. This is contraindicated in these infants because they are already hyperstimulated from the drug withdrawal process.
*Cognitive Level:* Application
*Nursing Process:* Implementation; *Test Plan:* PHYS

**10 Answer: 2** *Rationale:* Increasing OFC is an indication of increasing intracranial pressure, which could result from an IVH. It should be assessed in infants at risk for an IVH every 8 to 12 hours. Changes in blood pressure may also occur, but the changes may not be as noticeable and can be caused by many other problems. Changes in Moro reflex are not an indication of an IVH.
*Cognitive Level:* Analysis
*Nursing Process:* Assessment; *Test Plan:* PHYS

## *References*

Blake, W. W. & Murray, J. A. (1998). Heat balance. In Merenstein, G. B. & Gardner, S. L. (Eds.), *Handbook of neonatal intensive care* (4th ed.). St. Louis: Mosby, pp. 100–115.

Frank, C. G., Cooper, S. C., & Merenstein, G. B. (1998). Jaundice. In Merenstein, G. B. & Gardner, S. L. (Eds.), *Handbook of neonatal intensive care* (4th ed.). St. Louis: Mosby, pp. 393–412.

Gardner, S. L. & Lubcheno, L. O. (1998). The neonate and the environment: Impact on development. In Merenstein, G. B. & Gardner, S. L. (Eds.), *Handbook of neonatal intensive care* (4th ed.). St. Louis: Mosby, pp. 197–242.

Hagedorn, M. I., Gardner, S. L., & Abman, S. H. (1998). Respiratory diseases. In Merenstein, G. B. & Gardner, S. L. (Eds.), *Handbook of neonatal intensive care* (4th ed.). St. Louis: Mosby, pp. 437–499.

Lepley, C. J., Gardner, S. L., & Lubchenco, L. O. (1998). Initial nursery care. In Merenstein, G. B. & Gardner, S. L. (Eds.), *Handbook of neonatal intensive care* (4th ed.). St. Louis: Mosby, pp. 70–99.

McGowan, J. E., Hagerdorn, M. I., & Hay, W. W. (1998). Glucose homeostasis. In Merenstein, G. B. & Gardner, S. L. (Eds.), *Handbook of neonatal intensive care* (4th ed.). St. Louis: Mosby, pp. 259–274.

Merenstein, G. B., Adams, K., & Weisman, L. E. (1998). Infection in the neonate. In Merenstein, G. B. & Gardner, S. L. (Eds.), *Handbook of neonatal intensive care* (4th ed.). St. Louis: Mosby, pp. 413–436.

Moe, P. & Paige, P. L. (1998). In Merenstein, G. B. & Gardner, S. L. (Eds.), *Handbook of neonatal intensive care* (4th ed.). St. Louis: Mosby, pp. 571–603.

Niermeyer, S. & Clarke, S. (1998). Delivery room care. In Merenstein, G. B. & Gardner, S. L. (Eds.), *Handbook of neonatal intensive care* (4th ed.). St. Louis: Mosby pp. 46–69.

Olds, S. B., London, M. L., & Ladewig, P. A. (2000). *Maternal-newborn nursing: A family and community-based approach.* (6th ed.). Upper Saddle River, NJ: Prentice-Hall, Inc., pp. 705–759, 805–903.

Pierce, J. R. & Turner, B. S. (1998). Physiologic monitoring. In Merenstein, G. B. & Gardner, S. L. (Eds.), *Handbook of neonatal intensive care* (4th ed.). St. Louis: Mosby, pp. 116–128.

Pillitteri, A. (1999). *Maternal and child health nursing: Care of the childbearing and childrearing family* (3rd ed.). Philadelphia: Lippincott, pp. 562, 697–742.

Sherwen, L. N., Scoloveno, M. A., & Weingarten, C. T. (1999). *Maternity nursing: Care of the childbearing family* (3rd ed.). Stamford, CT: Appleton & Lange, pp. 962–963, 1019–1062, 1067–1111.

Siegel, R., Gardner, S. L., & Merenstein, G. B. (1998). Families in crisis: Theoretical and practical considerations. In Merenstein, G. B. & Gardner, S. L. (Eds.), *Handbook of neonatal intensive care* (4th ed.). St. Louis: Mosby, pp. 647–672.

Townsend, S. F., Johnson, C. B., & Hay, W. W. (1998). Enteral nutrition. In Merenstein, G. B. & Gardner, S. L. (Eds.), *Handbook of neonatal intensive care* (4th ed.). St. Louis: Mosby, pp. 275–299.

Weiner, S. M. & Finnegan, L. P. (1998). Drug withdrawal in the neonate. In Merenstein, G. B. & Gardner, S. L. (Eds.), *Handbook of neonatal intensive care* (4th ed.). St. Louis: Mosby, pp. 129–145.

## CHAPTER 14

# Issues of Loss and Grief in Maternity Nursing

Pamela Hamre, RN, CNM, MS
Deborah Bartnick, RN, MSN

## CHAPTER OUTLINE

Grieving

Perinatal Situations in which Grief
  is Expected

Phases of Bereavement

Nursing Care during the Grief
  Reaction

## OBJECTIVES

▊ Describe the parent's response to loss of a pregnancy.

▊ Describe the parent's response to infertility.

▊ Discuss parental grieving for the loss of the expected child.

▊ Discuss nursing interventions to foster healthy grieving in parents.

**[ Media Link ]**

Use the CD-ROM enclosed with this text, or log onto the address given to access the free, interactive Companion Website created for this series. The CD-ROM and Companion Website accompanying this book offer additional practice opportunities and information—NCLEX Review, Case Studies, Glossary, In Depth with NCLEX, and more.

**www.prenhall.com/hogan**

## REVIEW AT A GLANCE

**anticipatory grieving** *grieving done prior to and in preparation for the actual death*

**bereavement** *the subjective responses experienced after the death of a loved one*

**fetal anomaly** *abnormality of the fetus, can be genetic or nongenetic causation, may be detected prior to or not until after delivery*

**grief** *the total response to the emotional experience of a fetal loss; experienced by parents, siblings, grandparents, and other close friends and relatives*

**incongruent grieving** *when partners are in different stages of grief, can create additional stress within the family due to*

*perceived lack of support or understanding*

**infertility** *inability to conceive after 12 months of unprotected intercourse*

**intrauterine fetal demise (IUFD)** *fetal death from any cause that occurs in utero prior to the onset of labor*

**maceration** *the changes undergone by a dead fetus as it is retained in utero; characterized by reddening and loss of skin, as well as distortion of features over time*

**mourning** *the behavioral process through which grief eventually becomes resolved; influenced by culture, religion/spiritual practices, and customs; experienced by the parents of the infant*

*who has died as well as siblings, grandparents, other close friends and relatives*

**neonatal death** *death of a live-born fetus from any cause within the first month of life*

**regrieving** *renewed sense of grief that occurs at anniversaries of the fetal loss*

**stillbirth** *birth of a dead infant at greater than 20 weeks gestation*

**sudden infant death syndrome (SIDS)** *infant death without apparent cause after autopsy, death scene investigation, review of symptoms or illnesses the infant had prior to dying and any other pertinent medical history*

## *Pretest*

**1** The client states "Sometimes I feel like I left my baby somewhere, and can't remember where she is. Then I remember that she isn't alive." This is an example of:

(1) Anticipatory grieving.
(2) Disorientation.
(3) Reorganization.
(4) Searching and yearning.

**2** The father of a stillborn infant wants to hold the child. The nurse's best response is to:

(1) Encourage him to discuss this with his wife first.
(2) Dress the infant in a t-shirt and diaper and let him hold the child.
(3) Tell him that it would be better not to hold the child.
(4) Give him the photographs of the child that you took instead.

**3** The nurse determines that teaching about sudden infant death syndrome (SIDS) has been effective when the client states:

(1) "No definite cause of death is found at autopsy."
(2) "The cause is a brain malformation."
(3) "Breast-feeding causes sudden infant death syndrome."
(4) "Genetic disorders are the cause of SIDS."

**4** The nurse recognizes which of the following as somatic complaints during grieving?

(1) Tingling on the back of the neck and hearing a baby's cry.
(2) Heaviness in the chest and fatigue.
(3) Increased taste sensitivity and deep, restful sleep.
(4) Stiffness in the legs and arms.

**5** The client is returning to the clinic for her postpartal exam after having delivered a stillborn girl 6 weeks ago. She asks the nurse "When will I feel normal again?" The nurse's reply is based on knowledge that grief work takes:

(1) 2 to 3 months.
(2) A year or more.
(3) 4 to 6 months.
(4) Not more than 8 months.

**6** Anticipatory grieving may occur in which of the following situations?

(1) Sudden infant death syndrome (SIDS)
(2) Ectopic pregnancy
(3) Placental abruption during labor
(4) Fetal anomaly identified during pregnancy

7 Which of the following are tokens of rememberance that are appropriate to give to grieving parents?

(1) Lock of hair, footprints
(2) Baptism or naming
(3) Visit from chaplain
(4) Sympathy card from staff

8 The family is experiencing a fetal loss. Which of the following statements indicates that the nurse's teaching on the family's involvement in the birthing process has not been effective?

(1) We can have our child baptized.
(2) We can decide not to stay on the postpartal unit after the birth.
(3) We will be able to name our infant.
(4) We will have the child's funeral through the mortuary the hospital uses.

9 The nurse is making assignments for the next shift. The nurse assigns the same nurse to the family experiencing a fetal loss as cared for them yesterday because a positive relationship was established and continuity of care will:

(1) Decrease the need for the family to interact with the rest of the world.
(2) Increase support for the family.
(3) Prevent the family from needing to ask questions.
(4) Facilitate dependence on the nurse.

10 Which of the following would be useful in the diagnosis of an intrauterine fetal death?

(1) Chadwick's sign
(2) Piskacek's sign
(3) Spalding's sign
(4) Homan's sign

*See page 326 for Answers and Rationales.*

## I. Grieving

A. *Grief:* the total response to the emotional experience related to loss; manifested emotionally, somatically, and cognitively; associated with overwhelming distress or sorrow

B. *Bereavement:* the subjective responses experienced by a survivor of loss

C. *Mourning:* the behavioral process through which grief is eventually resolved; influenced by culture, religion, and customs; takes over 1 year

## II. Perinatal Situations in which Grief Is Expected

A. *Infertility*

1. Definition: lack of pregnancy after 12 months of unprotected intercourse

2. Incidence: 6.2 million people in the United States in 1998

3. Etiology: male factors, female factors, genetic factors, or unknown causation

4. When pregnancy has not happened spontaneously and infertility treatment has been sought, couples are experiencing physical, emotional, and financial stress; achieving pregnancy through treatment for infertility brings a sense of optimism to parents as their dream of parenting becomes a possibility; when the pregnancy ends through fetal death, parents must grieve the fetal loss as well as deal with the recent sense of optimism; this complex set of emotional issues is difficult for parents to resolve

B. **First trimester fetal loss**

1. 12 percent of pregnancies end in spontaneous abortion

2. Ectopic pregnancies (those occurring outside of the uterus) occur in 0.6 percent of pregnancies

3. Elective termination of pregnancy can also trigger a grief response and may be combined with guilt

C. *Fetal anomaly*

1. Incidence: 6.3 percent of all births result in fetal abnormality of genetic or nongenetic origin

2. Parents often grieve the loss of their "perfect child" when their baby is born with a congenital anomaly

3. The intensity of grief may be affected by the type and severity of the anomaly

4. Prenatally detected anomalies will allow for **anticipatory grieving,** which begins prior to the actual loss or death

D. *Neonatal death*

1. Definition: death within the first month of life

2. Incidence: 0.3 percent of newborns

3. Etiology: typically related to congenital defects (genetic and nongenetic), sepsis, prematurity, or sudden infant death syndrome

E. *Sudden infant death syndrome (SIDS)*

1. Sudden death of an infant under 1 year of age that remains unexplained after a complete investigation (autopsy, examination of the death scene, and review of the symptoms or illnesses the infant had prior to dying and any other pertinent medical history)

2. 3,000 infants per year die from sudden infant death syndrome

3. Higher incidence in nonwhite races, smokers, illegal drug users, and infants who sleep on their abdomens

D. *Stillbirth* or *intrauterine fetal demise (IUFD)*

1. Fetal demise in utero after 20 weeks gestation

2. Incidence: 33,000 babies are stillborn in the United States each year

3. Etiology: placental abruption and knots or entanglement in the umbilical cord are the common causes (1 percent of all births have knots in cord), however most often the cause of the stillbirth is unknown; fetal death can occur prenatally or during the intrapartal period

4. Most mothers spontaneously begin labor within 2 weeks after intrauterine fetal demise; if spontaneous labor does not ensue, the fetus can be coated in fibrin from the maternal circulation, leading to disseminated intravascular coagulopathy (DIC)

5. The first symptom of fetal death is absence of fetal movement

6. Stillborn infants will have dark red, peeling skin (**maceration**), soft and swollen-looking heads with overriding of the fetal skull bones (Spalding's sign), and a mouth that hangs open; the longer the fetus has been dead, the worse the maceration will become

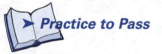

### III. Phases of Bereavement

**A. Responses of survivors of loss proceed through four phases (Table 14-1)**

**B. Shock and numbness**

1. Characterized by a feeling that "this is all a bad dream"; parents may have difficulty making decisions during this time

2. This phase predominates during the first 2 weeks following the loss

**C. Searching and yearning**

1. Parents search for answers and yearn for their infants; parents are preoccupied with thoughts about what happened, guilt about what they may have done or not done that caused the death, and the death itself; mothers may also experience irrational perceptions, such as phantom fetal movement, hearing a baby crying, and a feeling of heaviness in their arms, which may lead them to think they are "losing their minds"; this is a normal response as they psychologically search for their baby

2. This phase begins within a week of the loss and peaks between 2 weeks and 4 months after the loss, and is the longest phase of bereavement

**D. Disorientation**

1. Primary sign or symptom is depression; mourner may take on a sick role to legitimize their depression and avoid criticism; may lose appetite and not perform personal cares

2. This phase occurs during the first week after the loss, and will intensify and subside at intervals for months to years

3. **Regrieving** is a common phenomenon, especially during the anniversary of the child's birth and death, holidays, and any other time that reminds the parents of that child; this typically occurs for years after the loss, and perhaps for the lifetime of the parents; parents never "get over" the loss of a child

**E. Reorganization**

1. During this stage, the numbness wears off and the reality of the loss becomes real; the parents are better able to cope with new challenges, take better care of themselves, and can feel sadness that is not immobilizing

2. Can take 18 months to 2 years to achieve full resolution

**Practice to Pass**

One week after delivering a stillborn infant, the mother tells you that every time the doorbell rings she briefly thinks it is someone from the funeral home with her baby and they're going to tell her they made a mistake and her baby is just fine. What should your priority intervention be?

| Table 14-1 | Phase of Bereavement | Onset & Length | Symptoms |
|---|---|---|---|
| **Phases of Bereavement** | Shock and numbness | First 2 weeks after loss | Disbelief, difficulty making decisions |
| | Searching and yearning | Within 1 week of loss, peaks at 2 to 4 months | Preoccupation with causes of death and feelings of guilt |
| | Disorientation | First week after loss, recurs for months to years | Depression, appetite loss, decreased activities of daily living, regrieving on anniversaries |
| | Reorganization | Up to 18 months to 2 years | Numbness diminishes, loss becomes real, able to cope and take care of themselves |

## IV. Nursing Care during Perinatal Grief

**A. Assessment of factors affecting the grief reaction (see Table 14-2)**

1. Male-female differences

    a. In many cultures, women tend to express more symptoms of grief, such as crying, anger, and guilt, than men

    b. The pregnancy may initially be less real to the father because he does not directly experience the changes of pregnancy; this may affect his reaction to an early pregnancy loss

2. Previous losses

    a. A history of a previous pregnancy loss will affect the way parents react to subsequent losses; once the bereavement phases have been experienced and grief resolved, the grieving is more familiar emotional territory

    b. Parents who have had difficulty conceiving may experience additional grief: failure of the long-desired pregnancy and the optimism for the future it brought, as well as the loss of the child

    c. Other concurrent losses, such as divorce or death of another family member, may contribute to the intensity of grief

    d. Pregnancy loss is often the first death in the family that the parents experienced, so the death rituals and grief work will be unfamiliar

3. Timing of death

    a. When parents know the fetus has died prior to delivery, they will experience anticipatory grieving

    b. In most cases, death is sudden and unexpected

| Table 14-2 | Factor | Grief Reaction |
|---|---|---|
| **Factors Affecting Grief Reaction** | Male-female differences | Men: internalize their grief, want to get back to routine; early pregnancy may not seem real yet |
| | | Women: more expressive, cry more, and want to talk about the loss more; early pregnancy more real because of subjective changes in the body, and more likely to be grieved than in men |
| | Previous losses | Previous pregnancy loss will have an effect |
| | | Treatment for infertility will make grieving more complex |
| | | Concurrent losses (i.e., divorce, death of another family member) intensify the grieving |
| | | Pregnancy loss often the first death the couple has experienced |
| | Timing of death | Anticipatory grief if death is anticipated (i.e. diagnosis of lethal fetal anomaly) |
| | | Most often death sudden and unexpected |
| | Coping style | Couple's ability to evaluate, plan, and adjust to new situations will influence length of grief and progression through bereavement phases |
| | Cultural influences | Determine appropriate mourning behaviors (verbalization, facial expressions, clothing, who is present) |
| | | Religious/spiritual or cultural rituals and ceremonies may be held |
| | | Autopsy and when infant should be buried affected |
| | | Naming may be prohibited |
| | Support systems | Family, friends, religious community, social agencies assist grief work; stable relationship as a couple helpful |

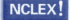

4. Coping styles

a. The parents' ability to evaluate, plan, and adjust to new situations will affect their ability to cope with a loss

b. Positive coping mechanisms should be encouraged

c. Reliance on alcohol or prescription sedatives should be discouraged to facilitate acceptance of the loss as real

5. Cultural influences

a. Verbalization and behavioral demonstrations of grief are determined by cultural norms, ranging from open wailing to stoic quietness; facial expressions and public crying will vary

b. Clothing color and style to be worn by parents and the dead infant may be culturally determined

c. Presence of extended or nuclear family and or friends may be culturally determined

d. Naming of the infant may be culturally determined

e. Religious or spiritual practices may include amulets, medallions, or other symbols placed on or near the infant; rituals and ceremonies may be desired

f. Timing of burial, autopsy, and organ donation may be culturally determined

6. Support systems

a. Intact and available support systems, such as family, friends, and religious, community or social agencies, can assist the parents in their grief work

b. A relationship in which the parents are supportive of each other is helpful

**B. Assessment of signs and symptoms of grief (see Table 14-3)**

1. Somatic (physiologic)

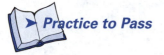

**Practice to Pass**

A Muslim woman has just given birth to a stillborn boy. What information do you need to plan culturally appropriate care for this family? Where can you obtain the information that you need?

| **Table 14-3** Signs and Symptoms of Grief | | | |
|---|---|---|---|
| **Somatic** | Gastrointestinal | Anorexia, weight loss, nausea/vomiting, overeating |
| | Respiratory | Sighing, hyperventilation |
| | Cardiovascular | Palpitations, chest heaviness |
| | Neuromuscular | Vertigo, headaches |
| **Behavioral** | Feelings | Guilt, sadness, anger and hostility, apathy, helplessness |
| | Preoccupation with deceased infant | Daydreams, fantasies, nightmares, arms ache to hold infant |
| | Interpersonal relationships | Withdrawal, decrease in sex drive, incongruent grieving |
| | Crying | Public or private |
| | Activities of daily living | Loss of concentration and poor memory, fatigue and exhaustion, insomnia or increased sleep time, decreased interest in grooming and dressing |
| **Siblings** | Up to age 6 | Death viewed as temporary & reversible, may think their negative thoughts caused the death |
| | Age 6—12 | View death as inevitable and irreversible |
| | Over age 12 | Think of death abstractly |
| **Grandparents** | Similar somatic and behavioral symptoms that parents experience | |

    **a.** Gastrointestinal

       1) Anorexia and weight loss, may persist for several months

       2) Nausea or vomiting, especially in shock and numbness phase

       3) Overeating

    **b.** Respiratory

       1) Hyperventilation, especially early in the grieving and at time of disclosure of the death

       2) Deep sighing respirations

    **c.** Cardiovascular

       1) Cardiac palpitations or "fluttering" in chest

       2) "Heavy" feeling in chest

    **d.** Neuromuscular

       1) Headaches, may persist as grief work continues

       2) Vertigo, especially with thoughts of the deceased and when death is first discovered

**2.** Behavioral (psychologic)

    **a.** Feelings

       1) Guilt over having somehow caused the death

       2) Sadness, can be overwhelming

       3) Anger and hostility toward self, partner, healthcare providers

       4) Apathy and inability to make decisions

       5) Helplessness

    **b.** Preoccupation with the lost infant

       1) Daydreams and fantasies, can manifest as hearing a baby cry

       2) Nightmares, often about forgetting the baby someplace; may be recurrent

       3) "Empty arms" and a longing to hold the baby

    **c.** Interpersonal relationships

       1) Decreased sexual interest, partner may not feel the same

       2) Withdrawal from social activities

       3) **Incongruent grieving:** partners may be in different phases of bereavement, leading to perceptions that the other is either malingering or unfeeling

    **d.** Crying: public and private, can be stimulated by minor occurrence

    **e.** Activities of daily living

       1) Loss of concentration and motivation are common, and may interfere with job performance

2) Fatigue and exhaustion, may or may not be associated with insomnia

3) Sleep changes: insomnia, poor quality sleep, or increased amount of time spent sleeping

4) Loss of interest in grooming and dressing leading to a disheveled appearance

3. Siblings

a. A child's reaction to the death of a sibling depends on the surviving child's developmental level and the response of the parents to the loss

b. The universal fear of childhood is the fear of separation and abandonment, and the child may fear the parents may also die

c. Through 6 years of age, children view death as temporary and reversible; children in this age group may feel guilty that their negative thoughts may have caused the death

d. Children 6 to 12 years of age view death as inevitable and irreversible

e. By 12 years of age, most children can think abstractly like an adult about death

4. Grandparents

a. Grandparents also grieve the loss of their grandchild and may experience many of the same signs and symptoms that the parents do

b. Grandparents also report a feeling of helplessness as they watch their child grieve

C. **Priority nursing diagnoses:** Anxiety; Anticipatory grieving; Dysfunctional grieving; Interrupted family processes; Compromised family coping; Situational low self-esteem; Ineffective coping; Spiritual distress

D. **Planning and implementation with grieving parents:** the nurse can respond in a variety of ways as shown in Table 14-4

1. Non-helpful responses

a. Maintaining the state of denial

1) Not acknowledging the pregnancy or loss

2) Using tranquilizers, sedatives, and other drugs makes the experience "dreamlike" for the mother and may prolong the denial and, therefore, the grieving process

3) Encouraging the parents not to cry or talk about their loss

b. Isolation

1) Not going into the client's room

2) Placing the client on a non-maternity floor against the couple's wishes

c. Prohibiting contact between infant and parents

1) Not encouraging the parents to see and hold their child encourages fantasies about what the child really looks like

2) These fantasies are always more frightening than reality

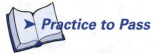

**► Practice to Pass**

The parents of a stillborn infant tell you that they are going to tell their 5-year-old son that his brother "went to sleep and is in heaven now." How should you respond?

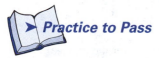

**► Practice to Pass**

A client is 34 weeks gestation and has come to the clinic because she hasn't felt the baby move today. When she arrives, the client says "I'm really afraid there's something wrong with my baby." How should you respond?

| Table 14-4 | What to do | Call the child by name |
|---|---|---|
| | | Cry with the family |
| **Responding to Grieving Parents** | | Attend the funeral or memorial service |
| | | Remember the family on their baby's due date, birthday, and death date anniversaries |
| | Remembrances you can give the family | Photographs |
| | | Lock of hair |
| | | Footprints and handprints |
| | | Baby ID band |
| | | Clothes the baby was photographed in |
| | What you can say | "I'm sorry." |
| | | "This must be hard for you." |
| | | "How are you doing with all of this?" |
| | What NOT to say | "At least it wasn't older." |
| | | "It was God's will." |
| | | "You can have other children." |
| | | "At least you have other children." |
| | | "Time will heal." |

**2.** Helpful responses

   **a.** Environment

   1) Parents should be allowed to choose whether they want to stay on the postpartal unit or another unit away from the nursery

   2) Provide a quiet, private setting to allow the parents to say hello and good-bye to their infant at the same time

   **b.** Supportive relationship

   1) Utilize an empathic manner when working with the family

   2) Provide consistency in nursing staff assignments and support from the nurse

   **c.** Information

   1) Parents should be told the child's prognosis as soon as possible

   2) Information may need to be repeated as parents will be in a state of shock and not hear all that is said the first time

   **d.** Encouraging expression of emotions

   1) Verbalizing thoughts and feelings provides an outlet for the intense feelings associated with grief

   2) Telling and reliving the experience is necessary to gain understanding and mastery over a frightening situation

   **e.** Seeing and touching

   1) Parents should be informed of the appearance of their infant so they can make the decision whether or not to see and touch their child

   2) Many parents are reluctant to see and touch their baby initially, but most of them state they are glad they did

3) Parents should be encouraged to spend as much time as they want with their infant; many parents will want to see their infant more than one time, if given the opportunity; this is the only chance they will ever have to see their child

4) The infant should be dressed like other infants on the unit (usually a diaper and T-shirt) and wrapped in a baby blanket; the nurse should stay in the room or close by for support

**f.** Remembrances

1) The nurse should take pictures of the infant both dressed in baby clothes and without clothes for the parents; the pictures should be offered to the parents; if the parents refuse the pictures, they should be told the pictures will be kept on the unit in case the parents change their mind; pictures help the parents accept their child's death and move forward in the grieving process

2) A lock of hair, one of the baby's identification bracelets, and handprints and footprints can also be obtained and given to the parents

**g.** Open visitation should be encouraged

**h.** Autopsy

1) Knowing why the infant died may help parents resolve the guilt that is common after a child dies

2) Permission to do an autopsy should be obtained after the parents have had a chance to deal with the reality of the death

3) Some religious faiths prohibit autopsy

**i.** Religious or spiritual practices or ceremonies

1) Families may wish to have the baby baptized or participate in other religious or spiritual sacraments, ceremonies, or rituals

2) A visit from the hospital chaplain should be offered to the family, or clergy from the family's religious community should be contacted by hospital staff, if desired by the parents

3) The death of a child is often the first experience that parents have with death; the hospital staff should contact the funeral home of the parents' choice and make beginning arrangements; someone knowledgeable about the options available should discuss them with the parents

**j.** Anticipatory guidance

1) Parents should be contacted periodically to provide support; this is especially important at the anniversary of the due date (with early pregnancy losses) and the birth and death dates

2) Support groups may help parents cope with the death of their child; provide written information on support groups to the family prior to discharge

**E. Evaluation**

**1.** Family members express their feelings about the death of the child

**2.** The family participates in the decision to see, hold, or engage in other ceremonies or rituals regarding their baby

**NCLEX!**

► *Practice to Pass*

A client delivered a stillborn infant 3 hours ago. You bring the infant to her so she can see and touch him. She asks if she can give her baby a bath. How should you respond?

3. The family knows what community resources are available, if they choose to use them

4. The family moves through the grieving process

**Case Study**

A client experienced a complete placental abruption during labor and delivered a stillborn infant following an emergency cesarean section. The client is married and has two other children, ages 10 and 6.

❶ The couple is reluctant to see their infant. How would you explain this infant's appearance to them?

❷ What should be considered when assigning this client to a room after delivery?

❸ The parents state they aren't sure how to explain this to their other children. What should you tell them?

❹ You overhear the client's mother tell her, "I'll bet you'll be feeling better in no time." What should you do?

❺ Two weeks later the client calls and states she feels like she's "going crazy" because she occasionally hears a baby cry, but when she looks for the baby she never finds it. How should you respond?

*For suggested responses, see pages 341–342.*

## Posttest

**1** The partner of a woman experiencing induction of labor for an intrauterine fetal death should be:

(1) Included for support and to facilitate the partner's acceptance of the fetal death as real.
(2) Included to decrease misunderstanding of medical procedures by the mother.
(3) Excluded to prevent the additional emotional strain of the birth on the partner.
(4) Excluded to help understand that another child can be conceived soon and thus forget this death.

**2** Which of the following statements indicates to the nurse that the client is expressing somatic symptoms of the grieving process?

(1) "If our doctor hadn't insisted on doing that extra bloodwork our baby would be alive now."
(2) "I told God I'd never again smoke another cigarette if our baby could just be born alive."
(3) "I feel nauseated and don't want to eat. Please take the tray out of my room."
(4) "My mother can't stop crying. She says she feels like she failed me by letting this happen to me."

**3** The plan of care for the pregnant client who experienced an unexplained intrauterine fetal demise during her last pregnancy should include:

(1) Education on the causes of intrauterine fetal demise given to both parents.
(2) Encouragement to think positively and not dwell on the previous fetal loss.
(3) Support for increased fears as this fetus reaches the gestational age of the previous fetal loss.
(4) Facilitation of grieving of the lost fetus through carrying a photo and a lock of hair at all times.

**4** The client had a stillborn infant at term. She is in the clinic for her postpartal exam. Her husband has accompanied her. The nurse would expect:

(1) Both parents to be expressing their grief in the same way.
(2) Concordant coping mechanisms being exhibited by the parents.
(3) The parents to be in the same grief work stage.
(4) Differences between how each of the parents is grieving.

**5** The mother of a stillborn infant tells the nurse that she feels like she is missing a part of herself. The nurse understands that this is unrelated to:

(1) Parents simultaneously grieving and resolving their attachment to the lost infant.
(2) The unborn child having been incorporated into a mother's physical and emotional being.
(3) A significant loss of self-esteem that often occurs with both parents after perinatal loss.
(4) Mothers of stillborns finding a way to justify their desire to become pregnant again.

**6** The client has an infant with a neural tube defect. Which of the following strategies will facilitate anticipatory grieving during the pregnancy?

(1) Quietly and consistently encourage the family to terminate the pregnancy.
(2) Protect the family from information about what effects the defect will have on their child.
(3) Promote inner-strength and avoiding asking for help from others after the child is born.
(4) Educate the client as to realistic expectations of the medical care the child will receive after birth.

**7** The family has just received the amniocentesis report that their daughter has trisomy 21 (Down syndrome). Which statement is the father most likely to initially make?"

(1) "There has to be some mistake. These are someone else's results."
(2) "If I donate money to the hospital, will you redo the test?"
(3) "Which one of you idiot incompetents mixed up the results?"
(4) "This is difficult, but we'll get through it together.

**8** The client has just given birth to full-term twins. One twin was stillborn. You know that this family will need to:

(1) Simultaneously grieve the loss of one infant while forming an attachment to the other.
(2) Be passive in accepting the death in order to form an attachment to the living infant.
(3) Control their emotions to prevent undue stress for the surviving twin.
(4) Minimize the time spent with the dead infant to facilitate attachment with the survivor.

**9** Bereavement after a fetal demise in utero can be facilitated through:

(1) Protecting the parents from having to see the dead fetus.
(2) Culturally determined naming and burial practices.
(3) Encouraging the client to tell the older children nothing.
(4) Avoiding the financial stress of an autopsy.

**10** The client has given birth to a full-term stillborn male as a result of placental abruption. The grandparents have come to visit. The nurse expects the grandparents to:

(1) Exhibit apathy about the fetal loss.
(2) Experience a more intense grief reaction than the parents.
(3) Avoid talking about the dead fetus.
(4) Go through the same grief phases as the parents.

*See pages 326–327 for Answers and Rationales.*

## Answers and Rationales

### Pretest

**1  Answer: 4** *Rationale:* During the searching and yearning phase of grieving, parents yearn for their deceased infants, are preoccupied with thoughts of the lost infant, and will have physical manifestations such as aching arms, or looking for the infant.
*Cognitive Level:* Application
*Nursing Process:* Assessment; *Test Plan:* PSYC

**2  Answer: 2** *Rationale:* Holding a stillborn helps the family to accept the infant's death as real, and thus facilitate the grieving process.
*Cognitive Level:* Application
*Nursing Process:* Implementation; *Test Plan:* PSYC

**3  Answer: 1** *Rationale:* Autopsy rules out other causes of death, but in cases of SIDS, autopsy findings are normal.
*Cognitive Level:* Application
*Nursing Process:* Evaluation; *Test Plan:* PSYC

**4  Answer: 2** *Rationale:* Somatic complaints during the grieving process include sighing, weight loss, decreased appetite, restless sleep, fatigue, choking, shortness of breath, throat or chest tightness, abdominal pain, weakness in the legs or generalized weakness.
*Cognitive Level:* Application
*Nursing Process:* Assessment; *Test Plan:* PSYC

**5  Answer: 2** *Rationale:* The stages of grief must be worked through in order to resolve a fetal loss. This process takes about a year for most people.
*Cognitive Level:* Application
*Nursing Process:* Assessment; *Test Plan:* PSYC

**6  Answer: 4** *Rationale:* Anticipatory grieving is grieving that starts prior to the actual loss. When a fetal anomaly is identified by ultrasound during the pregnancy, the parents begin to grieve the loss of the perfect child prior to the child's birth.
*Cognitive Level:* Analysis
*Nursing Process:* Assessment; *Test Plan:* PSYC

**7  Answer: 1** *Rationale:* Tokens of remembrance such as a lock of hair, photos, card with infant's footprints or handprints help the parents accept the reality of their infant's death and facilitate the grieving process.
*Cognitive Level:* Application
*Nursing Process:* Planning; *Test Plan:* PSYC

**8  Answer: 4** *Rationale:* Parents have options for nearly all decisions regarding their delivery and post-partal care, including whether or not to use sedatives during labor, naming the infant, rituals or religious rites or sacraments, and which funeral home to plan or hold the funeral or memorial service. The hospital staff can facilitate the mortuary's involvement, but should not recommend one over another or tell the family that the hospital endorses one.
*Cognitive Level:* Application
*Nursing Process:* Evaluation; *Test Plan:* PSYC

**9  Answer: 2** *Rationale:* Continuity of care increases support through trust and familiarity. A new nurse assigned to this family would not know and understand the details of the loss and would have to take extra time in obtaining a history that could otherwise be used to assess for coping with the loss.
*Cognitive Level:* Application
*Nursing Process:* Planning; *Test Plan:* PSYC

**10  Answer: 3** *Rationale:* Spalding's sign is overriding of the fetal cranial bones as seen on ultrasound, which occurs as a result of the decreased tissue turgor that occurs after death.
*Cognitive Level:* Assessment
*Nursing Process:* Assessment; *Test Plan:* PSYC

### Posttest

**1  Answer: 1** *Rationale:* Involvement in the labor and birth process will help facilitate moving out of the denial stage, and help facilitate that this death of their child was real. The partner is often a good source of support for the mother during the pain of labor.
*Cognitive Level:* Application
*Nursing Process:* Planning; *Test Plan:* PSYC

**2  Answer: 3** *Rationale:* Somatic symptoms of grief can be expresed in any physiologic system of the body. Common gastrointestinal symptoms include nausea, vomiting, anorexia, weight loss, or overeating. The other options do not include physiologic symptoms.
*Cognitive Level:* Application
*Nursing Process:* Analysis; *Test Plan:* PSYC

**3  Answer: 3** *Rationale:* Parents report increased stress around the time of the previous fetal loss during subsequent pregnancies. The nurse should ask open-ended questions to determine the parents' stress level and grieving, and provide support as indicated.
*Cognitive Level:* Application
*Nursing Process:* Planning; *Test Plan:* PSYC

**4   Answer: 4** *Rationale:* The parents will often be in different stages of grief, using different coping mechanisms, and expressing their grief differently. Women tend to be more verbal in their grieving, while men tend to be more internalizing with their grief. The nurse's role is to facilitate communication between the parents and let them know that these differences are both normal and expected.
*Cognitive Level:* Application
*Nursing Process:* Assessment; *Test Plan:* PSYC

**5   Answer: 4** *Rationale:* Loss of self-esteem is reported by both parents after fetal loss. During pregnancy, the fetus is incorporated into the pregnant woman's view of self both physically and emotionally, and a fetal loss is often viewed as a loss of a body part similar to an amputation. Parents form an attachment to the unborn child during pregnancy, and must terminate this attachment when the child is stillborn while also grieving the death of their child.
*Cognitive Level:* Application
*Nursing Process:* Assessment; *Test Plan:* PSYC

**6   Answer: 4** *Rationale:* Anticipatory grieving is grief work that takes place prior to the actual loss. In this case, the family will grieve the loss of a perfect child. Providing factual information on what the child will look like and what medical interventions will be necessary, along with support facilitate this grief work.
*Cognitive Level:* Application
*Nursing Process:* Assessment; *Test Plan:* PSYC

**7   Answer: 1** *Rationale:* This is a statement that indicates shock and numbness, the first stage of the grieving process.
*Cognitive Level:* Application
*Nursing Process:* Assessment; *Test Plan:* PSYC

**8   Answer: 1** *Rationale:* The loss of one twin with the survival of the other creates a complex psychological situation. The family must go through the grief work associated with the fetal loss while simultaneously beginning attachment with the surviving infant. These mothers are at higher risk for a pathological grief reaction because of the complexity of the task.
*Cognitive Level:* Application
*Nursing Process:* Planning; *Test Plan:* PSYC

**9   Answer: 2** *Rationale:* Parents need to see and hold their infant to accept the reality of the child's birth and death. Naming the child and having the newborn baptized or participating in other religious ceremonies or rituals also facilitates grief work and acceptance of this loss. Older children must have the death explained to them in developmentally appropriate terms. Autopsy can sometimes provide an answer to the cause of the fetal death, and should be undertaken, if the parents request it or if law requires it.
*Cognitive Level:* Application
*Nursing Process:* Planning; *Test Plan:* PSYC

**10   Answer: 4** *Rationale:* Grandparents grieve the loss of the grandchild as well as feel pain at the suffering of their child in response to the loss.
*Cognitive Level:* Application
*Nursing Process:* Planning; *Test Plan:* PSYC

## References

Armstrong, D. (2001). Exploring fathers' experiences of pregnancy after a prior perinatal loss. *American Journal of Maternal Child Nursing 26*(3): 134–147.

Bryar, S. H. (1997). One day you're pregnant and one day you're not: Pregnancy interruption for fetal anomalies. *Journal of Obstetrics, Gynecological, and Neonatal Nursing 26*(5): 559–566.

Cote-Arsenault, D. & Mahlangu, N. (1999). Impact of perinatal loss on the subsequent pregnancy and self: Women's experiences. *Journal of Obstetrics, Gynecological, and Neonatal Nursing 28*(3): 274–282.

Cote-Arsenault, D. (1999). Pregnancy after loss. *Journal of Obstetrics, Gynecological, and Neonatal Nursing 28*(1): 13–14.

de Montigny, F., Beaudet, L., & Dumas, L. (1999). A baby has died: The impact of perinatal loss on family social networks.

*Journal of Obstetrics, Gynecological, and Neonatal Nursing 28*(2): 151–156.

Detraux, J., Gillot-deVries, F., Eynde Vanden, S., Courtois, A., & Desmet, A. (1998). Psychological impact of the announcement of a fetal abnormality on pregnant women and on professionals. *Annals of the New York Academy of Sciences 847*: 210–219.

Dickason, E., Silverman, B., & Kaplan, J. (1998). *Maternal-infant nursing care* (3rd ed.). St. Louis: Mosby, pp. 716–719.

Hutti, M.H., dePacheco, M., & Smith, M. (1998). A study of miscarriage: Development and validation of the perinatal grief intensity scale. *Journal of Obstetrics, Gynecological, and Neonatal Nursing 27*(5): 547–555.

Kavanaugh, K. (1997). Parents' experience surrounding the death of a newborn whose birth is at the margin of viability. *Journal of Obstetrics, Gynecological, and Neonatal Nursing 26* (1): 43–51.

Kozier, B., Erb, K., Wilkinson, J., & Van Leuven, K. (1998). *Fundamentals of nursing* (Updated 5th ed.). Menlo Park, CA: Addison Wesley Longman, pp. 856–865.

Lowdermilk, D., Perry, S., & Boback, I. (2000). *Maternity and women's health care* (7th ed.). St. Louis: Mosby.

McKinney, E., Ashwill, J., Murray, S., James, S., Gorrie, T., & Droske, S. (2000). *Maternal-child nursing.* Philadelphia: W. B. Saunders, pp. 1224–1225.

NIH Sudden Infant Death Syndrome Fact Sheet, retrieved June 17, 2001. *http://www.nichd.nih.gov/publications/pubs/ sidsfact.htm.*

Olds, S., London, M., & Ladewig, P. (2000). *Maternal newborn nursing* (6th ed.). Upper Saddle River, NJ: Prentice-Hall, Inc., pp. 633–634.

Pilliteri, A. (1999). *Maternal and child health nursing* (3rd ed.). Philadelphia: Lippincott, pp. 691–692.

Radestad, I., Steineck, G., Nordin, C., & Sjogren, B. (1996). Psychological complications after stillbirth—influence of

memories and immediate management: population-based study. *British Medical Journal 312*(7045): 1505–1508.

Robertson, P., & Kavanaugh, K. (1998). Supporting parents during and after a pregnancy subsequent to a perinatal loss. *Journal of Perinatal and Neonatal Nursing 12*(2): 63–60.

Rybarik, F. (1996). Perinatal grieving. *Journal of Obstetrics, Gynecological, and Neonatal Nursing 25*(9): 731.

Sherwen, L., Scoloveno, M., & Weingarten, C. (1999). *Maternity nursing: Care of the childbearing family* (3rd ed.). Stamford, CT: Appleton & Lange, p. 315.

Vance, J. C., Najman, J. M., Thearle, M. J., Embelton, G., Foster, W. J., & Boyle, F. M. (1995). Psychological changes in parents eight months after the loss of an infant from stillbirth, neonatal death, or sudden infant death syndrome—A longitudinal study. *Pediatrics 96*(5): 933–939.

Varney, H. (1997). *Varney's midwifery* (3rd ed.). Sudbury, MA: Jones & Bartlett, p. 632.

Wallerstedt, C., & Higgins, P. (1996). Facilitating perinatal grieving between the mother and the father. *Journal of Obstetrics, Gynecological, and Neonatal Nursing 25*(5): 389–394.

Wolf-Gabor, S. (1997). The individuality of grief. *AWHONN Lifelines 1*(2): 72–71.

# Appendix

➤ *Practice to Pass Suggested Answers*

## Chapter 1

Page 5: *Solution*—This nurse should be terminated as individual and institutional standards of care as well as national standards of care were violated. Through an educational program the nurse would have learned the proper way to administer medications: checking each medication against the physician's order at least three times, giving medications to one client at a time, and then charting the medications that had been administered. The institution's policies and procedure were violated, as within the policy would be a procedure for correct administration of medications. These policies and procedures are developed for the clients' safety and well being and would be reviewed by national organizations that accredit hospitals and other health care institutions. The nurse violated national standards, as reasonable and diligent practice of the registered nurse within all regions would take more care in administering and documenting medications.

Page 14: *Solution*—While the decision to forego surgery may be considered negligent in the eyes of the law and unwise and inappropriate from a medical perspective, it is ethically justifiable. The nurse could refer the issue to the institution's ethics committee or use an ethical decision-making framework (MORAL) to guide discussions between the interested parties, the parents and healthcare professionals.

Page 15: *Solution*—The nurse manager will need to help the nursery nurses identify their own cultural beliefs, personal biases, attitudes, stereotypes, and prejudices. Then the nurses will need to learn about the cultures of the clients. As the nurses become more familiar with the cultural ways of their clients, the nurses can become more sensitive to the clients and hopefully overcome many of the cultural conflicts.

Page 20: *Solution*—The nurse needs to recognize that the client may not be the primary care provider for the infant when they go home, especially if the client will be returning to school. The nurse should include the grandmothers in the teaching, acknowledging their expertise and letting them share it with the client. The nurse could use the opportunity to educate the grandmothers and the client about current childbearing and childrearing practices to promote the health of all family members.

Page 26: *Solution*—Explain to your friend the different levels of care available for expectant mothers and the philosophical differences between physicians and advanced practice nurses. Since this is her first pregnancy and if she is low risk, you might encourage her to see someone who will provide a great deal of education throughout the pregnancy and encourage her and the family to be actively involved in the process.

## Chapter 2

Page 42: *Solution*—The basal body temperature is most accurate when taken upon awakening from the longest stretch of sleep a woman gets in a day *prior* to arising. The client should be instructed to follow her usual sleep-wake routine, and take her temperature every day before she gets out of bed, regardless of what time she awakens.

Page 42: *Solution*—A hysterosalpingogram utilizes an iodine-based dye, which is then instilled into the uterus and fallopian tubes. Shellfish allergy is a risk factor for anaphylactic reaction. The nurse's role is to verbally inform the physician performing the examination of the allergy, and to make certain it is clearly marked on the chart and on the client's allergy wristband.

**329**

Page 43: *Solution*—Lack of sperm in the ejaculate does not always indicate lack of sperm production. Blockage of the vas deferens or epidydimis will prohibit the sperm from being ejaculated. A testicular biopsy will be performed to detect the presence of sperm deeper within the epidydimis. If sperm are found, they can be obtained via needle aspiration, and then fertilization can be facilitated via intrauterine insemination, GIFT, in vitro fertilization, or sperm insertion into the ova. If no sperm are present, the couple will need to use donor sperm artificial insemination to achieve pregnancy.

Page 43: *Solution*—Infertility treatments can create stress for a couple through a number of factors: cost of the treatments, time away from work for appointments, necessity of having intercourse at prescribed times, need for the male to masturbate for semen analysis or sperm samples, anticipatory grieving for the inability to conceive spontaneously, family and social pressures to have children, and medications used to induce ovulation that can create moodiness in women. Marital difficulties may manifest themselves as impotence, lack of interest in sexual intercourse, communication difficulties, and many others. The role of the nurse is to assess the couple's communication with each other, the need for further information regarding infertility treatments, and the need for professional counseling. Many couples find that attending a support group for infertile couples helps a great deal, and the nurse should provide the couple with information on such groups. Most important is to acknowledge that the stress response of both of the individuals and the couple together is normal and expected during the stressful time of infertility treatments.

Page 44: *Solution*—Ovulation induction medications are given on a daily basis beginning around day 5 of the menstrual cycle. Daily ultrasound examinations that require an office visit may be necessary beginning around midcycle to monitor ovarian follicle production and maturation, and for timing of hCG administration to stimulate final maturation. Egg retrieval is performed when several follicles are mature, after which the client must rest for about 2 hours. Embryo reinsertion is performed 42 to 72 hours later; zygotes are reinserted 18 to 24 hours later. In either case, the client should restrict her activities to bed rest for 12 to 24 hours after the procedure is performed. No further clinic visits will be needed for about 14 days, when pregnancy testing or ultrasound examination will be undertaken if menses do not begin.

## Chapter 3

Page 53: *Solution*—A teaching plan for a client with low literacy skills can be effectively modified through the use of less printed instructions and greater use of models and diagrams with reinforcement through verbal instructions. Clients should be given the opportunity to see and handle the method selected for contraception, demonstrating the correct usage, and verbally restating pertinent information to verify understanding.

Page 57: *Solution*—Fertility awareness methods of contraception are based on identification of the fertile period, which surrounds the time of ovulation, and the avoidance of unprotected inter-course during this period to prevent pregnancy. Ovulation usually occurs about 14 days prior to the next menses and physical signs can be used in addition to a menstrual calendar to indicate the release of the ovum. Primary indicators of ovulation include basal body temperature and changes in the cervical mucus. Basal body temperature typically drops just prior to ovulation, then rises and remains elevated until 2 to 3 days prior to the next menses. Cervical mucus becomes thin, clear, watery, slippery, and stretchable at the time of ovulation. Secondary indicators of ovulation include increased libido, abdominal bloating, midcycle abdominal pain or mittleschmerz, breast or pelvic tenderness, a feeling of pelvic or vulvar fullness, slight dilatation of the cervical os, and the softer cervix is located higher in the vagina.

Page 62: *Solution*—Because the diaphragm covers the cervix and remains in place for up to 4 hours prior to intercourse and at least 6 hours following coitus, the risk of infection is a possibility. By teaching the woman to remove the diaphragm at least once in a 24-hour period, the incidence of toxic shock syndrome can be reduced. Use of the diaphragm should also be avoided during the menstrual period or when any abnormal vaginal discharge is present. If the client experiences any warning signs of toxic shock syndrome such as elevation of temperature >100.4°F, diarrhea and vomiting, weakness and faintness, muscle aches, sore throat, or sunburn-type rash, the woman should contact the healthcare provider immediately.

Page 67: *Solution*—The nurse should first determine what type of oral contraceptive pill, progestin-only or combination estrogen-progestin, the woman is taking and which week in the menstrual cycle the woman is in. If the woman is using progestin-only pills, every pill is an active pill. She should take the next pill at the regular time and use a back-up method for the remainder of the cycle. If the woman is using combination pills and is in week 1 or 2 of the cycle, she should take 2 pills a day for 2 days, finish the cycle, and use a back-up method. If she is in the 3rd week of the cycle and uses combination pills, she should take 1 pill a day until Sunday, start a new pack of pills on Sunday, and use a back-up method for 1 week.

Page 71: *Solution*—The nurse should inquire what method of contraception the woman is currently using or has used in the past and with what degree of success in preventing pregnancy. The nurse should explore if the woman is dissatisfied with the method itself, is experiencing side effects, and what the woman's plans are for future childbearing. If the woman desires no further pregnancies, it may be appropriate to discuss permanent sterilization through tubal ligation or vasectomy for the male partner. If pregnancy is desired in the future, alternative methods of contraception should be explored.

## Chapter 4

Page 80: *Solution*—It requires two recessive genes to develop PKU. Therefore, a mother with PKU carries these two genes. Although the father does not have PKU, he may be a carrier having one of the recessive genes. If he is a carrier, the possible combinations of genes are PKU/no PKU, PKU/no PKU, PKU/PKU, and PKU/PKU. There is a 50 percent chance of having a child with PKU and a 50 percent chance that the child will be a carrier. If the father is not a carrier, the possible genetic combinations are all PKU/no PKU. No children will have PKU, but all will be carriers.

Page 81: *Solution*—Humans possess 23 pairs of chromosomes for a total of 46 chromosomes. Each parent contributes 23 chromosomes that are paired during the union of the sperm and ovum. Trisomy 21 is a chromosome condition seen when the 21st chromosome has three chromosomes rather than the usual two. The third chromosome often forms before fertilization even occurs. The ovum may have two chromosomes 21 instead of one because the cells did not separate as expected. When this ovum joins with a sperm, the extra chromosome is included.

Page 81: *Solution*—The nurse educates the client by defining and describing anencephaly in a sensitive manner. The nurse validates client understanding of the seriousness of the condition and expectations for the pregnancy. She reviews the client's options and possible outcomes for each option while being sensitive to the client's social, cultural, and religious beliefs. Questions are asked and answered in a nonjudgmental manner. Decisions regarding the pregnancy belong to the client only. The nurse maintains confidentiality.

Page 83: *Solution*—If the couple is trying to achieve a pregnancy it is important that the clients understand the viability of sperm and ova. An ovum released during ovulation is capable of being fertilized for 24 hours. Sperm survive for 48 to 72 hours in the female genital tract but are most capable of fertilization 24 hours after ejaculation. To achieve fertilization, the couple should have intercourse no earlier than 24 hours prior to ovulation and no later than 24 hours after ovulation.

Page 84: *Solution*—Monozygotic twins are often called identical twins. They are identical in that they have the same genetic code. Since chromosomes determine gender, they will always be the same sex and have similar physical characteristics. Identical twins occur at random when a fertilized ovum separates very early in the pregnancy to form two identical zygotes. They may share placentas and amniotic sacs. Dizygotic twins are not identical and are also called fraternal twins. They occur when the mother releases two ova during ovulation and they are fertilized by two different sperm. They carry different genetic codes so they may be different sexes and physical characteristics. They are related genetically the same way any sibling is related. They usually have separate placentas and amniotic sacs. The tendency to have dizygotic twins does run in families.

Page 94: *Solution*—The ductus arteriosus connects the pulmonary artery to the aorta in the fetus to allow blood to bypass the fetal lung. The lung receives little circulation in the fetus because it is not a unit for gas exchange. If the ductus arteriosus remains patent in the newborn there is a potential for the infant's circulation to continue bypassing the lung. Once out of the uterus the infant depends on the lungs as a unit of gas exchange. If blood bypasses the lungs, this cannot take place.

Page 95: *Solution*—The embryo is a stage of development from 2 to 8 weeks gestation characterized by cell multiplication and specialization. All of the body's tissues and organs are formed during this time although they are immature. The embryo may not have a human external appearance. The fetal stage is from 8 weeks gestation until birth. This is a time of growth and maturation of tissues and organs. The fetus takes on a very human appearance.

## Chapter 5

Page 107: *Solution*—The nurse should begin by assessing what the mother is thinking and feeling. Questions such as, "What are you feeling now that you have seen your baby?" or "You seem upset; how are you feeling about your pregnancy?" might help to clarify the situation. The nurse can affirm the mother's feeling by telling her that most women have ambivalent feelings toward pregnancy, even if the pregnancy is planned. Explaining to the mother that pregnancy is a developmental challenge resulting in stress and anxiety for the woman and her family will help her realize that her response is not abnormal or unusual.

Page 108: *Solution*—The nurse should begin by assessing what the woman knows about prenatal care, as she may be uninformed or have been misinformed by relatives or friends, as well as her reasons for not planning to participate in prenatal care. Then the nurse can take the opportunity to teach her the purposes of prenatal care including assessment of well-being of both mother and baby; screening, prevention or management of any problems that may develop; and opportunities for education related to childbirth, nutrition, management of the discomforts of pregnancy, and parenting. Barriers to prenatal care such as money, transportation, and childcare can be explored with the mother. The nurse may be able to make referrals to help the mother overcome any barriers that are impacting her care.

Page 109: *Solution*—The nurse can share information on what classes are available and the content of these classes. By assessing the mother's goals and expectations for this pregnancy, the nurse may be able to direct the mother or other members of her family to a class that is helpful. New information since her last delivery may be available, or specialized classes, such as those designed for siblings or grandparents, may be useful.

Page 112: *Solution*—According to her menstrual history, the client is about 8 weeks pregnant. This means it is probably too early to heart the fetal heartbeat with a Doppler device or fetoscope or to palpate fetal movement. The only way to positively diagnose pregnancy at this point is to visualize the fetus by ultrasound. This can be done as early as 2 to 3 weeks after conception.

Page 113: *Solution*—The nurse should begin by explaining that when the client lies on her back, the weight of the pregnant uterus presses on major blood vessels and decreases the amount of blood returning to the heart. This compromises oxygen supply to both the mother and the fetus, should be avoided, and probably explains the feeling of faintness. The nurse should suggest that the mother try positioning herself with pillows for back support, between her legs, and or for her upper arm when she sleeps on her side. If the mother must sleep on her back, she could try elevating her upper body or putting a pillow under her right hip.

Page 115: *Solution*—Assuming the client's weight was within normal limits before she became pregnant, the nurse should begin by affirming the woman's concerns about her weight. The client and the nurse should review the client's dietary history and preferences and then work together to develop a plan for lunches and snacks that include increased amounts of fruits and vegetables with decreased fried foods. This might involve bringing lunch and snacks from home or making better food choices at restaurants.

Page 116: *Solution*—The nurse should begin by assessing former and current family roles and expectations. The nurse can help the mother determine what support systems are available and what types of help would best relieve the situation. The nurse can then help the mother develop a plan for getting needed help from her husband, extended family, or other sources.

## Chapter 6

Page 125: *Solution*— "The problem was probably caused by your mother's blood type or Rh status and that these factors are hereditary. Your blood type and Rh will be checked in the laboratory work that is done at the first prenatal visit. If it is determined that you have Rh negative blood or a blood group which places your baby at increased risk for problems, these findings will be explained to you and follow-up assessments will be done."

Page 127: *Solution*—Several of the TORCH infections cause severe problems for the fetus but only minor signs or symptoms in adults and it is possible to have the infection without knowing it. Routine testing of all pregnant women can help to identify women who have had an infection, women with a current infection and no symptoms, or women at risk for an infection because of lack of immunity.

Page 128: *Solution*—The human immunodeficiency virus (HIV) is transmitted through exchange of body fluids including semen, blood, or vaginal secretions and can be passed in this manner from any person to another. Women are the group of people showing the greatest rise in incidence, and transmission is usually through heterosexual contact. Testing of pregnant women is especially important, since the woman may not know she is infected. The virus can cross the placenta and infect the baby or it can be passed to the newborn in breast milk. Early diagnosis of the disease is not only important to the woman, but treatment during pregnancy decreases the incidence of the baby contracted the infection before birth.

Page 130: *Solution*—"Testing your urine at every visit is an important assessment of your health during pregnancy and can tell us if problems are developing. If we found sugar in your urine, it could mean you are developing gestational diabetes. If we found protein in your urine, it could indicate pregnancy induced hyper-

tension. White blood cells or nitrites in the urine can indicate an infection."

Page 133: *Solution*— "This test provides information about how your baby's heart rate reacts when the baby is active and gives an indication of the current well-being of the baby. Typically, when a baby is active, moving, and receiving enough oxygen, the heart rate will speed up. The contractions of labor provide an additional source of stress to the baby. Because this test does not involve uterine contractions, it does not give any information about how well the baby will tolerate labor."

## Chapter 7

Page 148: *Solution*—The narcotic antagonist properties of Stadol will block the effects of the methadone causing narcotic withdrawal symptoms in the addicted client. A better choice for this client would be epidural analgesia.

Page 149: *Solution*—Universal blood and body fluid precautions should be implemented with all clients. The nurse should avoid contact with maternal blood by wearing gloves and using other protective devices as needed. The mother should be instructed to wash her hands after pericare and before caring for her infant. She should be advised to formula-feed her baby to avoid passing the virus through breast milk.

Page 156: *Solution*—The nurse should be supportive without offering false hope. The client should be given accurate information with time allowed for questions and expression of feelings. Communication techniques such as empathy, reflection, and providing information about the grief process are most appropriate after perinatal loss. The loss should not be minimized in any way.

Page 159: *Solution*—The client needs to be evaluated closely for possible placental abruption. She should be placed on a fetal monitor and baseline FHR, variability, and any accelerations or decelerations noted. Uterine activity should be palpated as well as monitored. The client should be instructed to report any abdominal pain or vaginal bleeding. Ultrasound may be used to identify an abruption.

Page 160: *Solution*—The goal of nursing care with a prolapsed cord is to relieve pressure on the cord. The client needs to be immediately placed in the knee-chest position in the bed. The nurse places a sterile gloved hand into the vagina to hold the fetal presenting part off of the cord and calls for help to prepare for a cesarean birth. A multigravida with premature SROM may be at high risk for prolapsed cord because the fetus may not engage until labor starts.

## Chapter 8

Page 171: *Solution*—This is a late deceleration, which is always ominous. Nursing interventions are aimed at increasing oxygenation of the fetus through facilitating utero-placental transport. If the client is in a supine position, she should be repositioned to the left lateral position to improve utero-placental perfusion. If the client is hypotensive, increase the IV fluid rate or start an IV. Oxygen should be administered by mask at 7 to 10 liters per minute. If the contractions are being augmented or induced, decrease uterine stimuli by turning off or decreasing the oxytocin. Findings should be documented, fetal monitoring should be continuously maintained and assessed, and the healthcare provider notified.

Page 172: *Solution*—The intrauterine pressure catheter (IUPC) detects the strength of uterine contractions, measured in mm of Hg just like blood pressure. IUPCs are used when inducing labor or when labor is not progressing as quickly as expected to determine if augmentation of contractions is needed. External contraction monitoring could also be used but it cannot accurately measure contraction strength and may not accurately detect contractions if the fetus is transverse, the client is either very thin or obese, or the woman or fetus frequently change positions.

Page 173: *Solution*—The attitude, or relationship of fetal parts to one another, of the fetus in a frank breech position demonstrates flexion of the hips with extension of the knees The lie is longitudinal with the cephalocaudal axis of the fetus parallel to the cephalocaudal axis of the mother. Presentation refers to the part of fetus entering the pelvis first. In this case, the breech, or buttocks are presenting first. The position, RSA, indicates the fetal sacrum is presenting with the back of the fetus toward the right anterior portion of the maternal pelvis.

Page 178: *Solution*—The nurse should teach the client that episiotomies are sometimes performed in the case of fetal distress or when the healthcare provider suspects that lacerations may occur. Because each birth is unique, it is not possible to predict in advance which clients will need episiotomies or sustain lacerations during delivery. The nurse should reassure the client that the healthcare provider will try to prevent serious lacerations and will perform an episiotomy only if necessary. The client also needs reassurance that should she need an episiotomy or experience a laceration, adequate anesthesia will be provided so that the repair will not be painful.

Page 180: *Solution*—Nonpharmocologic methods of pain relief appropriate for this client include hydrotherapy through soaking in a tub or sitting or standing in the shower; breathing techniques; relaxation techniques which may be facilitated through massage, listening to relaxing music, imagery, or visualization; position changes as dictated by the location of the client's pain or walking; and therapeutic touch or support from the presence of the nurse or other support person. Pharmacologic options appropriate for this stage of labor would include intrathecal narcotics or epidural placement. It is critical to ascertain that informed consent has been obtained before intrathecal or epidural analgesia is performed, so that the client is aware of the potential side effects. It is too early for IV administration of a narcotic agent because labor progress may be slowed.

## Chapter 9

Page 191: *Solution*—It is best to tell the client that forceps may leave a red mark or a bruise on the face that will go away in a few days. Sometimes there is slight swelling and often the baby's head will seem misshapen because it molds or conforms to the shape of the birth canal. Clients who have not been forewarned may be worried about the appearance of their baby right after delivery.

Page 194: *Solution*—As you begin the assessment, visualize the fetus lying in the abdomen. In a breech presentation, the examiner should find a much firmer, rounded fetal pole in the fundus (the fetal head), as opposed to the softer irregular shape of the feet and buttocks. The fetal head floating in the uterine fundus is also ballottable (bounceable or easily moveable between the examiner's hands). During the third and fourth maneuvers (palpating the lower uterine segment and determining engagement of the presenting part), the examiner will note a softer, irregular, and wider fetal pole as opposed to the firm and rounded fetal head. An additional finding to help confirm suspicion of breech presentation is the location of fetal heart tones above the umbilicus (in an upper quadrant).

Page 196: *Solution*—Using lay terminology, tell the client that the fetal monitor indicates that something needs to be done to improve blood supply to the placenta so there will be more oxygen available to the baby. Lying on the side improves blood circulation to the placenta and to the baby, so there is a better oxygen supply. It is better to lie on either side, rather than on the back, but the left side has been shown to be the best position for good circulation to the baby.

Page 204: *Solution*—"If your baby's birth can be delayed about 3 or 4 weeks, it would be best. Even though all the baby's organs are formed, they are still not functioning at a mature level. This is especially true of the lungs. Many babies who are born before 37 weeks have problems with breathing (respiratory distress). Every day that your baby stays inside you helps make sure that he or she is developed enough to do live outside your body without help."

Page 205: *Solution*—As with any precipitate birth, do not leave the patient alone. Send for help. If time allows, obtain a towel or blanket and put on sterile gloves. Feet and/or buttocks may appear at the introitus and can deliver through an incomplete cervix, setting the stage for entrapment of the fetal head. Therefore, allow the delivery to proceed slowly. Observe for cord prolapse. Encourage the woman to pant or blow to decrease the urge to push. If the client is more comfortable on her side, allow her to stay in that position until the fetal abdomen begins to deliver. At that point, reposition the mother and raise the infant's trunk and legs upward to facilitate delivery of the head. The infant's head must be delivered quickly to prevent asphyxia. Applying slight pressure above the symphysis, may help speed delivery of the head. The major risks of vaginal delivery of a breech infant are cord prolapse, head entrapment, and birth injury.

Page 2100: *Solution*—The most common causes of emergency cesarean section are dystocia or difficult labor, which is most often caused by the baby's head being too large for the size of the bony pelvis (cephalopelvic disproportion), fetal distress, and breech presentation. None of these factors can be controlled by the mother, therefore, avoiding an emergency cesarean section may not be possible. The only thing that a woman can do is to maintain her health throughout the prenatal period and to preserve her strength and well-being during labor. The outcome, a healthy baby, is more important than the method of delivery. It is important to learn about cesarean delivery in case your baby needs to be delivered in this way.

## Chapter 10

Page 222: *Solution*—It is not unusual for a client's white blood cell count to rise as high as 30,000/mm$^3$ during the first few days after delivery. However, the nurse should always assess for signs of infection such as fever, increased uterine pain or tenderness, foul-smelling lochia, or frequency, burning, and urgency with urination.

Page 222: *Solution*—It is true that women who are breast-feeding are less likely to ovulate and may have more difficulty conceiving while breast-feeding, but they can still become pregnant again. Although it is used as a birth control method in some Third World countries, breast-feeding is only considered effective if the woman breast-feeds exclusively and nurses throughout the night. It is not generally recommended for women in the United States as a method of birth control because other reliable and safe methods are readily available.

Page 224: *Solution*—The nurse must be careful to avoid contact with blood and body fluids. Because there is a chance of exposure to lochia and other body fluids while assessing the perineum, gloves should be worn during this part of the assessment.

Page 225: *Solution*—The nurse should first assess the front of the perineum with the client on her back and her legs apart. Then the nurse should have the client turn onto her side and stand behind the client to examine the back portion of the perineum and anus. The client should draw the upper leg toward the chest and the nurse should life the upper buttock to improve visualization.

Page 228: *Solution*—Breast-milk production is based on supply and demand. The more the breasts are stimulated, the more milk they will produce. The mother will need to drink additional fluids and will have additional nutritional needs of 200 to 500 kcal per baby. The mother may choose to nurse both babies at the same time to allow herself more rest between feedings or she may feed one baby at a time in sequence. Mothers who breast-feed simultaneously may wish to experiment with positions and often need help getting the babies to latch on or be removed from the breast. Cultural considerations are also important to the care of this client. Warm fluids may be more acceptable than cold to restore balance and food preferences should be respected. Hmong women find expressing or pumping the breasts unac-

ceptable, but combining breast- and bottle-feeding is a common feeding practice.

## Chapter 11

Page 239: *Solution*—In assessing the client, her birth history indicates she is at risk for several complications. She delivered a large-for-gestational age infant that could cause overstretching of the uterus resulting in uterine atony. Lacerations of the genital tract are associated with forceps-assisted births. Macrosomia and operative delivery both increase the likelihood of hematoma, which can result from birth trauma. All three of the identified risk factors increase the likelihood of early postpartum hemorrhage for this client.

Upon physical assessment, the nurse might find a boggy uterus, expelled clots, and visible, bright red bleeding. If a laceration were present, the bleeding would appear as a steady stream or trickle in the presence of a firm uterus. Bleeding from a hematoma is not readily visible as blood is collected in the tissues and can be located anywhere in the genital tract that has been subjected to trauma during birth. The client may complain of extreme pain or pressure, and may be unable to void.

Page 243: *Solution*—Following delivery, subinvolution is the failure of the uterus to return to its normal size. subinvolution of the placental site due to retained placental tissue is the most frequent cause of late postpartum hemorrhage occurring within 1 to 2 weeks after childbirth. Symptoms may include fundal height greater than expected, lochia that fails to progress from rubra to serosa to alba normally, and lochia rubra that persists longer than 2 weeks. Women may also report scant brown lochia or irregular heavy vaginal bleeding. If infection is a cause, there may be leukorrhea, backache, or foul-smelling lochia.

Page 250: *Solution*—Preventing mastitis is easier than treating it. Mothers should be instructed in correct breast-feeding techniques before discharge. The nurse or lactation consultant should assist new mothers with breast-feeding as soon as possible following delivery.

In this case, the client probably has a low-grade fever that is coinciding with her breast milk coming in. the difference between breast fullness and engorgement should be defined. With engorgement, the breasts are hard, painful, and appear taut and shiny. Nursing is difficult for the infant and painful to the mother. To relieve engorgement the client should hand-express some of the milk. A warm, moist cloth can be placed over the breast and the woman can massage her breast to stimulate let down or use a manual pump to express some of the milk. This relieves the pressure, which will allow the infant to latch on to the breast more successfully. The mother should be encouraged to wear a well-fitting and supportive nursing bra 24 hours a day to prevent discomfort from the increased weight of the breast.

The client should be provided instructions on symptoms of mastitis which appear suddenly and include: fever greater than 100.4°F, headache, flu-like symptoms, and a warm, reddened, painful areas of the breast, usually in the upper outer-quadrant accompanied by enlarged and tender axillary lymph nodes. The client should contact her healthcare provider immediately if she suspects mastitis. Ten percent of all cases of mastitis will result in a breast abscess requiring incision and drainage. Mastitis should be treated with a 10-day course of antibiotics and non-steroidal anti-inflammatory drugs (NSAIDs) as needed, increased fluid intake, rest, local applications of heat and cold, and the breasts should be emptied frequently either by nursing or pumping.

Page 253: *Solution*—Thromboembolic disease may occur during the antepartum period, but it is considered more of a postpartum problem. Risk factors include history of thromboembolic disease, varicosities, anemia, obesity, increased maternal age, high parity, and anesthesia or surgery with resultant venous stasis. The client should be assessed for signs of pain, edema, color and temperature changes, and peripheral pulses. With the client's knee flexed, Homan's sign should be assessed by dorsiflexing the client's foot. Pain in the foot or leg is a positive Homan's sign and may be indicative of a thromboembolic condition. Absence or differences in peripheral pulses should also be noted and may be indicative of altered circulation. The client should be instructed not to massage her leg or get out of bed until the nurse discusses the client's condition with her healthcare provider.

Page 255: *Solution*—Adjustment reaction with depressed mood (baby blues) is accompanied by feeling overwhelmed, unable to cope, fatigued, anxious, irritable and oversensitive. Episodic tearfulness without an identifiable reason is a key feature. Symptoms of postpartum psychosis include agitation, hyperactivity, insomnia, labile mood, confusion, irrationality, difficulty remembering or concentrating, poor judgment, delusions, and hallucinations. Postpartum major mood disorder, or postpartum depression, is characterized by sadness, frequent crying, insomnia, appetite change, difficulty concentrating and making decisions, feelings of worthlessness, obsessive thoughts of inadequacy as a person and parent, lack of interest in usual activities, and lack of concern about personal appearance. Persistent anxiety contributes to the woman's feeling out of control, and irritability and hostility toward others, including the newborn, may be evident.

## Chapter 12

Page 267: *Solution*— "Those small white spots are called milia. They are plugged sebaceous or sweat glands and are normal in newborns. They will disappear without treatment in a few weeks."

Page 268: *Solution*—Posture: breech deliveries and a dislocated hip may affect the ability to perform the leg and hip maneuvers required for the gestational age assessment. A fractured clavicle will not allow the arm and shoulder maneuvers. Sole creases: assessment must be performed within the first few hours after birth. After 2 hours, the edema of tissues present in most new-

borns begins to resolve and creases appear; these creases do not have the same predictive value as those assessed before resolution of newborn edema. Breast bud tissue: there may be accelerated development in a large-for-gestational age newborn and there may be less tissue development in a small-for-gestational age newborn.

Page 269: *Solution*—Newborns usually assume a flexed position as it allows less body surface to be exposed to the environment, thereby preserving body heat. The infant has also been in a flexed position while in the uterus and prefers to maintain a position that is familiar and comfortable.

Page 272: *Solution*—When mothers choose not to bottle-feed, the American Academy of Pediatrics recommends the infant be given only formula for the first 6 months and then formula plus the addition of solid food for the remainder of the first year of life to reduce the possibility of the infant developing allergies. Cow's milk is more difficult for the newborn to digest because the protein molecules are much larger, resulting in vomiting or diarrhea.

Page 274: *Solution*—The mother can listen for audible swallowing by the 3rd or 4th day, check the infant for one wet diaper the 1st day, two wet diapers the 2nd day, and so on until the infant is having seven or more wet diapers per 24-hour period. As the breast milk supply increases, so will the amount of wet diapers. Mother can inspect the infant's mouth after a feeding to look for signs of colostrum (a white-yellowish thick substance). If the newborn is quiet for 1 1/2 hours after a feeding, this can indicate satiation. The mother can try to express colostrum or milk from her breast to validate lactation and provide reassurance that nutrition is available for her infant.

## Chapter 13

Page 285: *Solution*—The initial response should always be to look at the infant first, because occasionally the monitor is not accurately measuring the saturation. If the infant is pink and active, assess the probe site and possibly reposition it. However, if the infant is not pink begin the steps of resuscitation: airway, breathing, and compressions. Remember to treat the client, not the machine.

Page 295: *Solution*—If meconium is present in the amniotic fluid, the infant is at risk for meconium aspiration syndrome (MAS). The infant's airway should be thoroughly suctioned prior to delivery of the shoulders. The infant should be placed under a radiant warmer and the vocal cords visualized with a laryngoscope. If there is meconium present it should be suctioned out. When the cords are clear of meconium, respiratory effort can be stimulated and resuscitation can proceed if necessary.

Page 301: *Solution*—HIV has been isolated in the breastmilk of mothers who are HIV-positive. The risk of transmission to the newborn is not clear. Mothers in the US have access to nutritious formula supplements, which are not readily available in many underdeveloped countries. For this reason, the Center for Disease

Control (CDC) has recommended that HIV-positive women in the US should not breast feed. In underdeveloped countries, the risk of severe malnutrition and death is significant for infants who are not breastfed. It is felt that even though there is a risk the infant will contract HIV from the breast milk of an HIV-positive woman, the risk of severe malnutrition is even greater. Therefore, HIV-positive women in these countries are encouraged to breast feed.

Page 302: *Solution*—This means that if this infant were in an open crib, he most likely would be experiencing hypothermia. Hypothermia is a common sign of early sepsis and should be evaluated closely.

Page 307: *Solution*—Clients with chronic diabetes are at risk for vascular disease. This can include the blood vessels of the uterus, which would decrease the blood flow to the placenta during pregnancy, resulting in decreased growth in the fetus and an infant who is small for gestational age (SGA).

## Chapter 14

Page 317: *Solution*—Reassure the mother that what she is experiencing is normal and indicates of the searching and yearning phase of bereavement. Although disturbing, this will pass as the client moves toward reorganization.

Page 319: *Solution*—You need to explore Muslim requirements and customs regarding infant death. If the client speaks English,

gently ask her or a family member if there are specific timelines to be adhered to regarding burial, if autopsy is desired, and what you need to do when you care for the infant. If the client does not speak English, obtain the services of a trained medical interpreter. Consulting a sourcebook on nursing care in other cultures can also be helpful, but the nurse must avoid assuming what is presented is true for all families. Clarify the accuracy of the information with this specific family before intervening to assure cultural competence.

Page 321: *Solution*—Children under 6 do not understand the abstract nature of death yet. Additionally, they may believe that negative feelings they had about the new baby caused the fetal death. Comparing death to sleeping can be confusing to young children, and should be avoided so that the child does not fear going to sleep himself because he might also die.

Page 321: *Solution*—Respond therapeutically, asking "Tell me what you think might be wrong." Then either obtain a doppler and listen for fetal heart tones or ask the healthcare provider to listen for fetal heart tones. If listening is inadequate to verify fetal heart tones, an ultrasound may be used to document the heart beat and fetal movement.

Page 323: *Solution*—Allow the parents of a stillborn to perform whatever cares they desire, including bathing, dressing, applying lotion, combing the hair, etc. Provide for privacy for the clients while they bathe their infant, and encourage the parents to explore the fingers, toes and body just as parents of a liveborn child will do.

## ➤ Case Study Suggested Answers

### Chapter 1

1. Because the child was not conceived with the hope that the stem cells would genetically match their son, there are not as many ethical issues as there would be with a planned conception. An ethical framework could be used to identify the ethical concerns and address the issues.

2. Hindus consider organ donation and the giving of blood and blood products acceptable practices, therefore, harvesting stem cells to donate to another would also be an acceptable practice. The specific views and values of the family involved need to be explored to validate the acceptability of this practice.

3. Sons are very significant to Asian Indians. The son is the one to inherit, to provide for the parents in their old age, and to participate in the ritual of death and mourning that guarantees the passage of the parent into Heaven. The birth of a son, especially as a first born, significantly improves his mother's status within the family.

4. In many cultures, the extended family plays a significant role during the postpartal period. A grandmother will gener-

ally come for an extended stay to help with the running of the household.

5. The nurse should realize that the issue of stem cell harvesting and birth of a daughter could have significant cultural meaning. As the client is being admitted, the nurse should explore the couple's cultural beliefs, sharing them with other staff, and supporting the couple's plans. This might also be an opportunity for the nurse to develop cultural awareness about Asian Indian Hindu families.

### Chapter 2

1. You will obtain a full medical and surgical history. Has she ever had any surgery (especially abdominal or pelvic surgery)? Does she have any medical problems? Has she ever had to be hospitalized, and if so, why? Has she had pelvic infections such as PID or sexually transmitted infections such as gonorrhea or chlamydia? Has she had recent weight loss or gain? What medications, vitamins, and herbs does she take? Does she have any allergies? When did her menses begin, and what is her cycle frequency, length, and flow? What contraceptive methods has she used, when did

she use them, and has she had any problems with the methods?

2. You will obtain a full medical and surgical history. Has he ever had any surgery? Does he have any medical problems? Has he ever had to be hospitalized, and if so, why? Has he had sexually transmitted infections such as gonorrhea or chlamydia? Has he had recent weight loss or gain? What medications, vitamins, and herbs does he take? Does he have any allergies? In addition, you will need to ask if he has ever had trauma to his scrotum and/or genitals, whether he had mumps, and if so, when?

3. You should describe the need to detect abnormalities in either of the couple, which may require discussion about their sexual practices, physical examination, blood testing, semen analysis, hysterosalpingogram, and post-coital examination.

4. How often is the couple having intercourse, and when in the menstrual cycle? What positions do they use? Does the husband have any difficulty with either premature ejaculation or impotence?

5. Women after the age of about 35 tend to ovulate less regularly, and are more likely to have anovulatory menstrual cycles. Therefore, she is more likely to be prescribed ovulation induction medications. For unknown reasons, IVF is less successful in women after their mid-30s. However, by no means does her age indicate that the couple will not be able to become pregnant.

## Chapter 3

1. While oral contraceptives are a safe and effective method, they are not indicated for every woman. A woman with a history of thromboembolic or cardiovascular disorders, breast cancer, or estrogen-dependent neoplasms should not use combination pills. Combination oral contraceptives are also contraindicated for women who are currently pregnant, lactating of less than 6 weeks duration, smoking more than 20 cigarettes per day, are over 35 years old, have focal headaches with neurological symptoms, have had recent leg surgery or prolonged immobility, have hypertension greater than 160/100, or diabetes mellitus of more than 20 years duration with vascular disease.

2. The advantages of birth control pills include menstrual periods which are more regular and predictable, a decrease in menstrual flow and premenstrual symptoms, and provide a safe, effective contraceptive method which can be used until menopause for women who do not smoke.

3. Disadvantages include no protection against sexually transmitted infections, the need to remember to take a pill each day at the same time, decreased effectiveness of the birth control pill when taken with some other drugs which are anticonvulsants, antifungals, or antibiotics, and decreased effectiveness of insulin or oral anticoagulants when taken with oral contraceptives. If progestin-only pills are used, they are more likely to cause irregular bleeding or amenorrhea, and if the client conceives, the risk of ectopic pregnancy is increased.

4. Most clients are advised to begin the cycle of pills on the Sunday following the first day of the menstrual period and take one pill at the same time each day. A back-up method of contraception is usually advised for the first cycle of pills until the contraceptive effect of the oral contraceptives is established. If pills are missed, the client is advised to contact the health care provider for specific instructions based on the type of oral contraceptive provided, the number of pills missed, and the time in the cycle. Clients should always be advised that a mechanical method of contraception should be used to provide protection against sexually transmitted infections.

5. The client should be taught the acronym ACHES to represent the warning signs related to the use of oral contraceptives. These include: abdominal pain; chest pain, cough and/or shortness of breath; headaches, dizziness, weakness of numbness; eye problems, such as blurring or change in vision, and problems with speech; and severe leg, calf, and/or thigh pain. If any of these signs develop, the client should be instructed to contact the healthcare provider immediately.

## Chapter 4

1. The pre-embryonic period spans 2 weeks, the time from fertilization until the zygote is embedded in the uterus. There are three significant events of the pre-embryonic period, cellular multiplication, travel through the fallopian tube into the uterus, and implantation. The fertilized ovum, or zygote, divides rapidly in a process called cleavage. It takes on a mulberry-like shape and is called a morula. The morula has a solid inner mass called the blastocyst and an outer layer that will become the placental tissue. It takes 3 to 4 days for the blastocyst to make its journey from the fallopian tube to the uterus. It floats in the uterus for another 4 to 5 days. The uterus prepares for pregnancy with each monthly menstrual cycle. The uterine lining after ovulation is thick and vascular. Uterine glands secrete nourishment used by the blastocyst before it implants. The blastocyst burrows into this rich lining, now called decidua, 7 to 9 days after fertilization. The outer layer of the blastocyst develops finger-like projections that imbed in the decidua. These projections are called villi that later become the placenta. Once implanted, the blastocyst begins the process of differentiation by developing three layers of tissue from which all body tissue is derived. All of these events occur in the first 2 weeks after fertilization, a time prior to when most women have not even had a missed period or realize they are pregnant. If the pregnancy is lost during this time, the woman most likely will not realize she is even pregnant.

2. Weeks 2 through 8 are called the embryonic stage. During this time, cells are changing to become the various organ systems that make up the human. This process is called organogenesis. Because organogenesis occurs very rapidly, the embryo is extremely vulnerable to anything that interferes with this process. Should that occur, a birth defect or

miscarriage may result. Such interferences are called teratogens. They include chemicals, radiation, and micro-organisms. Since organogenesis begins before most women realize they are pregnant, it is important that women avoid potential teratogens if they are attempting to become pregnant.

3. While many congenital anomalies are genetic, others may be caused by teratogens in the first 8 weeks of pregnancy, or, as in many cases, there may be no identifiable cause. As childbearing age increases, the risk of having a child with a chromosome anomaly such as Down syndrome increases. Genetic testing procedures and genetic counseling are available for parents concerned about genetic disease. The nurse informs the class how to receive a referral if desired.

4. The fetus has the potential to survive outside of the womb after 23 weeks gestation provided the infant receives intensive care. At this time the lung's small air sacs, called alveoli, are beginning to form. This is also the time when the capillaries are close enough to the lung to allow oxygen exchange. While survival is a possibility it is still unlikely since every body system is immature.

5. First trimester: All body organs are formed but immature. The fetus has a human appearance. The heart is beating and the fetus is moving. Facial features are present although the eyelids are fused. Genitalia are identifiable. Length is 3.2 inches and weight is 1.6 ounces.

   Second trimester: The fetus has the potential for life outside of the womb with intensive care. Its length is 11.2 inches and weight is 1 pound, 10 ounces. The fetus has hair on its head, eyelashes, and eyebrows. It is covered with downy hair called lanugo and a cheesy protective coating called vernix caseosa. Fetal movement is clearly felt by the mother. The skin is red and wrinkled with little fat deposit. Testes are not descended. The eyelids are closed but will open shortly.

   Third trimester: After 38 weeks the fetus is considered term. The length is 18 to 21 inches. The weight is 6 pounds, 10 ounces to 7 pounds, 15 ounces. The fetus has the appearance of a newborn consistent with race. Lanugo and vernix caseosa are mostly gone. Fat deposits give the body a plump appearance. Fingernails and toenails are present.

## Chapter 5

1. The nurse should assess for factors possibly affecting the GI system such as the client's dietary intake, especially with regard to fruit and vegetables, fiber and spicy foods; use of stool softeners, laxatives, or antacids; and timing of food intake. Factors affecting lower-extremity swelling such as rest and activity patterns should be assessed.

2. With regard to GI function, the nurse should inspect the anus for the presence of hemorrhoids. Lower extremities should be assessed for varicose veins. The client should also be assessed for signs and symptoms of pregnancy-induced hypertension such as elevated blood pressure, protein in the urine, and swelling other than in the lower extremities.

3. Nursing diagnoses could include Mild anxiety, Body image disturbance, Constipation, Risk for aspiration, or Altered comfort.

4. The nurse should assure the client that all of these symptoms, while not life-threatening, can affect her function and comfort, are commonly associated with pregnancy, and can be treated. To manage heartburn, the client could avoid lying down after eating, avoid fatty or fried foods, eat smaller and more frequent meals, and take a low-sodium antacid, if needed. To minimize constipation and the development of hemorrhoids, the woman could increase her fluid intake to at least 2000 mL per day; increase her intake of fruits, vegetables, and fiber; participate in daily exercise; allow sufficient time for bowel function; and use stool softeners, if needed. To decrease or prevent ankle edema, the client could avoid prolonged standing or sitting, dorsiflex the feet frequently, avoid tight bands or garters around the legs, and elevate the feet and legs during frequent rest periods.

5. The nurse should encourage the client to call the healthcare provider's office if these symptoms are not relieved by the measures suggested. When the woman returns for her next prenatal visit, these problems should be assessed and, if needed, further management should be considered.

## Chapter 6

1. Because the mother's age is greater than 35 years, her fetus is at increased risk for Down syndrome (trisomy 21).

2. This client should be offered an amniocentesis or chorionic villus sampling for genetic testing that would indicate chromosomal problems such as Down syndrome.

3. Chorionic villus sampling can be done earlier in gestation. This provides information more quickly, decreases the amount of time the client has to wait or worry about the results and provides for earlier and safer options for pregnancy termination, if the client so desires.

4. Having chromosomal information can decrease worry concerning the condition of the fetus and result in a less stressful pregnancy. If there is a problem, being aware of it may affect decisions regarding delivery site, health care providers needed for mother or baby, and postpartal plans. It also provides a period of adjustment for the family prior to delivery.

5. Potential maternal complications from amniocentesis include hemorrhage, infection, preterm labor, abruptio placentae, inadvertent damage to the intestines and/or bladder, and amniotic fluid leakage or embolism. Potential fetal complications include death, hemorrhage, infection, and direct injury from the needle. Complications occur in less than 1% of cases. Potential maternal complications from chorionic villus sampling include vaginal spotting or bleeding, miscarriage, rupture of membranes and chorioamnionitis. Limb anomalies of the fetus have been reported when the procedure is done before 10 weeks gestation but this complication is very rare.

## Chapter 7

1. Other assessments for the severe preeclamptic client include: temperature every 4 hours unless membranes are ruptured; hourly blood pressure, pulse and respirations, deep tendon reflexes (DTRs) with clonus assessment, assessment of edema, intake and urine output with assessment for proteinuria, and assessment of the presence of headaches, visual changes or epigastric pain. The fetus needs to be continuously monitored.

2. The severe preeclamptic client is at risk for seizures (eclampsia), pulmonary edema, abruption of the placenta, HELLP syndrome, DIC, hepatic hematoma with possible rupture, cerebral vascular accident (CVA), and possible acute renal tubular necrosis.

3. The client with severe preeclampsia should be given IV magnesium sulfate to decrease the likelihood of seizures, and possibly antihypertensive medications. Since this client is at 42 weeks gestation, she will probably also have oxytocin (Pitocin) to induce labor since delivery is the only cure for PIH.

4. This fetus is at risk for intrauterine growth retardation (IUGR) resulting in an small-for-gestational age (SGA) infant, and chronic hypoxia because of the underlying vasospasm creating damage to the placental vasculature. The infant is also almost postterm (greater than 42 weeks) and may have meconium stained amniotic fluid. This fetus may not have the reserves and placental resources needed to tolerate labor.

5. The client and her family should be given honest, simple explanations about the condition, the plan of care, and all interventions. Family may be asked to limit visitors and noise to decrease central nervous system irritability.

## Chapter 8

1. During the active phase of the first stage of labor and with intact membranes, the maternal temperature is assessed every 4 hours unless it is elevated >99.6°F. Blood pressure, pulse, and respirations are assessed every hour, if normal. Fetal status is being continuously monitored electronically. The nurse should review the monitor tracing and document her findings in the client's record every 30 minutes if the client is low-risk or every 15 minutes if the client is high-risk or non-reassuring findings are determined.

2. With a posterior position the hard occiput of the fetus is against the maternal sacrum, which causes pressure and pain in the low back. Additionally, the woman may feel discomfort in the region of the symphysis pubis from the cervical dilatation that is occurring.

3. Nonpharmacologic methods to promote comfort for a woman in active labor with intact membranes and a posterior position include: positioning the client in anything except a supine or semi-Fowler's position to keep the weight of the fetus off her low back. Walking, hydrotherapy, music, relaxation, visualization, and breathing techniques may be helpful. Reassurance and support may also increase com-

fort. Pharmacologic options that could be offered include IV narcotics, intrathecal narcotics, and epidural block. The client's desires, beliefs, and cultural preferences should be assessed when planning for increased comfort during labor.

4. The contractions can be expected to become stronger and last longer. In transition, contractions may also become more frequent. As delivery becomes more imminent, anxiety, irritability, and restlessness may increase and the woman may experience a normal but intense sensation of pressure with contractions. The client may find it more difficult to understand directions; experience hiccuping, belching, nausea, or vomiting; perspire more; or experience rectal pressure or the uncontrollable urge to bear down. During the second stage, the woman may feel relief and a regained sense of control when she can push in response to the urge to bear down with contractions. As the fetus descends and the perineum distends, the client may feel pain and a burning sensation. Following delivery, nausea and vomiting usually cease, the woman may be hungry or thirsty, and may experience a shaking chill associated with the end of the physical exertion of labor. The client should be reassured that she will not be left alone and that the nurse will be available to provide comfort and support in coping with the stress of labor.

5. Some healthcare providers advocate electronic monitoring only for pregnant women at high risk for complications. Others recommend continuous monitoring for all women in labor as a means to provide a constant and objective assessment of the fetal response to the stress of contractions. Even though the client's pregnancy has been uneventful, there is no guarantee that labor and delivery will also proceed normally. Constant surveillance can detect changes in fetal well-being earlier so interventions can be implemented more effectively.

## Chapter 9

1. Assess the contraction frequency, duration, and intensity, and compare this to previous contractions. A common cause of nonprogressive labor is hypotonic uterine dysfunction or poor contraction quality. In addition, assess fetal and maternal response to contractions to detect distress in the fetus and tension and anxiety in the mother. Maternal psyche can also impact labor progress.

2. The small triangular fontanel is the posterior fontanel. This means that the presentation is occiput and the position (toward mother's back and right side) is right occiput posterior (ROP).

3. Explain to the husband that there are several possible causes of prolonged labor. The most common reasons are decreased contraction quality, shape of the mother's pelvic bones, and the way the baby is positioned. You might say, "Your baby seems to be in a 'facing-upward' position that is more difficult to deliver than the usual 'facing-downward' position. This is called a posterior position. It may take your

wife a little longer to deliver, but there doesn't seem to be any signs of a health problem for the baby right now."

4. Reassuring the client and repositioning her on her left side (opposite the fetal back) may help with rotation of the fetal head from ROP to an occiput anterior (OA) position. Continue to assess contractions and maternal response to contractions. Encourage relaxation. Laboring in a position on hands and knees for several contractions, pelvic rocking, and assuming a tailor sitting position have been reported to be helpful for rotation and descent of the fetus.

5. Yes, the physician should be notified. Although there are no signs of fetal distress, the physician needs to know about the client's lack of progress, contraction status, and fetal position. Augmentation of labor with oxytocin (Pitocin) may be ordered to correct hypotonic uterine dysfunction. Continuous assessment of contractions, fetal heart rate, maternal response, and labor progress is warranted.

## Chapter 10

1. Other important information to gather about this client would include: gravida, para, length of labor and type of delivery, how long membranes were ruptured before delivery, blood type and Rh, baseline vital signs, findings from last postpartal physical assessment, time of the last voiding, medications received during labor and delivery, and if she has received analgesia since birth.

2. If her vital signs are normal and stable, the client should first be assisted to sit on the side of the bed and then gradually adjust to a standing position. The nurse assists the woman to ambulate slowly to the bathroom making sure the woman has feeling and control of her legs prior to ambulation. It is normal for new mothers to experience a trickle of lochia the first time they stand after delivery, caused by pooling in the uterus and vagina, and the nurse should anticipate and teach the woman about this. If the client becomes weak or dizzy, she should be encouraged to sit down immediately. The nurse should stay with the client until she returns to bed.

3. Postpartum women may have difficulty voiding the first time after delivery. The sensation of a full bladder or the urge to void may be decreased and the woman may feel uncomfortable with another person present. The nurse should reassure the woman this is normal and that the nurse's presence is to protect the woman's safety, not to invade her privacy. The nurse should first try interventions to encourage voiding such as running water in the bathroom, putting the woman's hands in warm water, or pouring warm water over the perineum. The client could try again to urinate after a short time. If the client's bladder is distended, the uterus displaced, or 6 hours have elapsed since delivery, the client will be need to be catheterized.

4. Clients may experience a mild elevation in body temperature shortly after delivery related to dehydration. Bradycardia after delivery is common to 50 to 70 beats per minute and the blood pressure is within normal range. The nurse

should continue to monitor the vital signs and encourage oral fluids, unless contraindicated. The nurse may suspect the fever is related to dehydration, however, the client should also be assessed for signs of infection. If signs of infection are identified or the temperature reaches 101°F, the physician should be notified.

5. New parents typically want to see and hold their new baby immediately after delivery. Mothers often speak in quiet, high-pitched tones and call the baby by name. Eye contact is usually established with the en face position. Touch is typically progressive beginning with fingertip exploration of the extremities, then palmar contact with larger body areas, and finally the newborn is enfolded with the whole hand and arm and held closely cradled to the mother's body. The mother may identify characteristics of family members present in the infant. The mother should respond to newborn cues, attempt to meet the infant's needs and show general concern for the baby's well-being.

## Chapter 11

1. The client's risk factors for a postpartal infection, especially an infection of the abdominal wound or lining of the uterus, include the following:
   * Cesarean delivery places her at risk because it is an invasive procedure.
   * Prolonged rupture of membranes allows organisms from the non-sterile vagina to reach the uterus.
   * An unsuccessful course of labor predisposes the client to infection because of fatigue, possible use of internal monitoring, and increased likelihood of vaginal examinations to determine progress, or lack of progress, in labor.

2. Ongoing nursing assessments necessary to identify an infection include the following:
   * Monitoring vital signs every 4 hours, especially temperature.
   * Wound assessment using REEDA to determine redness, edema, ecchymosis, discharge and approximation of skin edges.
   * Monitoring laboratory results, especially WBCs, Hgb, and Hct.
   * Assessment of lochia: observing for amount, color, and odor.
   * Assessment of malaise, lethargy, chills: subtle signs of infection.

3. The definition of puerperal infection is a fever of greater than 100.4°F that occurs on 2 out of 10 days after the first 24 hours following childbirth.

4. The first step is to identify the location of the infection and the organism causing the infection so that appropriate antibiotic therapy can be initiated. This information is usually obtained through cultures of any wound drainage, lochia or urine prior to the administration of antibiotics.

5. Pertinent nursing diagnoses could include:
   * Risk for injury related to further spread of infection

- Pain related to the presence of infection
- Knowledge deficit related to lack of information about condition and its treatment
- Risk for altered parenting related to delayed parent-infant attachment secondary to woman's malaise and other symptoms of infection
- Ineffective breast-feeding related to delayed interaction with infant secondary to symptoms of infection

## Chapter 12

1. The first assessment reveals that the client's blood pressure was elevated one hour after delivery. This may indicate the mother is experiencing pain and negatively impacts her desire to hold or feed her infant at this time.

2. Asking her an open-ended question about how she is feeling may reveal that she is experiencing pain or that she is disappointed or fatigued after her cesarean delivery. You explain to the mother that her comfort and readiness are essential to breast-feeding success. You reassure the mother that she can begin breast-feeding at a later time. You tell her that you will take Andrew to the nursery now but will bring him back to her when she is rested, more comfortable and you will be available to assist her when she is ready to initiate breast-feeding.

3. You should take the baby to the mother when she requests him. If she does not request the baby, the nurse should offer to do so at frequent intervals and provide information about his status while mother and baby are separated.

4. Begin with simple instructions and offer to stay with the mother and baby to provide assistance. Your initial focus should be a position of comfort to hold the infant and initiate breast-feeding if the mother is ready. Suggest the side-lying position which may be the most comfortable for a cesarean-delivered mother with an abdominal incision. Place the infant so that the mother can use the hand that does not have an intravenous infusion. Use pillows to position and support mother's body in good alignment and use a rolled-up baby blanket to keep the infant directly facing his mother, not rolling partially onto his back.

5. The priorities for promoting a positive breast-feeding experience for this mother and baby are flexibility, continued patient education, follow-up by telephone or a home visit and referral to a lactation consultant or public health nurse, if indicated.

## Chapter 13

1. Client history would include any pertinent prenatal or labor/delivery history (i.e., maternal diabetes, infectious diseases, prolonged rupture of membranes, fetal distress, etc.), Apgar scores, and birth weight. Current information would include respiratory status, oxygen therapy, oxygen saturation reading and any other unexpected findings.

2. The initial priority of care for this infant is to establish and maintain an airway. Another high priority need for this infant is thermoregulation. Fluid balance, risk of infection, nutrition and bonding are additional nursing problems appropriate for this patient.

3. Oxygen given in high doses over a prolonged period of time can increase the risk of retinopathy of prematurity (ROP). Oxygen should not be withheld from infants but administered cautiously, using the minimal amount to meet the infant's oxygenation needs. If the infant is not receiving enough oxygen, cells within the body will begin to die, including brain cells. This could result in permanent neurologic damage. It is also known that hypoxia increases the risk of necrotizing enterocolitis (NEC), which can be life-threatening.

4. It is important to promote bonding. Encourage the parents to visit as much as possible. Parents can bring personal items for the baby, such as pictures, small toys, etc. Parents are often initially afraid to touch their preterm baby because they're afraid they will hurt the infant. Encourage parents to touch the baby, stroke the hand or foot, and hold the newborn, if the condition allows. When the baby is stable, parents can be encouraged to do "kangaroo care," where they put the unclothed baby on their bare chest to allow for skin-to-skin contact for short periods of time. Preterm infants need developmental stimulation, just like a term baby, but may need shorter periods of interaction. The baby should be positioned in a fetal position in the isolette or radiant warmer to provide a sense of security as well as limit loss of body heat.

5. The mother should be encouraged to breast feed, although the baby will not be able to nurse until the suck/swallow reflex is established and the newborn is strong enough to nurse. Until that time, the mother should pump her breasts every 2–3 hours while awake, save the milk in small amounts in Playtex Nurser bags, and freeze it. The milk can then be given to the baby during tube feedings. This will also stimulate milk production in the mother. Breast milk is easier to digest and contains valuable immunoglobulins which can help prevent infection in the baby.

## Chapter 14

1. The infant will be pale and bluish. The muscle tone will be very floppy, making the baby feel limp like a rag doll. The mouth may droop open.

2. Ask the client if she would like to be on the postpartum unit, or on another unit. If on the postpartum unit, assign her to a room that is away from the nursery. Try to assign consistent caregivers to increase support to the family.

3. Children age 6 and under do not yet understand what death is, or that it is permanent, but may feel responsible for the death if they had negative feelings toward the expected infant. School-age children understand that death is inevitable and permanent. It is best to explain that the baby died while it was being born, giving details of the placental abruption

only if the children ask about it or if the children are used to talking about body parts and functions.

4. Gently tell the client while the mother is still in the room that although she will recover from surgery over the next few weeks, her grieving will take up to 2 years to completely resolve. Give the client written information on the phases of bereavement, as well as on infant loss support groups.

5. Listen to the client's concerns. Provide empathy through therapeutic communication. Reassure the client that hearing a baby's cry after a fetal loss is a common and completely normal occurrence. It indicates being in the searching and yearning phase of bereavement. These sensations will gradually fade with time. Encourage the client to read the information on grieving that was given to her in the hospital or consider joining a support group.

# Credits

## Chapter 2

**Fig. 2-1**  Art, From *Maternal-Newborn Nursing: A Family and Community Approach*, by Sally B. Olds, Marcia L. London, Patricia Wieland Ladewig, Edition 6, © 2000 by Prentice-Hall, Inc., Upper Saddle River, New Jersey; Page 127, Fig. 6-5.

**Fig. 2-2**  © Prentice Hall Health, Upper Saddle River, New Jersey.

## Chapter 3

**Fig. 3-1**  Art, From *Maternal-Newborn Nursing: A Family and Community Approach*, by Sally B. Olds, Marcia L. London, Patricia Wieland Ladewig, Edition 6, © 2000 by Prentice-Hall, Inc., Upper Saddle River, New Jersey; Page 48, Fig. 3-4.

**Fig. 3-2**  Art, From *Maternal-Newborn Nursing: A Family and Community Approach*, by Sally B. Olds, Marcia L. London, Patricia Wieland Ladewig, Edition 6, © 2000 by Prentice-Hall, Inc., Upper Saddle River, New Jersey; Page 49, Fig. 3-5.

**Fig. 3-3**  Art, From *Maternal-Newborn Nursing: A Family and Community Approach*, by Sally B. Olds, Marcia L. London, Patricia Wieland Ladewig, Edition 6, © 2000 by Prentice-Hall, Inc., Upper Saddle River, New Jersey; Page 49, Fig. 3-6.

## Chapter 4

**Fig. 4-1**  Art, From *Maternal-Newborn Nursing: A Family and Community Approach*, by Sally B. Olds, Marcia L. London, Patricia Wieland Ladewig, Edition 6, © 2000 by Prentice-Hall, Inc., Upper Saddle River, New Jersey; Page 158, Fig. 7-7a.

**Fig. 4-2**  Art, From *Maternal-Newborn Nursing: A Family and Community Approach*, by Sally B. Olds, Marcia L. London, Patricia Wieland Ladewig, Edition 6, © 2000 by Prentice-Hall, Inc., Upper Saddle River, New Jersey; Page 164, Fig. 7-15.

**Fig. 4-3**  Art, From *Maternal-Newborn Nursing: A Family and Community Approach*, by Sally B. Olds, Marcia L. London, Patricia Wieland Ladewig, Edition 6, © 2000 by Prentice-Hall, Inc., Upper Saddle River, New Jersey; Page 167, Fig. 7-16.

**Table 4-1**  From *Maternal-Newborn Nursing: A Family and Community Approach*, by Sally B. Olds, Marcia L. London, Patricia Wieland Ladewig, Edition 6, © 2000 by Prentice-Hall, Inc., Upper Saddle River, New Jersey; Page 168-169, Table 7-2. *Sources:* Sadler TW: *Langman's Medical Embryology*, 7th ed. Baltimore: Williams & Wilkins, 1995; and Moore KL, Persand TVN: *The Developing Human: Clinically Oriented Embryology*, 6th ed. Philadelphia: Saunders, 1998.

**Table 4-2**  From *Maternal-Newborn Nursing: A Family and Community Approach*, by Sally B. Olds, Marcia L. London, Patricia Wieland Ladewig, Edition 6, © 2000 by Prentice-Hall, Inc., Upper Saddle River, New Jersey; Page 174, Table 7-3.

## Chapter 5

**Fig. 5-1**  Art, From *Maternal-Newborn Nursing: A Family and Community Approach*, by Sally B. Olds, Marcia L. London, Patricia Wieland Ladewig, Edition 6, © 2000 by Prentice-Hall, Inc., Upper Saddle River, New Jersey; Page 236, Fig. 10-6; Artist: Kristin Mount.

**Fig. 5-2**  Art, From *Maternal-Newborn Nursing: A Family and Community Approach*, by Sally B. Olds, Marcia L. London, Patricia Wieland Ladewig, Edition 6, © 2000 by Prentice-Hall, Inc., Upper Saddle River, New Jersey; Page 231, Fig. 10-3.

## Chapter 6

**Fig. 6-1**  Art, From *Maternal-Newborn Nursing: A Family and Community Approach*, by Sally B. Olds, Marcia L. London, Patricia Wieland Ladewig, Edition 6, © 2000 by Prentice-Hall, Inc., Upper Saddle River, New Jersey; Page 456, Fig. 17-17.

**Fig. 6-2**  Art, From *Maternal-Newborn Nursing: A Family and Community Approach*, by Sally B. Olds, Marcia L. London, Patricia Wieland Ladewig, Edition 6, © 2000 by Prentice-Hall, Inc., Upper Saddle River, New Jersey; Page 458, Fig. 17-19.

## Chapter 7

**Fig. 7-1**  Art, From *Maternal-Newborn Nursing: A Family and Community Approach*, by Sally B. Olds, Marcia L. London, Patricia Wieland Ladewig, Edition 6, © 2000 by Prentice-Hall, Inc., Upper Saddle River, New Jersey; Page 638, Fig. 22-18; Precision Graphics.

**Fig. 7-2**  Art, From *Maternal-Newborn Nursing: A Family and Community Approach*, by Sally B. Olds, Marcia L. London, Patricia

Wieland Ladewig, Edition 6, © 2000 by Prentice-Hall, Inc., Upper Saddle River, New Jersey; Page 235, Fig. 22-17; Precision Graphics.

## Chapter 8

**Fig. 8-1**    Art, From *Maternal-Newborn Nursing: A Family and Community Approach*, by Sally B. Olds, Marcia L. London, Patricia Wieland Ladewig, Edition 6, © 2000 by Prentice-Hall, Inc., Upper Saddle River, New Jersey; Page 478, Fig. 18-7; Precision Graphics.

**Fig. 8-2**    Art, © Prentice Hall Health, Upper Saddle River, New Jersey.

## Chapter 9

**Fig. 9-1**    Art, From *Maternal-Newborn Nursing: A Family and Community Approach*, by Sally B. Olds, Marcia L. London, Patricia Wieland Ladewig, Edition 6, © 2000 by Prentice-Hall, Inc., Upper Saddle River, New Jersey; Page 621, Fig. 22-11; Precision Graphics.

**Fig. 9-2**    Art, From *Maternal-Newborn Nursing: A Family and Community Approach*, by Sally B. Olds, Marcia L. London, Patricia Wieland Ladewig, Edition 6, © 2000 by Prentice-Hall, Inc., Upper Saddle River, New Jersey; Page 623, Fig. 22-12; Precision Graphics.

**Fig. 9-3**    Art, From *Maternal-Newborn Nursing: A Family and Community Approach*, by Sally B. Olds, Marcia L. London, Patricia Wieland Ladewig, Edition 6, © 2000 by Prentice-Hall, Inc., Upper Saddle River, New Jersey; Page 625, Fig. 22-13; Precision Graphics.

## Chapter 10

**Fig. 10-1**    Art, From *Maternal-Newborn Nursing: A Family and Community Approach*, by Sally B. Olds, Marcia L. London, Patricia Wieland Ladewig, Edition 6, © 2000 by Prentice-Hall, Inc., Upper Saddle River, New Jersey; Page 908, Fig. 30-1; Artist: Kristin Mount.

**Fig. 10-2**    Art, From *Maternal-Newborn Nursing: A Family and Community Approach*, by Sally B. Olds, Marcia L. London, Patricia Wieland Ladewig, Edition 6, © 2000 by Prentice-Hall, Inc., Upper Saddle River, New Jersey; Page 922, Fig. 30-5; Precision Graphics.

**Fig. 10-3**    Photo, From *Maternal-Newborn Nursing: A Family and Community Approach*, by Sally B. Olds, Marcia L. London, Patricia

Wieland Ladewig, Edition 6, © 2000 by Prentice-Hall, Inc., Upper Saddle River, New Jersey; Page 999, Fig. 33-3; © Elena Dorfman / Addison Wesley Longman.

## Chapter 11

**Fig. 11-1**    © Prentice Hall Health, Upper Saddle River, New Jersey.

**Fig. 11-2**    Art, From *Maternal-Newborn Nursing: A Family and Community Approach*, by Sally B. Olds, Marcia L. London, Patricia Wieland Ladewig, Edition 6, © 2000 by Prentice-Hall, Inc., Upper Saddle River, New Jersey; Page 576, Fig. 20-11; Precision Graphics.

**Table 11-1**    From *Maternal-Newborn Nursing: A Family and Community Approach*, by Sally B. Olds, Marcia L. London, Patricia Wieland Ladewig, Edition 6, © 2000 by Prentice-Hall, Inc., Upper Saddle River, New Jersey; Page 983, Table 33-1.

**Table 11-2**    From *Maternity Nursing: Care of the Childbearing Family,* by Laurie N. Sherwen, Mary Ann Scoloveno, Carol Toussie Weingarten, Medial Edition, © 2001 by Prentice-Hall, Inc., Upper Saddle River, New Jersey; Page 900, Table 29-3.

## Chapter 12

**Fig. 12-1**    Art, From *Maternal-Newborn Nursing: A Family and Community Approach*, by Sally B. Olds, Marcia L. London, Patricia Wieland Ladewig, Edition 6, © 2000 by Prentice-Hall, Inc., Upper Saddle River, New Jersey; Page 790, Fig. 27-6. Adapted from Lawrence RA: *Breastfeeding: A Guide for Medical Profession*, 4th Edition. St. Louis: Mosby, 1994, p. 219. Permission Granted.

## Chapter 13

**Fig. 13-1**    Art, From *Maternal-Newborn Nursing: A Family and Community Approach*, by Sally B. Olds, Marcia L. London, Patricia Wieland Ladewig, Edition 6, © 2000 by Prentice-Hall, Inc., Upper Saddle River, New Jersey; Page 886, Fig. 29-13; Artist: Nea Hanscomb.

**Fig. 13-2**    Art, From *Maternal-Newborn Nursing: A Family and Community Approach*, by Sally B. Olds, Marcia L. London, Patricia Wieland Ladewig, Edition 6, © 2000 by Prentice-Hall, Inc., Upper Saddle River, New Jersey; Page 866, Fig. 29-13, Precision Graphics.

# Index